Metabolism of Xenobiotics

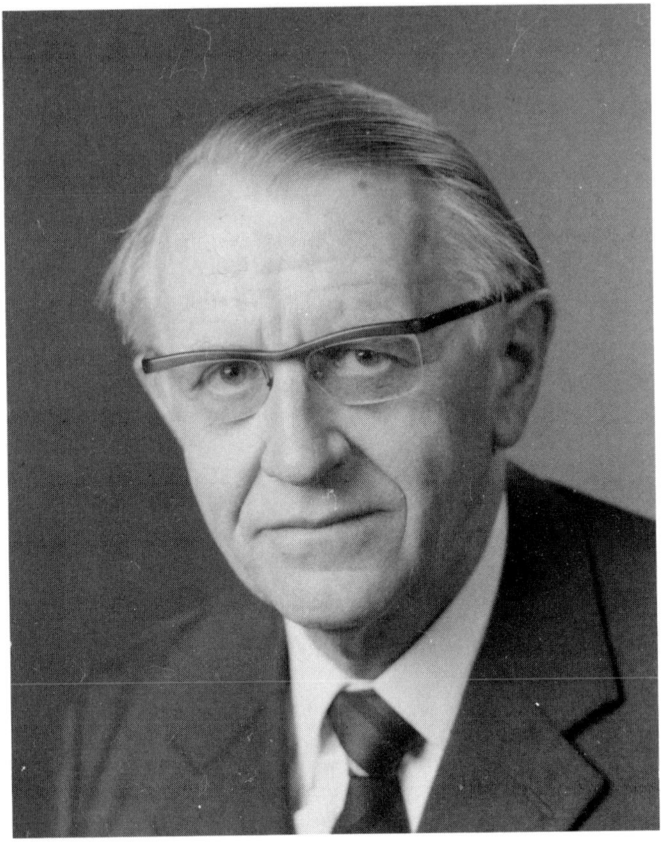

Herbert Remmer

This volume is dedicated by the International Society for the Study of Xenobiotics to Professor Dr Herbert Remmer, in recognition of his leading role in the development of biochemical pharmacology and toxicology in Europe, in particular his elucidation of the phenomena and enzymology of drug-metabolizing enzyme induction.

Metabolism of Xenobiotics

Edited by

J.W. Gorrod
Kings College (Chelsea), University of London, UK

H. Oelschläger
Johann Wolfgang Goethe-Universität, Frankfurt, FR Germany

J. Caldwell
St Mary's Hospital Medical School, London UK

Taylor & Francis
London · New York · Philadelphia
1988

UK Taylor & Francis Ltd, 4 John St, London WC1N 2ET

USA Taylor & Francis Inc., 242 Cherry St, Philadelphia,
PA 19106-1906

British Library Cataloguing in Publication Data

Metabolism of Xenobiotics.
1. Xenobiotics
I. Gorrod, J.W. II. Oelschläger, H.
III. Caldwell, John, *1947-*
574.1'33 QP529

ISBN 0-85066-360-1

Printed in Great Britain by Taylor & Francis (Printers) Ltd.
Basingstoke, Hants

CONTENTS

PREFACE

The papers presented in this volume originated from the 2nd European Meeting of ISSX held in Frankfurt. They consist of authoritative overviews of certain specific topics and present state of the art concepts. Some authors have included recent research results presented against a wide background of information. In order to ensure that adequate cover was given of the topics, the senior Chairpersons were invited to expand their opening and closing remarks into a text. In most cases, this invitation was accepted and these articles have been included.

The volume clearly demonstrates the breadth of activities of the members of the society and is a fitting tribute to Professor Dr. H. Remmer.

J.W. Gorrod

1. Factors affecting xenobiotic disposition

Factors Affecting Xenobiotic Disposition: Storage and Accumulation: An Introduction

Robert L. Smith

Department of Pharmacology
St. Mary's Hospital Medical School
London W2 1PG

The first ISSX European Regional Meeting on Foreign Compound Metabolism was held at the University of Malta in February 1985. This particular Symposium was largely concerned with an overview of foreign compound metabolism in its broadest sense since it dealt with the disposition of a wide range of xenobiotic substances including drugs, chemical carcinogens, food additives, fragrance chemicals and detergent substances. The Malta meeting was also of particular note since at the same meeting Professor Eric Boyland was awarded an honorary degree by the University of Malta and a Symposium was devoted to his life-long interest namely, the metabolic fate of carcinogenic chemicals.

Since the first European Regional Meeting of ISSX had dealt with a global perspective of the range of xenobiotic substances that undergo metabolism it was felt that the second Regional Meeting should deal with more specific aspects of xenobiotic metabolism. Accordingly members of the Programme Committee were solicited for their views and advice as regards topics for the programme. The final programme which was put together by Professor Oelschläger, Professor Gorrod and myself represents a synthesis of the various advice that was received. Of particular note was the advice from some Councillors for ISSX to begin to deal with the question of "Alternatives to Whole Animals in Xenobiotic Research". The question of the use of living animals in biomedical research raises many problems - emotional, social and political in several countries at the present time and it is as well that ISSX should begin to grapple with what is a very difficult and contentious issue. We therefore decided to include a session on this subject under the Chairmanship of Professor Gillian Powell as a beginning for ISSX in this area.

With these few preliminary remarks I would now like to introduce the first session which has been dignified with the somewhat broad title of "Factors Affecting Xenobiotic Disposition". Perhaps, on reflection a more appropriate title would have been "Storage and Accumulation of Xenobiotic Substances" since this was the main thrust of this Symposium. The question of xenobiotic accumulation as with drug storage *in vivo* and the concentration of xenobiotic substances in food chains is very important and in many respects has not received the degree of attention the matter requires.

In recent years some important advances have been made with respect to our knowledge of the processes that underly xenobiotic accumulation in living systems. Of particular significance is our ability now to distinguish two types of mechanism which may be broadly classified as passive or active. In the former, accumulation occurs as a consequence of the physico-chemical properties of the xenobiotic substance and the exposed biological system as with the uptake of lipophilic substances into the adipose tissue storage sites. These passive aspects of foreign compound tissue accumulation are addressed by Professor Bickel and Dr. Mohr in their respective contributions. The second mechanism of xenobiotic accumulation is where active processes are involved such as the incorporation of xenobiotic substances into stable tissue macromolecules. This second aspect is dealt with by Dr. Hutson in his presentation on xenobiotic macromolecule conjugates. Finally, if xenobiotic accumulation is undesirable then the question arises as to whether or not it could be reduced if not avoided altogether. This then brings up the question of metabolically recalcitrant chemicals structure - activity relationships that determine metabolic inertness and how far the structural design and redesign of molecules can reduce accumulation and storage. This aspect has been addressed by Dr. Scheunert and Professor Korte in their paper entitled "Metabolically Resistant Chemicals".

The old concept that adipose tissue uptake and storage is a function of lipophilicity of the xenobiotic and partition into fat storage depots is now known to be too simplistic. Professor Bickel, in his paper shows how other factors besides lipophilicity including competition from other tissues, tissue perfusion rates all influence the accumulation of a xenobiotic in fat stores. In an attempt to introduce more quantitation in this field Professor Bickel has introduced the concept of an "adipose storage index; ASI" which relates the maximum concentration in adipose tissue reached after a single dose to the relative dose. The calculation of this index for about fifty lipophilic xenobiotics has clearly shown that adipose tissue storage is not merely a matter of lipid partition.

A very important aspect of tissue accumulation of drugs is that of drug-phospholipid interactions. The chronic administration of amphipathic compounds such as chlorphentermine, certain tricyclic antidepressants and amiodarone to experimental animals is associated with the appearance of phospholipid lysosome inclusion bodies. This phenomenon also occurs in man with drugs such as amiodarone. The appearance of such phospholipid inclusion bodies during the course of the animal toxicological evaluation of a new drug is not an infrequent occurrence and the interpretation of its significance, particularly as far as the human situation is concerned is troublesome.

In their paper on drug-phospholipid interactions, Dr. Mohr and Professor Lullmann while acknowledging the importance of phospholipid interactions from the point of view of influencing the pharmacokinetics of a drug they nevertheless go on to deal with a most important perspective, namely, the possible functional consequences of such interactions. Phospholipids are essential for the structure and function of the cell and are subject to cellular metabolism. An important question arises therefore as to the functional consequences of the incorporation within their structures of xenobiotic substances. Using techniques such as the adsorption of ^{45}Ca to lipid films and changes in phase-transition temperatures amphipathic compounds have been shown to alter the measured parameters suggesting that their inclusion in phospholipid membranes may not be an entirely innocent affair.

The 'active' aspect of tissue accumulation of xenobiotics is dealt with in the paper by Dr. Hutson. In this process the compound or a metabolite undergoes incorporation into a biological macromolecule such as a protein, nucleic acid or phospholipid. Such interactions, particularly with nucleic acids and proteins may be of critical importance from the point of view of toxic mechanisms. A most interesting aspect of xenobiotic tissue storage to emerge in recent years has been the recognition of the incorporation of various foreign compounds into tissue lipids particularly the hybrid triacylglycerols. Such hybrid triacylglycerols have been reported for phenoxybenzoic acid, acidic metabolites of cycloprate, fenoprofen and ibuprofen. Similarly, certain xenobiotic alcohols such as the tetrahydrocannabinols, dipyridamole and codeine are now well-known to form esters with long-chain fatty acids such as palmitic and stearic acid to name but a few. From the point of view of storage and accumulation it would appear that the formation of such hybrid triacylglycerols and long-chain fatty acid esters may be a major active factor in promoting tissue retention and the formation of xenobiotic residues. There may also be functional consequences but as Dr. Hutson has remarked there are currently more questions than answers regarding this point.

There is a general concensus that the accumulation and retention of a xenobiotic substance within biological systems is undesirable, although as pointed out earlier the functional consequences of such accumulation for most compounds is not yet clear. The question therefore arises as to how far chemicals can be structurally designed to avoid this problem. In their paper Dr. Scheunert and Professor Korte point out that metabolic resistance is specific to a functional group of a molecule rather than to the chemical structure of a compound as a whole. Examples of such metabolically recalcitrant groups are the organic carbon-halogen bond and the polycondensated aromatic structure. Chemicals containing such functions may nevertheless be metabolised quite readily if the molecule contains elsewhere within its structure other 'metabolisable' functions. It is argued that by the study of structure-persistence relationships it would be possible to overcome the problems of long-surviving chemical residues in the environment - due to metabolic recalcitrance - by the design of more readily degradeable ones.

In summary the last decade has seen some major advances, as outlined in this Symposium, in our understanding of the accumulation and storage of xenobiotics in living systems. Of particular importance has been the recognition and distinction between the role of passive and discrete active processes in xenobiotic accumulation. Furthermore, it is clear that there is scope to apply structural design to develop useful more readily metabolised compounds which are less likely to persist in the environment. Finally, it is also clear that we need to know rather more about the functional consequences of the tissue accumulation of xenobiotics.

ADIPOSE TISSUE STORAGE OF XENOBIOTICS

M. H. Bickel

Department of Pharmacology, University of Bern,
Friedbuehlstrasse 49, CH-3010 Bern, Switzerland

Xenobiotics absorbed into an organism are known to show an uneven distribution, often to an extreme degree. This fact reflects the complexities of higher organisms in which a xenobiotic is distributed by a perfusion system, has to overcome permeability barriers and, above all, encounters biomacromolecules such as proteins, nucleic acids, mucopolysaccharides, or lipids with widely varying affinities. Hence, one or several tissues can assume a storage or depot function for the compound, thereby influencing its pharmacokinetics and, as a consequence, its pharmacodynamics.

Adipose tissue must be considered an important potential storage tissue, since it contains an extremely high percentage of stored lipid in the form of triacylglycerol, and since its tissue mass in a mammalian body is only surpassed by skin and/or skeletal muscle. Several cases of pharmacodynamic consequences of adipose tissue storage are known:

- Termination of action (thiopental)
- Prolongation of action (volatile anesthetics)
- Prevention of toxicity (DDT, PCBs, TCDD)
- Risk of toxicity (mobilization of compound during "melting" of adipose tissue)

The old concept of adipose tissue storage

In the 1950s the short duration of action of thiopental was shown to be due to rapid redistribution into muscle and adipose tissue rather than to rapid metabolism (Brodie et al. 1952). The highly lipophilic DDT and related compounds were also shown to be stored in adipose tissue, but the less lipophilic pentobarbital and phenobarbital were not.

These observations led to the partition or lipophilicity concept of adipose tissue storage (Mark 1971). Indeed, the statement that lipophilic xenobiotics tend to be stored in adipose tissue is still found in most textbooks of pharmacology.

This concept is seriously disturbed if additional literature data on adipose tissue storage are collected. As is shown on Table 1 many xenobiotics of much higher lipophilicities (P = partition coefficient octanol/water) than thiopental are not stored in adipose tissue.

Table 1. Adipose tissue storage of a selection of model xenobiotics

Xenobiotic	Class	log P	Storage
Phenobarbital	acidic	1.4	-
Pentobarbital	"	2.1	-
Phenytoin	"	2.5	+
Thiopental	"	2.8	+
Phenylbutazone	"	3.3	-
Imipramine	basic	4.6	-
Chlorpromazine	"	5.3	-
DDE	neutral	5.8	+
2,4,5,2',4',5'-PCB	"	6.5	+
2,3,6,2',3',6'-PCB	"	6.5	-

PCB, polychlorinated biphenyl

However, these studies also show the need for a quantifiable criterion for adipose tissue storage or its absence. We therefore introduced an adipose storage index

$$ASI = \frac{c_{ad\ max}}{D_{rel}} \qquad (1)$$

where the numerator is the maximum concentration in adipose tissue reached after a single dose, and the denominator is the relative dose (Bickel 1984). In other words, ASI is the ratio of the concentration in adipose tissue and the fictitious concentration of the evenly distributed xenobiotic. Thus, values above unity indicate adipose tissue storage.

A major advantage of ASI is its being independent of the amount or proportion of adipose tissue.

From literature data we have calculated the ASI-values of about 50 lipophilic xenobiotics. A large number of compounds that are more lipophilic than thiopental had an ASI below unity, among them many acidic drugs, virtually all basic drugs, and even highly lipophilic neutral compounds. Thus, Table 1 depicts the situation correctly, and one must conclude that

$$ASI \neq f(\log P) \qquad (2)$$

and that adipose tissue storage of a xenobiotic is not simply a matter of lipid partition (Bickel 1984).

Studies with model compounds

The database mentioned above suggested in-depth studies of the pharmacokinetics in rats of selected model compounds which may be representative for certain types of adipose tissue storage. Thiopental, the classical "fat-seeker", is relatively rapidly redistributed into adipose tissue where it is transiently stored. This was first demonstrated by Brodie et al. (1952) and then confirmed by many authors including ourselves (Mühlebach et al., 1985). Phenylbutazone and imipramine represent acidic and basic lipophilic drugs which, in contrast to thiopental, are not stored in adipose tissue. It was demonstrated that even a loading of animals with maximum tolerated doses of imipramine over weeks will not result in adipose tissue storage (Bickel et al., 1983). Still another type is represented by the unmetabolizable PCB isomer, 2,4,5,2',4',5'-hexachlorobiphenyl (6-CB), which is highly stored in adipose tissue, however, at an extremely slow rate (Mühlebach et al., 1985). The characteristic differences of these model compounds are summarized in Table 2.

A dozen xenobiotics with log P-values between 0.25 and 6.5 were incubated in vitro with adipose tissue slices or isolated adipocytes. The uptake into these preparations was a clear-cut function of log P (Di Francesco & Bickel 1985). This demonstrates that, unlike in vivo, adipose tissue uptake in this in vitro situation is a simple lipid partition.

Table 2. Extent and duration of accumulation in adipose tissue after single doses

Xenobiotic	log P	ASI	$t_{ad\ max}$
Thiopental	2.8	4.1	1 hr
Phenylbutazone	3.3	0.5	1 hr
Imipramine	4.6	0.3	0.5 hr
DDE	5.8	3.7	17 hr
2,4,5,2',4',5'-PCB	6.5	10.0	5 weeks

ASI, adipose storage index, see text.
$t_{ad\ max}$, time of peak level in adipose tissue.

The difference between the in vitro and in vivo systems shown in Table 3 should theoretically provide a clue to a better understanding of the situation in vivo.

Table 3. How xenobiotics reach adipose tissue

System	Transport	Target(s)
in vitro	Diffusion	Adipose tissue (preparation)
Perfusion technique	Perfusion and capillary transport	Adipose tissue
in vivo	Perfusion and capillary transport	Adipose and other tissues

Indeed, using the technique of the isolated perfused rat adipose tissue it could be shown that imipramine and chlorpromazine, which are not stored in vivo, are even more rapidly taken up into isolated perfused adipose tissue than is thiopental (Gubser et al.,1986). This experiment clearly demonstrates that the lack of adipose tissue storage of drugs like imipramine cannot be due to a hypothetical permeability barrier between blood and adipose tissue. Rather, according to Table 3, the presence in vivo of other tissues in addition to adipose tissue must provide the key for an understanding of the differences between the situations in vivo and in vitro.

A new concept of adipose tissue storage

Accumulation and storage of xenobiotics in adipose tissue can be considered as a particular form of tissue binding. The process of distribution of a xenobiotic in the organism is being increasingly understood by the introduction of the parameter of tissue binding (Wilkinson 1983). In particular, distribution can be considered as the result of a competition between binding to plasma proteins and to tissue constituents which can be simulated by the technique of distribution dialysis (Bickel et al.,1987). Insight into distribution has also been helped by the introduction of physiological pharmacokinetic models (Rowland 1984; Lutz et al.,1984). The first of these models was applied to thiopental (Bischoff & Dedrick 1968). This drug is known to undergo a redistribution from blood to highly perfused viscera, to poorly perfused tissues like muscle and skin, and ultimately, to adipose tissue where maximum concentrations are reached about one hour after administration. This redistribution pattern is clearly flow-limited, i.e., determined by the perfusion rates of the individual tissues. Thiopental is a simple case in that it has high adipose tissue affinity which is not disturbed by a binding competition from plasma proteins or lean tissues (Bickel et al., 1987). However, with other xenobiotics the presence of lean tissues in vivo can impose a binding competition between adipose and lean tissues which is then superimposed to the flow limitation, i.e., to the fact that lean tissues are provided with 90 % of the drug-containing cardiac output, as compared to a mere 5 % for adipose tissue. Hence, lean tissue binding prevents adipose tissue accumulation in the case of imipramine or delays it in the case of 6-CB. Generally speaking, this kind of binding competition will strongly influence the appearance or non-appearance of a xenobiotic in adipose tissue.

Summary

Adipose tissue storage of xenobiotics is not simply a matter of lipophilicity and partition. Rather, it is a special case of a general theory of distribution, based on flow-limited physiological pharmacokinetic models, in which the binding competition between lean and adipose tissues becomes the chief determinant. This binding competition determines the rate of accumulation in adipose tissue which in turn determines whether and to what extent adipose tissue storage occurs. The molecular structure of the xenobiotic influences binding to lean tissues, whereas lipophilicity influences affinity to adipose tissue. This flow-limited binding competition model explains the different types of kinetic behavior of xenobiotics.

REFERENCES

Bickel M. H., 1984, Progress in Drug Research, 28, 273.

Bickel M. H., Graber B. E., & Moor M., 1983, Life Sciences, 33, 2025.

Bickel M. H., Raaflaub R. M., Hellmüller M., & Stauffer E. J., 1987, Journal of Pharmaceutical Sciences, 76, 68.

Bischoff K. B. & Dedrick R. L., 1968, Journal of Pharmaceutical Sciences, 57, 1346.

Brodie B., Bernstein E., & Mark L. C., 1952, Journal of Pharmacology and Experimental Therapeutics, 105, 421.

Di Francesco C. & Bickel M. H., 1985, Biochemical Pharmacology, 34, 3683.

Gubser R., Di Francesco C., & Bickel M. H., 1986, Journal of Pharmacology and Experimental Therapeutics, 237, 967.

Lutz R. J., Dedrick R. L., Tuey D., Sipes I. G., Anderson M. W., & Matthews H. B., 1984, Drug Metabolism and Disposition, 12, 527.

Mark L. C., 1971, Handbook of Experimental Pharmacology, 28/I, 258.

Mühlebach S., Wyss P. A., & Bickel M. H., 1985, Xenobiotica, 15, 485.

Rowland M., 1984, Drug Metabolism Reviews, 15, 55.

Wilkinson G. R., 1983, Drug Metabolism Reviews, 14, 427.

DRUG PHOSPHOLIPID INTERACTIONS

Heinz Lüllmann & Klaus Mohr

Department of Pharmacology
University of Kiel
Hospitalstr. 4, D-2300 Kiel, FRG

Introduction

In an aqueous environment, phospholipid-molecules are commonly arranged in bimolecular leaflets (for review see e.g. Lee 1975). These phospholipid bilayers form the matrix of cellular membranes and are thus present in abundance. Non-polar, polar, and amphiphilic drugs may bind to phospholipid bilayers. Non-polar drug-molecules, e.g. inhalational anaesthetics, intercalate in the hydrophobic interior of the membrane between the fatty acid chains. Polar drug-molecules interact with the polar phospholipid head-groups, e.g. aminoglycoside antibiotics bind to the surface of negatively charged phospholipids (Lüllmann & Vollmer 1982). Amphiphilic drugs contain both a polar and a non-polar part. The non-polar part commonly consists of an aromatic ring system, the polar part may be formed by an anionic group, e.g. a carboxyl residue as present in many analgetic and antiinflammatory drugs, or by a cationic residue, e.g. a protonized amino-group as present in local anaesthetic, antiarrhythmic or ß-adrenoceptor blocking drugs. Since the phosphate group of the phospholipids provides a negative charge, cationic amphiphilic drugs are especially prone to be taken up in phospholipid membranes. The cationic nitrogen is placed next to the anionic phosphate, the apolar ring system is directed towards the hydrophobic interior of the bilayer (Cerbon 1972, Yeagle et al. 1977, Herbette et al., 1983). The following considerations shall be focussed on the interaction of cationic amphiphilic drugs with phospholipids.

Interaction of cationic amphiphilic drugs with phospholipid membranes

The forces determining binding of catamphiphilic drugs to phospholipid bilayers were investigated in studies with liposomes prepared from various artificial phospholipids, e.g. phosphatidylserine, phosphatidylinositol, phosphatidic acid, phosphatidylcholine and phosphatidylglycerol (Lüllmann & Wehling 1979, Lüllmann et al., 1980, Hanpft & Mohr 1984). The binding affinity is determined by hydrophobic and electrostatic forces. The affinity of binding to a given phospholipid increases with increasing hydrophobicity of the drugs. Binding of the cationic drugs is higher in negatively charged phospholipids, e.g. phosphatidylserine, than in zwitterionic lipids, e.g. phosphatidylcholine. Additionally, the structural arrangement of the phospholipid-molecules has impact on the binding affinity, e.g. lipid-bilayers in the highly ordered gel state have been reported to bind less drug than in the less ordered liquid crystalline state (Singer 1977).

The consequences of the interaction of catamphiphilic drugs with phospholipid membranes can be looked upon under two aspects: firstly, its impact on the fate of the drug in the organism and secondly, its impact on the metabolism of phospholipids and on the functional properties of phospholipid bilayers.
It is immediately evident that accumulation of drug-molecules in the abundantly present cell membranes will affect the pharmacokinetics of the drug. The concentration of unbound drug is reduced, less drug-molecules are available both for the interaction with specific binding sites and for the entrance into the pathways of elimination. Consequently, the biologic activity will be diminished and the elimination will be retarded.

Also the phospholipids are subject to cellular metabolism, and furthermore, they are essential for the structure and the function of cell membranes.
The effect of drug-binding on phospholipid metabolism became evident in experiments on the pharmacokinetics of the anoretic drugs chlorphentermine and phentermine (Lüllmann et al., 1973). The tritiated compounds were chronically administered to rats by daily i.p. injection and the time-course of uptake into various tissues was followed. The tissue/blood ratios for the lungs are depicted in Fig.1. The tissue/blood ratio of phentermine remained constant over the experimental period, whereas chlorphentermine became increasingly accumulated with time. This finding suggested that the binding sites for chlorphentermine increased in number. Ultrastructural investigations supported this notion: chlorphentermine induced the formation of lysosomal inclusion bodies in various tissues, such as the lungs (Lüllmann-Rauch et al., 1972). These inclusion bodies consisted mainly of phospholipids (Schmien et al., 1974). Probably, the degradation of phospholipids by lysosomal phospholipases was impaired, because the enzymes did not accept the chlorphentermine-containing phospholipid membranes as an appropriate substrate. This drug-induced lipid-storage resembled inherited lipid-storage diseases known in human pathology. Several cationic amphiphilic drugs were found in the meantime to induce lipid-storage in experimental animals (for review see Lüllmann-Rauch 1979). In general, any cationic amphiphilic drug with affinity to phospholipids, which is not rapidly metabolized in the organism to a metabolite with less affinity, is likely to induce lipid-storage (Drenckhahn et al., 1976). Also in humans this effect was shown to occur

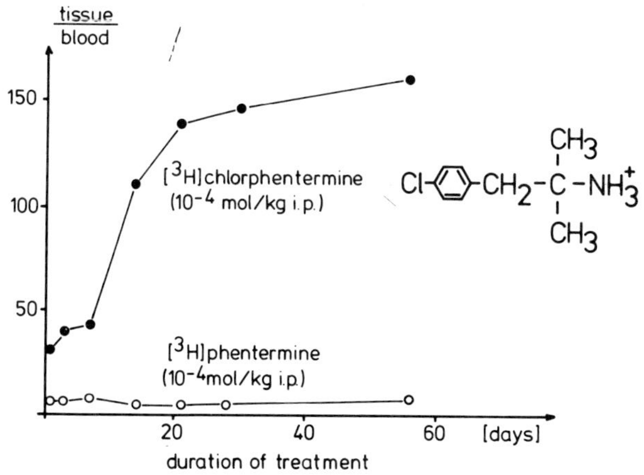

Fig.1: Accumulation of tritiated chlorphentermine and phentermine in the lungs of rats during chronic treatment with the indicated daily dosage (adapted from Lüllmann et al., 1973).

and to be of functional consequence. Some side effects encountered in drug therapy are explained by the formation of inclusion bodies: corneal opacities, observed under the treatment with the antiarrhythmic drug amiodarone, are caused by these particles (for review see Lüllmann-Rauch 1979).

In order to elucidate the possible consequences of the intercalation of cationic amphiphilic drugs into cell membranes a comparative study was performed. The potency of various cationic amphiphilic drugs to interact with artificial phospholipid membranes was determined and compared with the potency of the drugs to depress cardiac function.
The interaction of the drugs with the phospholipid polar head-group was studied in monolayers made of phosphatidylserine, using as an indicator of drug-binding the adsorption of ^{45}Ca to the lipid film. The method has been described in detail by Lüllmann et al. (1980). In short, the monolayer is spread over the surface of an aqueous buffer containing ^{45}Ca-ions and the adsorption of ^{45}Ca is measured by means of a *Geiger-*tube placed above the surface of the buffer solution (cf. inset Fig.2). The adsorption of ^{45}Ca is inhibited when cationic drugs are intercalated in the lipid layer and neutralize negative charges. As shown in Fig.2 for a number of ß-blockers, cationic amphiphilic drugs reduce ^{45}Ca-binding with different potency. Probably, the concentration response curves reflect the binding curves of the drugs to phosphatidylserine. The different potency of the drugs is indicated by different IC_{50}-values, i.e. the drug concentrations inhibiting ^{45}Ca-binding by 50%.

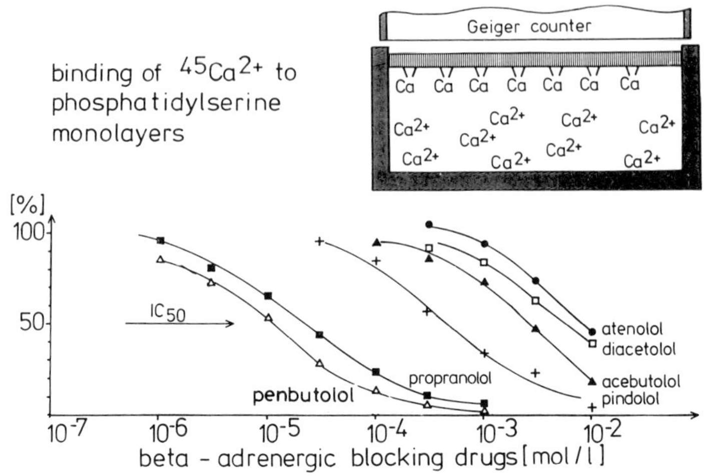

Fig.2: Inhibition of ^{45}Ca-binding to phosphatidylserine-monolayers by the indicated ß-blocking drugs. Binding of ^{45}Ca in the absence of a drug was set 100% (H. Weiß, unpublished).

The effect of drug-binding on the structural arrangement within the phospholipid membrane was studied by determining the drug effects on the phase-transition temperature (T_t) of liposomes made of dipalmitoyl-phosphatidic acid (DPPA). The temperature of the phase-transition from the gel into the liquid crystalline state was measured by means of differential scanning calorimetry. The method has been described in detail by Hanpft & Mohr (1985). In short, the endothermic heat flow occurring at the phase-transition is used to detect at which temperature the transition takes place. Original recordings obtained in an experiment with the ß-blocker propranolol are depicted in Fig.3. The drug induces an additional transition signal at a lower temperature. This signal indicates the transition in the drug-containing phospholipid domains (for a detailed delineation of this interpretation see Hanpft & Mohr 1985). The effectivity of the investigated drugs to depress T_t varied considerably. Probably, the individual effectivity depends on the molecular structure of a drug-molecule. Accordingly, each drug possesses its individual intrinsic activity to disturb the structural arrangement of the artificial phosphatidic acid membranes.

The cardiodepressant potency of the drugs was determined in guinea-pig atria. Spontaneously contracting whole atria were used to assess the

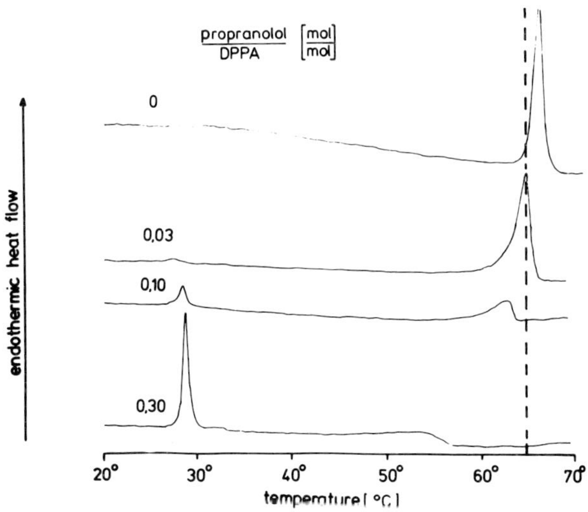

Fig.3: Effect of propranolol on the phase-transition temperature of liposomes made of dipalmitoylphosphatidic acid (DPPA). The thermograms were recorded by means of differential scanning calorimetry.

negative chronotropic potency of the drugs. The drugs were added cumulatively in increasing concentrations, each concentration present for 30min. The drug-concentrations required to reduce beat-frequency to 50% of the control value was taken as a measure of the negative chronotropic potency.

In Fig.4, the IC_{50}-values to inhibit spontaneous beat frequency are plotted versus the IC_{50}-values to reduce ^{45}Ca-binding to phosphatidylserine-monolayers and the ΔT_t-values to depress T_t of DPPA-liposomes.

In general, there was a good correlation between the potency of the drugs to interact with artificial phospholipid membranes and the potency to depress the frequency of contractions. The drugs fitted into the correlation, irrespective of whether being classified as antiarrhythmic, ß-blocking or local anaesthetic.

However, in both plots the Ca-antagonists verapamil and diltiazem revealed a stronger cardiodepressant potency than expected from their capability to affect the phospholipid membranes. Yet, this finding was not surprising, since these drugs are considered to interact specifically and with high affinity with Ca-channels, which are reported to be essential also for sinus node function (for reviews see Fleckenstein 1983, Godfraind 1986). Accordingly, both drugs were not included in the calculation of the correlation coefficients.

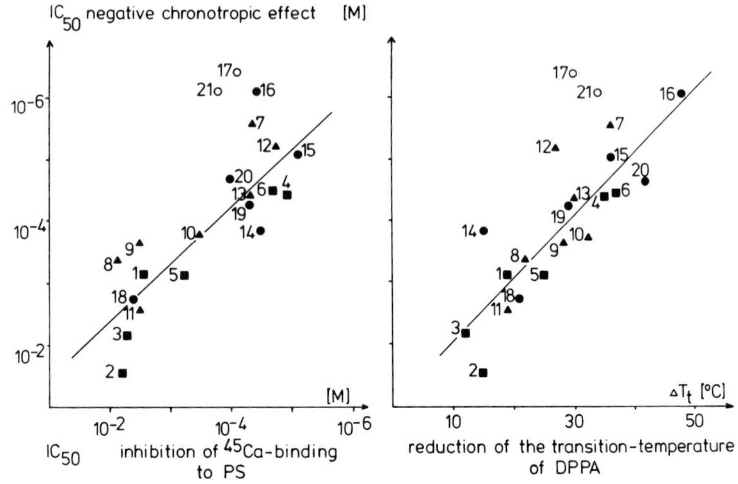

Fig.4: Correlations between the IC_{50}-concentrations to reduce the beat frequency of spontaneously contracting guinea-pig whole atria and the IC_{50}-concentrations to inhibit ^{45}Ca-binding to phosphatidylserine-monolayers or the drug-induced depression of the phase-transition temperature of DPPA-liposomes, respectively.
1-6 (squares): ß-blockers (1: acebutolol, 2: atenolol, 3: diacetolol, 4: penbutolol, 5: pindolol, 6: propranolol); 7-13 (triangles): antiarrhythmic drugs (7: aprindine, 8: disopyramide, 9: lidocaine, 10: mexiletine, 11: procainamide, 12: propafenone, 13: quinidine); 14-21 (circles): catamphiphilic drugs from various groups (14: chloroquine, 15: chlorpromazine, 16: dibucaine, 17: diltiazem, 18: procaine, 19: quinine, 20: tetracaine, 21: verapamil).
The Ca-antagonists diltiazem and verapamil were not included in the calculation of the regression line.

Interestingly, some drugs fitted well into one correlation but deviated from the regression line in the other correlation. The negative chronotropic potency of the local anaesthetic dibucaine was about 30fold higher than expected from its potency to inhibit ^{45}Ca-binding but corresponded to its effectivity to reduce to phase-transition temperature of DPPA. Conversely, the antiarrhythmic propafenone and the dicationic antimalarial chloroquine had a stronger cardiodepressant effect than predicted from their effectivity to reduce T_t, whereas the negative chronotropic action of propafenone matched its potency to inhibit Ca-binding and chloroquine acted even weaker than expected from its effect on phosphatidylserine. Accordingly, a multiple correlation including both the potency to inhibit ^{45}Ca-binding and the effectivity to depress T_t revealed an even better correlation coefficient (r=0.93) than the correlations depicted in Fig.4 (r=0.85 and r=0.84, resp.). Two interpretations can be derived from this finding: 1. The negative chronotropic potency of cationic amphiphilic compounds could be governed by both, the introduction of cationic charges into the head-group region of the phospholipid bilayer and the disordering effect on the arrangement of the phospholipid-molecules within the bilayer; 2. The negative chronotropic effect could depend only on the disordering effect of intercalated drug-molecules, but the extent of this effect is determined by a combination of both the intrinsic activity of a drug-molecule to disarrange the adjacent phospholipid-molecules (reflected by ΔT_t) and the number of drug-molecules bound to the phospholipid membrane at a given drug concentration, i.e. the binding affinity (reflected by IC_{50} to inhibit ^{45}Ca-binding).

The reduction of contraction frequency indicates a reduced rate of spontaneous depolarisation of the membrane potential in the sinus node cells. The pathways by which the ion currents cross the cell membrane are probably integral membrane proteins. Accordingly, the negative chronotropic action of cationic amphiphilic drugs should be expected to be evoked by an alteration of these ion channels. The question arises, whether this assumption is compatible with the notion that the phospholipid matrix of the sarcolemma is the binding site of these drugs.

The functional properties of integral membrane proteins are known to depend on the presence and the nature of the surrounding phospholipid matrix. The interdependence between the protein moiety and its phospholipid annulus has been studied for Na/K-ATPase, which is known to contain higher amounts of phosphatidylserine in its lipid environment. In order to test, whether the properties of this integral membrane protein may be altered by cationic amphiphilic drugs, [^{3}H]ouabain-binding to a cardiac Na/K-ATPase-preparation was measured in the presence of catamphiphilic compounds (Dunst et al., 1983). Since [^{3}H]ouabain binds to the receptor of cardiac glycosides located on the Na/K-ATPase protein, its binding serves as a sensitive indicator of alterations imposed on this protein. It was found that the drugs inhibited ouabain-binding via an allosteric mode of action. The potency of the drugs corresponded favourably with the affinity to bind to phosphatidylserine monolayers. Thus, the conclusion was drawn that the drugs bind to the phosphatidylserine annulus of Na/K-ATPase, thereby altering its properties, which in turn affected the properties of the integral membrane protein of Na/K-ATPase (Dunst et al., 1983).

Therefore, it seems possible that the negative chronotropic effect of cationic amphiphilic drugs may likewise be caused by an indirect effect on integral membrane proteins, i.e. ion channels, the effect arising from the incorporation of drug-molecules in the phospholipid matrix of the sarcolemma.

Conclusion

Drug phospholipid interactions do not only affect the pharmacokinetic properties of a drug, but have also impact on the metabolism and the function of phospholipid membranes. The intercalation of cationic amphiphilic drugs may inhibit intralysosomal phospholipid degradation and may give rise to the formation of inclusion bodies resembling those found in inherited lipid-storage diseases. Since the integrity of the phospholipid matrix of cell membranes is an essential prerequisite for cellular functions, the incorporation of drug molecules in the phospholipid bilayer may be expected to evoke a variety of biological effects, such as the cardiodepressant action. Some of these effects may be caused by an alteration of the function of integral membrane proteins mediated via drug-binding to the phospholipid annulus surrounding the membrane-integrated proteins.

References

Cerbon, J., 1972, Biochimica et Biophysica Acta, 290, 51

Dunst, J., Lüllmann, H. & Mohr, K., 1983, Biochemical Pharmacology, 32, 1595.

Drenckhahn, D., Kleine, L. & Lüllmann-Rauch, R., 1976, Laboratory Investigation, 35, 116

Fleckenstein, A., 1983, Calcium antagonism in heart and smooth muscle (John Wiley & Sons, New York, Chichester, Brisbane, Toronto, Singapore)

Godfraind, T., Miller, R. & Wibo, M., 1986, Pharmacological Reviews, 38, 321

Hanpft, R. & Mohr, K., 1984, Pharmazeutische Zeitung, 129, 21/2215

Hanpft, R. & Mohr, K., 1985, Biochimica et Biophysica Acta, 814, 156

Herbette, L., Katz, A.M. & Sturtevant, J.M., 1983, Molecular Pharmacology, 24, 259

Lee, A.G., 1975, Progress in Biophysics and Molecular Biology, 29, 5

Lüllmann, H. & Wehling, M., 1979, Biochemical Pharmacology, 28, 3409

Lüllmann, H., Plösch, H. & Ziegler, A., 1980, Biochemical Pharmacology, 29, 2969

Lüllmann, H. & Vollmer, B., 1982, Biochemical Pharmacology, 31, 3769

Lüllmann-Rauch, R., Reil, G.-H., Rossen, E. & Seiler, K.U., 1972, Virchows Archiv B, 11, 167

Lüllmann-Rauch, R., 1979, Drug-induced lysosomal storage disorders. In: Lysosomes, edited by J.T. Dingle, P.J. Jaques & I.H. Shaw (North-Holland Publishing Company, Amsterdam, New York, Oxford), p.49

Schmien, R., Seiler, K.-U. & Wassermann, O., 1974, Naunyn-Schmiedeberg's Archives of Pharmacology, 283, 331

Singer, M.A., 1977, Biochemical Pharmacology 26, 51

Yeagle, P.L., Hutton, W.C. & Martin, R.B. 1977, Biochimica et Biophysica Acta 465, 173

XENOBIOTIC-MACROMOLECULE CONJUGATES

D.H. Hutson

Shell Research Ltd., Sittingbourne,
Kent ME9 8AG, UK.

INTRODUCTION

The reaction of xenobiotics with tissue macromolecules *in vivo* may be an important factor affecting their disposition in animals. After a chemical has reacted with a macromolecule it may no longer have the same degree of bioavailability as does a low molecular weight xenobiotic. Its removal from the body depends on the exercise of limited options: (i) recognition of the abnormality by a surveillance system followed by either (a) excision of the xenobiotic fragment or (b) rejection and catabolism of the whole macromolecule, (ii) removal of the affected macromolecule by processes of natural turnover. The localisation of the xenobiotic on a macromolecule and its possibly delayed elimination from the body must always be regarded with concern. However, the consequences of macromolecular conjugation vary dramatically. The initiation of chemical carcinogenesis by the alkylation of DNA is an example of a serious consequence. On the other hand, the partial inhibition of a high capacity system is of much less importance, and may be of no consequence. The assessment of significance is a major concern and thus the explanation of an unexpected disposition of a chemical in terms of macromolecular conjugation answers only the first question. Xenobiotic-macromolecular conjugates must be viewed in the broader context of biochemical toxicology and not merely as products which explain unexpected disposition.

THE FORMATION OF XENOBIOTIC-MACROMOLECULE CONJUGATES

A macromolecular conjugate will be regarded, for this chapter, as a product of covalent reaction between a xenobiotic chemical (or one of its metabolites) with a centre in a large natural molecule such as a protein or a nucleic acid. The formation of macromolecular conjugates may be biochemical or chemical (i.e. relying on chemical reactivity of the xenobiotic). Frequently the process is a 2-stage one in which a reactive intermediate is formed biochemically; this then reacts spontaneously with tissue components. The most common types are formed by the alkylation by electrophilic xenobiotics of nucleophilic centres on macromolecules. These reactions can be regarded as analogies of the glutathione (GSH) conjugation process but without the catalysis. GSH is the most abundant and reactive biological nucleophile and responsible for much of the body's protection against soft electrophiles. The thiol groups and amino groups of proteins and certain nitrogen and oxygen atoms in nucleic acids are also sites of attack by electrophiles. As a very rough estimate, the relative amounts of reaction of these classes of macromolecules with soft electrophiles are: glutathione, 5,000; proteins, 100; RNA, 10; DNA, 1. Thus, whenever a mercapturic acid turns up in a metabolism study, the formation of macromolecular conjugates is also probably occurring, but often below the limit of detection. An important point to note about xenobiotic-macromolecule conjugates is that the chemical reactivity that drives the reaction is spent in the process, i.e. the xenobiotic (or its reactive intermediate) has shot its bolt. The major concern from this point on is the potentially altered function of the macromolecule or other response triggered by its presence. If the product is of no significance, then the reaction can be regarded as a detoxification.

Another covalent linkage involving the protein thiol group is the disulphide linkage exemplified by captopril (see below). These bonds are less stable than thioether and alkylamino (or imino) bonds, their formation being reversible in the presence of other thiol groups, those of GSH, for example. Conjugates can also be formed by the S, N or O-acylation of macromolecules. The acylating reagents are usually formed via Phase 1 biotransformation, but the reactivity of ester glucuronides (Phase 2 products) in this respect is a recently-discovered phenomenon (Stogniew and Fenselau, 1982). It may account for a number of low-level bound residues that are detected in studies of drugs, hormones and pesticides in farm animals.

The incorporation of xenobiotics into macromolecules via normal processes could also be regarded as a route to xenobiotic-macromolecule conjugates. Thus, the hybrid triacylglycerols and other xenobiotic lipids can also be classified as xenobiotic-macromolecule conjugates. Space does not allow a detailed discussion of these products but they are good examples of conjugates observed in metabolism studies because of unexpected distribution of residual radioactivity or delayed elimination from the body or both. The phenomenon, discovered only in the last ten years, has been reviewed recently by Fears (1985) and Quistad and Hutson (1986). The significance (toxicological and therapeutic) of the incorporation of xenobiotics into lipid biosynthesis is being studied at present but currently there are many more questions than answers.

The first macromolecular conjugate described below also stems from an unexpected disposition (of a herbicide). The further work undertaken to understand the reaction may afford a general approach to the problem of xenobiotic-macromolecule conjugates.

MACROMOLECULAR CONJUGATES FROM 2-METHYLMERCAPTO-s-TRIAZINES

During metabolic studies on a ^{14}C-labelled herbicidal s-triazine (cyanatryn,1) an unusual distribution of retained radioactivity was observed (Crawford et al., 1980), most of the 1% retained in the body 4 days after dosing being in the blood. The questions posed by this finding are detailed in Table 1. Because the retention was in blood, a relatively accessible material of relatively simple composition, the experimental approaches involved were somewhat easier than might be expected in other situations; however, the approach may be generally useful.

Using Table 1 for guidance, the following facts emerged: the radioactivity was due to a metabolite which could not be extracted (methanol) from the blood. It was associated with the erythrocyte content and could not be separated by chromatographic methods from haemoglobin (i.e. absorbance at 415 nm). It was attached to the globin moiety from which it could be released by gentle acid hydrolysis similar to that required to cleave an s-triazinyl-glutathione. The dose-dependency of formation indicated linearity between doses of 0.25 and 250 mg/kg (i.e. no threshold for the reaction was observed). The kinetics of accumulation (50 days to plateau) and depletion ($t_{\frac{1}{2}}$ 10-15 days) were in accord with a reaction with haemoglobin and removal of the product by normal destruction of haemoglobin. The structure of the conjugate was assumed to be globin, s- triazinylated at cysteine sulphur. Its formation could be modelled <u>in vitro</u> by S-oxygenation of the herbicide (with microsomal monooxygenase or m-chloroperbenzoic acid) and incubating the product with erythrocytes. The reaction

Table 1. Investigation of a retained xenobiotic

Is the xenobiotic unchanged or a metabolite?
Is the metabolite of low molecular weight?
If not, is it covalently bound to a macromolecule?
If a macromolecule:
Which class of macromolecule?
What is the dose-dependency of formation?
What are the kinetics of accumulation?
What are the kinetics of depletion?
What is the structure of the xenobiotic component?
What is the nature of the covalent bond?
Can the structure of the conjugate be inferred?
What is its mechanism of formation?
Is the function of the macromolecule altered?
Is this significant?
Could the macromolecule interfere with life processes?
Could it trigger the immune system?
Which other macromolecules may be targets?

in vivo or *in vitro* was apparently without effect on the oxygen-binding capacity of the haemoglobin. There was no evidence to suggest immunotoxicity and, therefore, the conjugate appeared to remain safely tucked away inside the erythrocyte. A further important consideration was that of species. The *in vitro* model indicated that rat haemoglobin was more reactive than that of man, rabbit or dog. In the light of the apparent lack of toxicological significance of the reaction, our major concern was for the potential of the *S*-oxide to react with DNA. This concern was allayed by (i) the non-mutagenicity of the *S*-oxide (ii) its lack of binding to DNA *in vitro* and (iii) immeasurable reaction of the herbicide with DNA *in vivo*. Hughes et al. (1981) and Hamboeck et al. (1981) reported similar results with the related *s*-triazine, simetryn, and extended the range of species studied to rat, mouse, guinea pig and chicken (reactive) and man, dog, cow, sheep and pig (relatively unreactive). Some excellent structural analysis revealed that the triazine group reacted at cysteine β-125 (one per haemoglobin tetramer) of rat. Surprisingly, the usually more reactive cysteine β-93 did not react. In conclusion, the reaction appeared to be of little significance to rat, did not occur in man and was not indicative of genotoxicity.

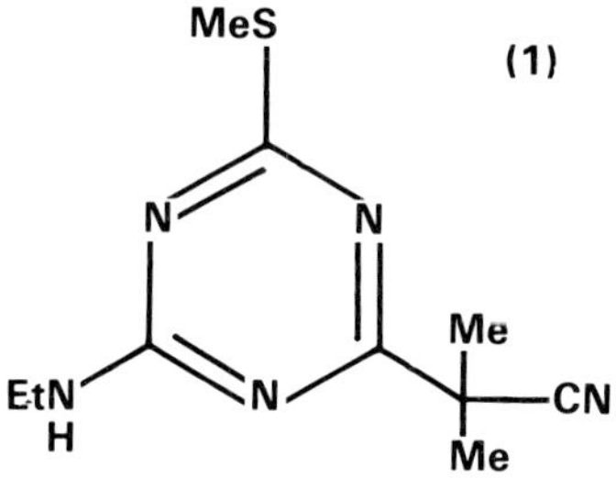

(1)

(2)

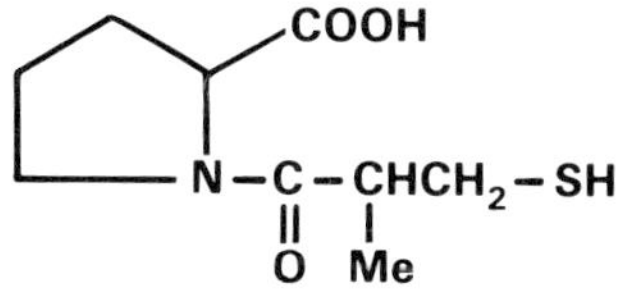

DRUG-PROTEIN CONJUGATES IN RELATION TO THE IMMUNE SYSTEM

When drug-macromolecule conjugates are formed and are available to the immune system they should function as haptens, trigger the formation of antibodies and may thus afford adverse reactions via an immunological mechanism (Park et al., 1987). This subject has received little attention from xenobiochemists until quite recently. The drug captopril (2) (used to treat hypertension and congestive heart failure) appears to afford such an immunotoxic reaction. Its chronic administration can lead to a variety of adverse reactions, the nature and time course of which are consistent with an immunological mechanism. Park and co-workers (1982) have carried out a series of studies which support this. Captopril is extensively bound to plasma albumin via a disulphide linkage. The conjugate has a relatively short half-life (70 min) being lost by interchange with other thiols including GSH (Yeung et al., 1983). Its immunogenicity has now been investigated in N.Z. white rabbits using heterologous proteins with captopril (CP) linked via amide and disulphide bonds (Yeung et al., 1985). Anti-CP antibody activity was readily detected (immunodiffusion) in the sera of rabbits immunised with amide-linked CP human serum albumin (23:1). The antigenic determinant in this case was CP and a lysine residue. Disulphide-linked CP afforded a weak antibody activity (detected by a sensitive ELISA method). The specificity of this activity was confirmed as being for CP-S-S-protein by its inhibition only by preincubation with CP-S-S-protein (the carriers alone and penicillamine-S-S-proteins did not inhibit). Thus, disulphide linked CP-protein conjugates are capable of immunogenicity under favourable experimental conditions and the ELISA method can now be used to test the situation in man. Many adverse drug reactions are ascribed to an immunological mechanism on the basis of clinical symptoms but in relatively few instances is the mechanism verified by the detection of either drug-induced antibody or sensitized cells of the immune system. However, antibodies to some 22 drugs have now been detected in humans (Park et al., 1987).

The reversible nature of the CP-S-S-protein conjugate has led to the suggestion (Drummer and Jarrott, 1984) that it may act as a Captopril prodrug, particularly when the captopril disulphide dimer (CP-S-S-CP) is dosed. The latter has a longer half-life than captopril and this could arise partly from equilibration of the dimer and protein conjugates.

Drug-protein conjugates are not necessarily very persistent in mammals. The CP conjugate has a half-life of about 70 min, possibly because of the lability of the disulphide bond. However, model conjugates of dinitrofluorobenzene (DNFB), i.e. dinitrophenylated (DNP-) proteins are catabolised quite rapidly. Thus, Kitteringham et al. (1985) prepared DNFB-conjugates with rat, rabbit and human albumins at several degrees of substitution (ratio DNFB: protein between 0.5 and 20) and studied their fate after i.v. administration to rats. The conjugates were cleared mainly through the liver and the DNP-moiety appeared in the bile and the urine as the novel amino acid conjugate N^2-acetyl-N^6-DNP-lysine. The shortest half-life (ca 1 hour) was obtained with the protein having the highest degree of DNP-substitution. A study in rabbits indicated that the clearance was not dependent on an immune mechanism and, furthermore, the DNP-protein conjugates did not appear to elicit an anti-DNP response when autologous protein conjugates were used.

MACROMOLECULAR CONJUGATES AND GENOTOXICITY

Perhaps the most serious consequence of the formation of xenobiotic-macromolecule conjugates is that initiated by the reactions of electrophiles with DNA. When these "conjugates" remain undetected by repair enzymes they may be free to malfunction, causing mutagenicity or carcinogenicity or both. The conjugates are never obvious, rather they must be sought out using xenobiotics labelled at high specific radioactivity and sophisticated analytical techniques operating at the nucleoside, nucleotide and the base level. These techniques must have a sensitivity of about 1 substitution per 10^8 or 10^9 bases. Simple reactions, like methylation, are difficult enough to deal with because of the profoundly different effects of the position of alkylation. Carcinogens requiring bioactivation present even more complex problems, from the relative simplicity of vinyl chloride to the complexity of benzo(a)pyrene (Huckle et al., 1986).

The detection of such chemical lesions remains almost as large a problem as interpreting their significance. The problem is particularly difficult in man, where access to DNA is very limited. The technique of using haemoglobin as a dose monitor for alkylating agents developed by Ehrenberg and co-workers (Calleman et al., 1978) leads us back into protein conjugates. Haemoglobin has a life-time of about 4 months in man and, provided that this value holds good for alkylated species, it can be used to monitor acute and chronic exposures. The technique was developed using alkylated cysteine and histidine residues but, currently, the N-alkylated-N-terminal valine residues afford the most useful products. These adducts are selectively and gently cleaved from the isolated haemoglobin using pentafluorophenyl isothiocyanate and measured by GC-MS (Tornqvist et al., 1987). This approach must, of course, be validated in experimental animals to ensure that there is a proportional relationship between the interaction with target organ DNA and with haemoglobin. Immunoassay techniques may be expected to make an increasing impact on the quantitation of these adducts both of DNA and protein. In addition, very sensitive ^{32}P-postlabelling methods for the detection of DNA adducts are becoming available which can be applied to a 1 ug sample of DNA (Randerath et al., 1985).

CONCLUSIONS

Xenobiotic macromolecule conjugates may be formed from xenobiotics or their intermediary metabolites by spontaneous chemical reactions or by enzyme-catalysed processes. A study of these conjugates is an essential part of the toxicological assessment of any xenobiotic giving rise to such products. However, the amount of conjugate formed and its persistence are far less important than the effect that the reaction has on the function of the parent macromolecule. Thus critical interactions can afford tissue necrosis, teratogenicity, mutagenicity and carcinogenicity. The altered macromolecule may be recognised by the immune system and in this way immune responses such as skin sensitisation and more serious systemic reactions may be developed. Where this does not happen, and when the function of the product is unaffected, interaction with the macromolecule may effect detoxification (by protecting more critical sites). Some substituted proteins appear to be catabolised quite effectively and the result of such interactions may be likened to a rather cumbersome analogue of glutathione and amino acid conjugation. However, the onus lies with the scientist to determine the significance of each macromolecular conjugate along the lines suggested in Table 1.

REFERENCES

Calleman, C.J., Ehrenberg, L., Jansson, B., Osterman-Golkar, S., Segerbäck, D., Svensson, S. & Wachtmeister, C.A., 1978, Journal of Environmental Pathology and Toxicology, 2, 427.

Crawford, M.J., Hutson, D.H., & Stoydin, G., 1980, Xenobiotica, 10, 169.

Drummer, O.H. & Jarrott, B., 1984, Biochemical Pharmacology, 33, 3567.

Fears, R., 1985, Progress in Lipid Research, 24, 177.

Hamboeck, H., Fischer, R.W., Di Iorio, E.E. & Winterhalter, K.H., 1981, Molecular Pharmacology, 20, 579.

Huckle, K.R., Smith, R.J., Watson, W.P. & Wright, A.S., 1986, Carcinogenesis, 7, 965.

Hughes, G.J., De Jong, C., Fischer, R.W., Winterhalter, K.H. & Wilson, K.J., 1981, Biochemical Journal, 199, 61.

Kitteringham, N.R., Maggs, J.L., Newby, S. & Park, B.K. 1985, Biochemical Pharmacology, 34, 1763.

Park, B.K., Coleman, J.W. & Kitteringham, N.R., 1987, Biochemical Pharmacology, 36, 581.

Park, B.K., Grabowski, P.S., Yeung, J.H.K. & Breckenridge, A.M., 1982, Biochemical Pharmacology, 31, 1755.

Quistad, G.B. & Hutson, D.H., 1986 in Xenobiotic Conjugation Chemistry, ACS Symposium Series No. 299, p. 204.

Randerath, K., Randerath, E., Agrawal, H.P., Gupta, R.C., Schurdak, M.E. & Reddy, M.V., 1985, Environmental Health Perspectives, 62, 57.

Stogniew, M. & Fenselau, C., 1982, Drug Metabolism and Disposition, 10, 609.

Tornqvist, M., Mowrer, J., Jenson, S. & Ehrenberg, L., 1987. Analytical Biochemistry, in press.

Yeung, J.H.K., Breckenridge, A.M. & Park, B.K., 1983, Biochemical Pharmacology, 32, 3619.

Yeung, J.H.K., Coleman, J.W. & Park, B.K., 1985, Biochemical Pharmacology, 34, 4005.

METABOLICALLY RESISTANT CHEMICALS

I. Scheunert & F. Korte

Gesellschaft für Strahlen- und Umweltforschung mbH München
Institut für Ökologische Chemie
Ingolstädter Landstr. 1, 8042 Neuherberg, FRG

INTRODUCTION

Only a limited number of xenobiotics can be fully metabolized and utilized as a source of carbon and energy for living organisms. Much more frequently, transformations of xenobiotics are due to cometabolism initiated by enzymes of animal or microbial origin.

Table 1 shows some primary enzymatic reactions of xenobiotic substances. The apparently great number of reactions, in principle, can be reduced to three reaction types: oxidation, reduction and hydrolysis. Some of the reactions listed are effected only by enzymes whose occurrence is rare, or limited to special environmental conditions. With regard to the multitude of chemical structures of man-made chemicals, it is obvious that many of them are resistant to metabolic processes.

Metabolic resistance is specific to a functional group of a molecule, rather than to the chemical compound as a whole. Chemicals with resistant functional groups may be transformed easily at other sites of the molecule; however, the transformation products still containing the resistant functional group continue to exist in the environment as metabolically resistant chemicals, even if they are conjugated and excreted by one or several species.

The polycondensed aromatic structure and the organic carbon-halogen bond are among the most wide-spread metabolically resistant molecular groups. In the following, some examples of metabolically resistant polychlorinated organic compounds are discussed.

Table 1. Primary enzymatic reactions of xenobiotic substances.

Reaction type	Examples	Chemicals transformed
Oxidations	C-Hydroxylation	Benzene derivatives, PCB, Benzo(a)pyren, DDT, Dieldrin
	Methyloxidation	Bromacil
	Epoxidation	Cyclodiene insecticides
	Ketone formation	Carbofuran
	ß-Oxidation	2,4-Dichlorophenoxy-alkanoic acids
	Sulfoxidation	Thioanisoles, Carboxin
	Phosphorothionate oxidation	Parathion
	C=C-cleavage	Cyclodiene insecticides, PCB, phthalates
	C-Dehydrogenation	Hexachlorocyclohexane
	N-Oxidation	Chlorinated anilines
Reductions	Reduction of keto groups	Acetophenone
	Reduction of azo groups	Azobenzene
	Reduction of nitro groups	Pentachloronitrobenzene, Parathion
	Reduction of N-oxides	Nicotinamid-N-oxide
	Reductive dechlorination	DDT, chlorinated benzene derivatives, Toxaphene
	C=C-reduction	DDMU (metabolite of DDT)
	C=C-reduction	Buturon
Hydrolytic reactions	Hydrolysis of carboxylic esters	Malathion, Kelevan, phthalates
	Hydrolysis of nitriles	2,4-Dichlorobenzoic acid nitrile
	Hydrolysis of amides	N-acetyl-2-aminofluorene
	Phosphate hydrolysis	Tri-o-tolyl-phosphate, Parathion
	Epoxide hydrolysis	Dieldrin
	Carbamate hydrolysis	Carbaryl

METABOLISM OF POLYCHLORINATED ORGANIC COMPOUNDS IN MAMMALS

The use of dieldrin as an insecticide was restricted or banned in most of the industrialized countries some years ago. Nevertheless, due to its metabolic resistance, it continues to occur in the environment including human food and human adipose tissue. Its two major metabolic products in mammals - the oxidative product 12-hydroxy-dieldrin and the hydrolytic product 4,5-aldrin trans-diol - are excreted by mammals in varying amounts depending on the animal species (Table 2). In both metabolites, the resistant carbon-chlorine bonds are unaffected, and after excretion by the mammal they remain in the environment as metabolically resistant chemicals.

Table 2. Metabolites of dieldrin excreted by various animals within 10 days after 0.5 mg/kg oral administration (in % of administered dose) (Müller et al., 1975).

Animal species		Dieldrin	12-OH-dieldrin	4,5-Aldrin-trans-diol
Mouse,	male	5.5	13.0	20.0
	female	3.2	7.5	26.0
Rat,	male	0.8	8.8	2.3
	female	2.8	4.6	2.4
Rabbit,	male	0.3	-	1.5
	female	0.5	0.2	2.0
Rhesus,	male	9.0	9.4	2.0
Chimpanzee,	female	3.2	2.0	1.1

The same applies to the metabolites of polychlorinated biphenyls, most of which are phenolic or methoxylated derivatives containing all of the chlorine atoms of the parent compounds. Among the metabolites of 2,3,7,8-tetrachlorodibenzo-p-dioxin, a contaminant which is released into the environment as a byproduct of chemical syntheses or of combustion processes, only a few products (Figure 1, III, IVa and b) have lost one of the four chlorine atoms.

The examples of ß-hexachlorocyclohexane, the most persistent of all HCH-isomers (Figure 2), and of hexachlorobenzene, one of the most persistent environmental chemicals (Figure 3), demonstrate that not only microorganisms but also mammals are able to break the organic C-Cl-bond.

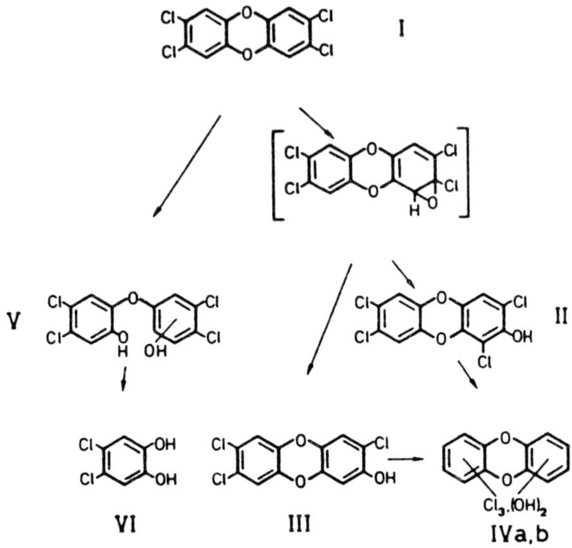

Figure 1. Proposed metabolic breakdown scheme of TCDD (Poiger et al., 1982).

For hexachlorobenzene, it has been shown that reductive dechlorination is catalyzed by an enzyme located in the microsomal fraction of liver, lung, kidney, and intestine of rats (Mehendale et al., 1975). However, when the metabolized portion of the total amount of xenobiotic in the body is minimal ($<$ 1 % after 7 days for hexachlorobenzene in rats), these reactions do not have any quantitative significance.

BEHAVIOUR OF METABOLICALLY RESISTANT CHEMICALS IN THE ENVIRONMENT

When released into the environment, metabolically resistant chemicals and their resistant metabolites get into natural cycles and join the pool of persistent natural compounds. Table 3 shows that they are also resistant to degradation in technical waste composting processes or in garden composting. After the composting time, they are recovered unchanged, to the extent of more than 80-90 %. In the case of heptachlor, the higher amount of conversion products was mostly due to a metabolite - heptachlor

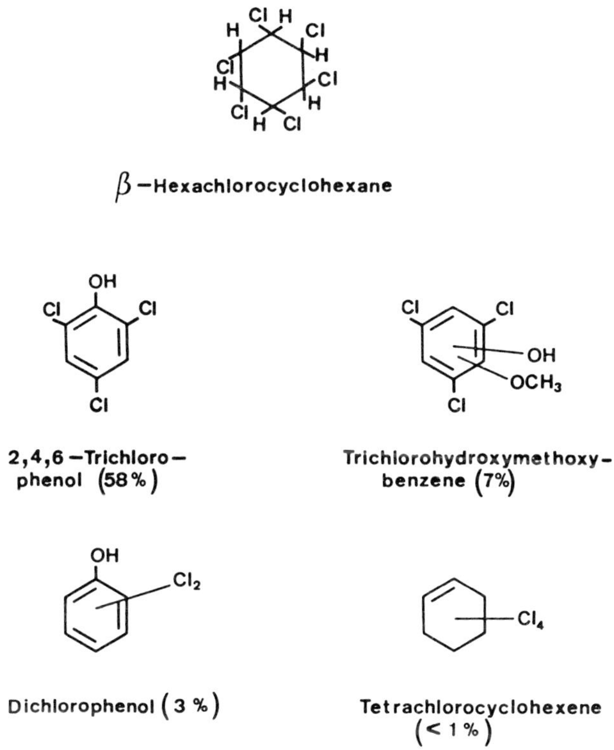

Figure 2. Metabolites of ß-hexachloro[^{14}C]cyclohexane isolated from rat urine (in % of radioactivity excreted in urine) (Lay et al., 1981).

epoxide - which is even more persistent than the parent compound. For 4-chloroaniline, the "conversion products" mostly consisted of unextractable material bound to natural organic matter.

Polycondensed aromatics of natural origin, lignin and humic substances are examples of resistant natural products in the environment. These are slowly transformed and degraded over longer time periods. Similarly, resistant man-made chemicals undergo measurable but very slow mineralization to carbon dioxide.

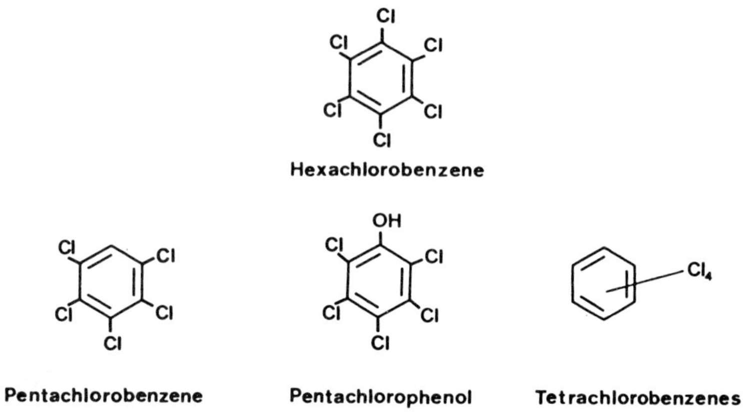

Figure 3. Metabolites of hexachlorobenzene isolated from urine of rats and Rhesus monkeys (Mehendale et al., 1975; Rozman et al., 1978).

Table 3. Degradation of resistant chemicals in waste composting processes (Müller & Korte 1975; Müller et al., 1974; Weber 1987).

Chemical	Composting process	%* Recovered unchanged
Aldrin	Simulation of technical waste composting (1 week)	83
Dieldrin	"	86
Heptachlor	"	60
Benzo-(a)-pyrene	"	93
2,2'-Dichlorobiphenyl	"	97
4-Chloroaniline	"	70
Hexachlorobenzene	Garden composting (7 weeks)	96

* % of initially applied dose

CONCLUSIONS

In order to overcome the problems of long-living chemicals in the environment, metabolically resistant xenobiotics should be replaced by degradable ones. This may be achieved by studying structure-persistence relationships. Some examples of such relationships known thus far are given in Table 4. Further correlations of this kind should be studied and evaluated for use in the synthesis of new products having more favourable structure characteristics.

Table 4. Correlation of metabolic resistance of chemicals with structure characteristics.

Less resistant	More resistant
Unbranched alkyl groups	Branched alkyl groups
Alkenes	Alkanes
Alkanes	Aromatics
Benzene derivatives	Triazines
Aromatics with less substituents	Aromatics with more substituents
Alkyl-substituted aromatics	Halogen-substituted aromatics
Aromatics with less halogen substituents	Aromatics with more halogen substituents
o,p'-DDT	p,p'-DDT
DDT-analogs with one free p-position	DDT-analogs with two substituted p-positions
PCBs with adjacent free p- and m-positions	PCBs with adjacent substituted p- and m-positions

REFERENCES

Lay, J.P., Klein, W. & Korte, F., 1981, Journal of Environmental Science and Health, Part B, 16, 227.

Mehendale, H.M., Fields, M. & Matthews, H.B., 1975, Journal of Agricultural and Food Chemistry, 23, 261.

Müller, W.P. & Korte, F., 1975, Chemosphere, 4, 195.

Müller, W., Nohynek, G., Woods, G., Korte, F. & Coulston, F., 1975, Chemosphere, 4, 89.

Müller, W., Rohleder, H., Klein, W. & Korte, F., 1974, Modellstudie zur Abfallbeseitigung - Verhalten repräsentativer xenobiotischer Substanzen bei der Müllkompostierung, GSF-Bericht Ö 104 (Gesellschaft für Strahlen- und Umweltforschung mbH München).

Poiger, H., Buser, H.-R., Weber, H., Zweifel, M. & Schlatter, Ch., 1982, Experientia, 38, 484.

Rozman, K., Müller, W.F., Coulston, F. & Korte, F., 1978, Chemosphere, 7, 177.

Weber, B., 1987, Verhalten von ^{14}C-markierten Umweltchemikalien bei der Herstellung von Gartenkompost, Doctoral Thesis (Technical University of München) (in preparation).

2. Non-‘P-450’ enzymes on xenobiotic oxidation

Drug Oxidation by Non P-450 Enzymes

V. ULLRICH

Faculty of Biology, University of Konstanz, FRG

Meetings on drug metabolism are usually devoted almost exclusively to cytochrome P-450 catalysed transformations. This seems justified since more than 90% of the average drug is converted by a cytochrome P-450 pathway. Only one other monooxygenase, the flavin-dependent monooxygenase for sulfur or nitrogen oxidations, is usually considered to be relevant and will be treated in depth in this section.

In considering the significance of the three groups of "non-P-450-oxidations" one has to classify the peroxidase-type of oxidations as the potentially most hazardous group of reactions. The radical intermediates in this pathway have not only been postulated but can also be measured by ESR. Although the potential toxicity seems to be clear the actualcases in which toxic effects can be pinpointed to the action of peroxidases are scarce. There is still the often cited case of acetaminophen and phenacetin which, by their common phenolic metabolite, may interfere with the cyclooxygenase-peroxidase reaction and thus may be responsible for kidney damage.

The two other groups of oxidases - the FAD-dependent monoxygenases and xanthine and aldehyde oxidases - clearly belong to pathways of detoxication and only with certain substrates toxic side effects may arise. With regard to these substrate specifities they seem to occupy metabolic niches since they can handle substrates for cytochrome P-450-dependent monooxygenations. Compounds with amino and sulphur groups and also with phosphorus can be metabolized by the FAD-monooxygenase. The different substrate specifities between monooxygenases and xanthine or aldehyde oxidases is partly based on chemistry since in monooxygenases the mechanism involves an electrophilic attack at the carbon whereas the oxidases require a nucleophilic addition at an unsaturated carbon.

Thanks to the availability of the ^{18}O-isotope we know that hydroxyl groups in drug metabolites can also be derived from water by the action of dehydrogenating enzymes which catalyze also a subsequent addition of water to the double-bond. Xanthine oxidase and aldehyde oxidase are examples in which molydbenum at the catalytic site plays an essential part in the mechanism. The significance of both enzymes is still under debate, and one contribution in this section will deal with this aspect.

Together with the cytochrome P-450 isoenzymes, the flavin-dependent monooxygenase and the two molybdenum-containing oxidases form the bulk of phase I drug oxidazing enzymes and all of them act on special subgroups of drugs in a well-defined stoichiometry and with a distinct product pattern. However, there are also drug oxidations known which have varying stoichiometries, ill-defined products and even their enzymatic structure is difficult to assess. They play only a minor quantitative role, but as they have the potential to yield reactive metabolites they should concern us because of their potential toxic effects.

Substrates for this group of drug oxidations are mostly phenols or other derivatives with reducing properties, and the mechanisms of oxidation are essentially one-electron oxidations causing the formation of radical intermediates. These may cause covalent binding or oxidative stress symptoms since subsequent chain reactions involving lipid peroxidation may arise. For example, a simple chemical like benzene, may be converted to phenol or catechols or arene oxide as the only primary metabolites, but it may be toxic because of secondary oxidations to phenoxy radicals. The enzymes responsible for these deleterious effects are predominantly peroxidases, but also non-enzymic oxidations by cellular oxygen radicals may occur.

The examples of pteridine-based drugs and their degradation or activation by monoamine oxidase lend support to a growing significance of "non-P-450-oxidations" the more we derive drugs from biologically related molecules. In cases where there is an overlap with the P-450-monooxygenases, a biochemical differentiation based on specific inhibitors or on different inactivation kinetics in the presence of NADPH will be very helpful.

Especially for the peroxidatic drug oxidation a word of caution seems to be appropriate. Because of their largely unknown nature these reactions seem to be ubiquitous and their physiological conditions are difficult to define. Very often in vitro assays are set up and in optimizing the reactions one gradually arrives at non-physiological conditions. One may easily exceed the physiological hydrogen peroxide concentrations or use substrate levels which never accumulate in vivo. Also the antioxidant potential of the intact cell may not allow oxidations that one sees in vitro. Nevertheless, peroxidatic reactions do occur and have to be studied since even a small percentage of such a pathway can cause side-effects or adverse reactions of a drug. This is documented in the first paper, dealing with the cyclooxygenase pathway and the co-oxidation of drugs.

Peroxidase-catalyzed metabolic activation of xenobiotics

ROGER LARSSON, JEAN BOUTIN AND PETER MOLDÉUS

Department of Toxicology, Karolinska Institutet
S-104 01 Stockholm, Sweden

A number of different peroxidases have been discovered in mammalian tissues distinct from the peroxidase activities of hemoproteins such as hemoglobin, myoglobin and catalase.

These peroxidases include prostaglandin synthase, probably the most important peroxidase and found in a variety of tissues such as kidney, lung, intestine, spleen and blood vessels (Samuelsson et al. 1978). Other peroxidases in this group include lactoperoxidase found for example in mammary glands (Jellinck and Cleveland 1977), myeloperoxidase found in white blood cells like neutrophils, peritoneal macrophages, bone marrow cells and liver Kupffer cells (Kalyanaraman and Sohnie 1985) and the tissue specific peroxidases thyroid peroxidase (Strum and Karnovsky 1970), intestinal peroxidase (Venkatachalam et al. 1970) and uterine peroxidase (Kumura et al. 1983).

The mechanism of peroxidase reactions in general, apart from myeloperoxidase-catalyzed oxidation of chloride to hypochlorite, appears to proceed by the scheme below involving the peroxidase intermediates, compounds I and II (Mason and Chignell 1981):

$$\text{Peroxidase} + H_2O_2 \longrightarrow \text{Compound I}$$
$$\text{Compound I} + RH_2 \longrightarrow \text{Compound II} + \dot{R}H_2^+$$
$$\text{Compound II} + RH_2 \longrightarrow \text{Peroxidase} + \dot{R}H_2^+$$

The role of the peroxide cofactor is to oxidize the heme-iron in the peroxidase enzyme from its +III resting oxidation state to that of +V thus generating compound I. Compound I can be reduced by two sequential one-electron transfer processes resulting in the regeneration of the peroxidase heme-iron resting state and two one-electron deficient substrate molecule free radicals. Reduction can also occur through a direct transfer of two electrons not involving formation of free radical intermediates. Different types of reactive free radicals can be produced by the action of mammalian peroxidases and it has been proposed that a free radical activation route may be important for toxicity of certain xenobiotics in extrahepatic tissues.

For example, the bone marrow toxicity of benzene may be as a result of in situ oxidation of phenol by myeloperoxidase since this tissue contains only very small amounts of cytochrome P-450 (Sawahata and Neal 1982). Of the chemicals containing the phenol structure, the peroxidative metabolism of the synthetic estrogen diethylstilbestrol (DES) has been studied most intensely. The genital tract tumors which have been observed in young women exposed to DES in utero has been proposed to result from activation of DES by uterine peroxidase (Metzler and McLachlan 1978).

The carcinogenicity of several N-hydroxyl-N-acetylaminoarenes like 2-hydroxyacetylaminofluorene towards subcutaneous tissue correlates inversely with the stability of their nitroxides. Nitroxides are formed from the N-hydroxy compounds in a variety of peroxidase reactions involving the lactoperoxidase and myeloperoxidase systems (Bartsch et al. 1971).

As already mentioned the most important peroxidase reaction involved in the metabolic activation of xenobiotics is probably the one catalyzed by prostaglandin synthase (PGS) (Marnett and Eling 1983, Eling et al. 1983). PGS catalyzes the oxygenation of polyunsaturated fatty acids to hydroxy endoperoxides (Samuelsson et al. 1978). The preferential substrate _in vivo_ is arachidonic acid (AA). PGS contains two activities. The fatty acid cyclooxygenase activity catalyzes the oxygenation of AA to a hydroperoxy endoperoxide (PGG_2), while the hydroperoxidase activity catalyses the reduction of PGG_2 to the hydroxy endoperoxide (PGH_2) (Miyamoto et al. 1976, O'Brien and Rahimtula 1976). PGH_2 represents a branching point in the metabolism of AA and it can undergo tissue specific metabolism to various prostaglandins, thromboxanes and prostacyclins. The cyclooxygenase activity of PGS is inhibited by nonsteroidal antiinflammatory agents such as indomethacin and acetylsalicylic acid (Vane 1971), while there are no known specific inhibitors of the hydroperoxidase activity.

It is thus the hydroperoxidase activity of PGS that catalyzes the metabolism (co-oxidation) of xenobiotics. As already indicated the PGS catalyzed co-oxidation often results in the formation of reactive products and a number of xenobiotics have been shown to be co-oxidized to reactive products. These include the aromatic amines benzidine, 2-aminofluorene and 4-aminobiphenyl, the phenols acetaminophen and diethylstilbestrol, the polycyclic aromatic hydrocarbons benzo(1)pyrene 7,8-dihydroxy-7,8-dihydrobenzopyrene and 7,12-dimethylbenzanthrazene and the miscellaneous FANFT (N-[4-(5-nitro-2-furyl)-thiazolyl]formamide) (for review see Marnett and Eling 1983, Eling et al. 1983).

We have in our laboratory studied the peroxidase catalyzed metabolism of an aromatic amine, p-phenetidine. Phenetidine is a major metabolite of phenacetin, an analgesic and anti-pyretic drug, which is known to cause toxic lesions in the kidney and the lower urinary tract (Hultengren et al. 1965). Phenetidine is an excellent peroxidase substrate and PGS as well as horse radish peroxidase (HRP) mediated metabolism of phenetidine has been demonstrated to result in the formation of a free radical intermediate and of several secondary products (Ross et al. 1985,1). This metabolism also results in extensive protein binding (Andersson et al. 1983), DNA binding (Andersson et al. 1984) and induction of DNA single strand breaks (Andersson et al. 1982). In addition to the free radical intermediate two reactive secondary products of p-phenetidine have been identified. These are the two dimers N-(4-ethoxyphenyl)-p-benzoquinone di-imine and N-(4-ethoxyphenyl)-p-benzoquinone imine (NEPBQI) (Larsson et al. 1984, Ross et al. 1985). The formation of the quinone di-imine dimer is presumably mediated through a head to tail coupling of two p-phenetidine radical intermediates with concomitant loss of ethanol. NEPBQI is then rather slowly formed from the quinone di-imine dimer through hydrolysis with elimination of ammonia. Both the dimers bind to protein as well as to nucleophiles such as GSH. NEPBQI does not however bind to DNA or induce DNA single strand breaks (Larsson et al. 1986). The DNA binding and damage thus appear to be caused by either the radical intermediate, the quinone di-imine dimer or an unidentified product. DNA binding of radical intermediates has been demonstrated for chlorpromazine (Ohnishi and McConnell 1965) and 2-aminofluorene (Krauss and Eling 1985). Free radicals are however primarily oxidizing species and the DNA binding during peroxidase catalyzed oxidation of p-phenetidine is more likely to be caused by a secondary reactive product possibly the quinone di-imine dimer. Support for the involvement of the di-imine dimer comes from results using benzidine. During metabolism by

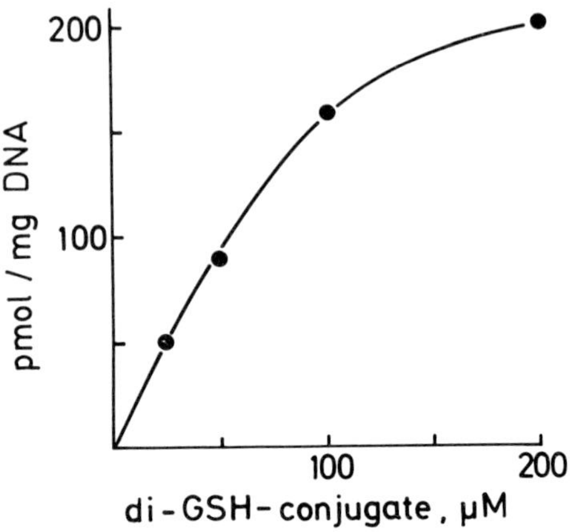

Figure 1. Binding of a di-glutathione conjugate of NEPBQI to DNA.

PGS benzidine extensively binds to DNA (Kadlubar et al. 1982, Zenzer et al. 1980). The mechanism of the peroxidase mediated interaction of benzidine with DNA appears to be distinct from the nitrenium ion mechanism elucidated for arylamides such as 2-acetylaminofluorene. A benzidine-DNA adduct identified as N-(deoxyguanosin-8-yl)-benzidine has thus been isolated , which is probably formed by benzidine di-imine binding (Yamazoe et al. 1986).

An interesting aspect of the peroxidase mediated DNA binding of p-phenetidine is the several fold enhanced binding which occurs when GSH is present in the incubation medium (Andersson et al. 1984). This enhanced DNA binding is in contrast to protein binding which is prevented by GSH (Andersson et al. 1983). In the presence of GSH a number of glutathione conjugates are formed, in addition to a glutathionyl radical intermediate, which is generated through the interaction of GSH with the p-phenetidine radical (Ross et al. 1983,3). We have identified mono-glutathione conjugates of the guinone di-imine dimer and NEPBQI as well as two di-glutathione conjugates of the same products. In addition to these four at least three other conjugates are formed (Ross et al. 1985,2). The isolated conjugates may exist in both oxidized and reduced forms and can be easily interconverted by redox processes (Larsson et al. 1986).

Table 1. DNA binding of glutathione conjugates formed after peroxidase catalyzed metabolism of p-phenetidine.

Conditions	DNA binding pmol/mg DNA
p-[2.6-^{14}C]-Phenetidine	490 ± 90
p-[ethyl-1-^{14}C]-Phenetidine	220 ± 30

Experimental conditions: 500 μM p-phenetidine (1 μCi/mmol), 0.2 μg/ml HRP and 1 mM H_2O_2 were incubated for 60 minutes. 500 μM GSH was then added and allowed to react for 5 minutes. DNA was then added and precipitated after 30 minutes.

We have since investigated whether the glutathione conjugates of the reactive p-phenetidine dimers could be responsible for the enhanced DNA binding which is observed in the presence of GSH. We have thus found that both the mono- and di- glutathione conjugates of NEPBQI bind to DNA. In Figure 1 such a binding to calf thymus DNA is demonstrated for the di-glutathione conjugate. The exact nature and mechanism of the DNA binding is not yet known but it is most probably the oxidized conjugate which is responsible for the binding.

Further support for the involvement of glutathione conjugates of the two reactive dimers in the GSH dependent enhancement of DNA binding during peroxidase catalyzed activation of p-phenetidine comes from experiments using ring and ethyl labeled p-phenetidine. In the presence of GSH a 2:1 DNA binding ratio is observed during HRP catalyzed metabolism of p-phenetidine (Table 1). Since one ethyl group is lost during formation of the quinone di-imine dimer this result thus strongly indicate that GSH conjugates of the quinone di-imine dimer and/or NEPBQI is responsible for the major part of the peroxidase mediated DNA binding of p-phenetidine in the presence of GSH.

The significance of the interaction of the glutathione conjugates with DNA for <u>in vivo</u> effects of p-phenetidine or phenacetin is not known but is presently under investigation. The interaction of glutathione conjugates with DNA may also be of importance for other type of xenobiotics undergoing metabolic activation by peroxidases or other enzyme system.

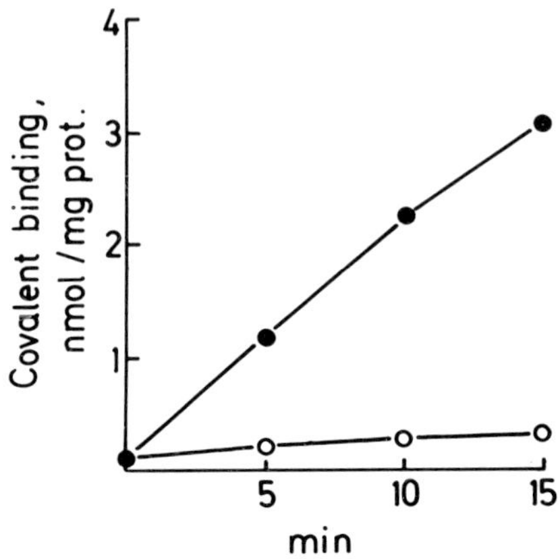

Figure 2. TPA dependent binding of p-phenetidine to protein in human leukocytes. Open symbols: No TPA added.

Table 2. TPA dependent binding of p-phenetidine to protein in human leukocytes.

Conditions	DNA binding nmol/10^6cells/15 minutes
p-[2.6-^{14}C]-Phenetidine	2.7
p-[ethyl-1-^{14}C]-Phenetidine	1.65
No TPA	0.39

Experimental conditions: Incubation contained $4x10^6$ cells/ml, 100 μM p-phenetidine (1 μCi/mmol) and 33 μM TPA.

We have also studied the metabolic activation of p-phenetidine in human leukocytes. As can be seen from the results presented in Figure 2 tetradecanoylphorbol-12,13-acetate (TPA) stimulates the formation of protein binding product(s) in these cells. The metabolic activation is most probably catalyzed by myeloperoxidase. Whether myeloperoxidase catalyzes a conventional peroxidase reaction or a mechanism involving hypochlorite is not known. However, results which supports a similar reaction mechanism as for the HRP and PGS catalyzed reactions are presented in Table 2. In this table protein binding of ring and ethyl labeled p-phenetidine is compared and a ratio close to 2:1 is obtained. These results are in agreement with what has been observed using HRP or PGS.

If the leukocyte catalyzed activation of p-phenetidine is of any importance for the toxicity of phenacetin is of course doubtful. The importance of myeloperoxidase catalyzed activation of other xenobiotics may however be of significance.

Supported by a grant from the Swedish Medical Research Council.

REFERENCES

Andersson, B., Nordenskjöld, M., Rahimtula, A. & Moldéus, P., 1982, Molec. Pharmacol., 22, 479.

Andersson, B., Larsson, R., Rahimtula, A. & Moldéus, P., 1983, Biochem. Pharmacol., 32, 1045.

Andersson, B., Larsson, R., Rahimtula, A. & Moldéus, P., 1984, Carcinogenesis, 5, 161.

Bartsch, H., Miller, J.A. & Miller, E.G., 1972, Biochim. Biophys. Acta, 273, 40.

Eling, T., Boyd, J., Reed, G., Mason, R. & Sivarajah, K., 1983, Drug. Metab. Rev., 14, 219.

Hultengren, N., Lagergren, C. & Ljungqvist, A., 1965, Acta Chim. Scand., 130, 314.

Jellinck, P.H. & Cleveland, S., 1977, Can. J. Biochem., 56, 203.

Kadlubar, F.F., Frederick, C.B., Weis, C.C. & Zenzer, T.V., Biochem. Biophys. Res. Commun., 108, 253.

Kalyanaraman, B. & Sohnie, P.G., 1985, J. Clinical Invest., 75, 1618.

Krauss, R.S. & Eling, T.E., 1985, Cancer Res., 45, 1680.

Kumura, S., Elce, J.S. & Jellinck, P.H., 1983, Biochem. J., 213, 165.

Larsson, R., Ross, D., Nordenskjöld, M., Lindeke, B., Olsson, L.-I. & Moldéus, P., 1984, Chem.-Biol. Interact., 52, 1.

Larsson, R., Lindquist, T., Lindeke, B. & Moldéus, P., 1986, Chem.-Biol. Interact., 60, 317.

Marnett, L.J. & Eling, T.E., 1983, In Reviews in Biochemical Toxicology V (Hodgson, E., Bend, J.R., Philpot, R.M., eds) Elsevier, New York, p. 135.

Mason, R.P. & Chignell, C.F., 1981, Pharm. Rev., 33, 189.
Metzler, M. & McLachlan, J.A., 1978, Biochem. Biophys. Res. Commun., 85, 874.
Miyamoto, T., Ogino, N., Yamamoto, S. & Hayaishi, O., 1976, J. Biol. Chem., 251, 2629.
O'Brien, P.J., Rahimtula, A., 1976, Biochem. Biophys. Res. Commun., 70, 832.
Ohnishi, S. & McConnell, H.M., 1965, J. Am. Chem. Soc., 87, 2293.
Ross, D., Larsson, R., Andersson, B., Nilsson, U., Lindquist, T., Lindeke, B & Moldéus, P., 1985(1). Biochem. Pharmacol., 34, 343.
Ross, D., Larsson, R., Norbeck, K., Ryhage, R. & Moldéus, P., 1985(2), Molec. Pharmacol., 27, 277.
Ross, D., Norbeck, K. & Moldéus, P., 1985(3), J. Biol. Chem., 260, 15028.
Samuelsson, B., Goldyne, M., Granström, E., Hamberg, M., Hammarström, S. & Malmsten, C., 1978, Annu. Rev. Biochem., 47, 997.
Sawahata, I. & Neal, R.A., 1982, Biochem. Biophys. Res. Commun., 109, 988.
Strum, J.M. & Karnovsky, M.J., 1970, J. Cell. Biol., 44, 655.
Vane, J.R., 1971, Nature, 231, 232.
Venkatachalam, M.A., Soltani, M.H. & Fahimi, H.D., 1970, J. Cell. Biol., 46, 168.
Yamazoe, Y., Roth, R.W. & Kadlubar, F.F., 1986, Carcinogenesis, 7, 179.
Zenzer, T.V., Mattammal, M.B., Armbrecht, H.J. & Davis, B.B., 1980, Cancer Res., 40, 2839.

Molybdenum Hydroxylases

C. BEEDHAM

School of Pharmaceutical Chemistry, University of Bradford, Bradford, West Yorkshire BD7 1DP, UK

INTRODUCTION

There are a number of molybdenum-containing enzymes including sulphite oxidase and nitrogenase but those which are important in carbon oxidation are aldehyde oxidase (AO) and xanthine oxidase (XO) /dehydrogenase. Both enzymes catalyse the oxidation of a wide range of aldehydes and N-heterocycles. Although purines such as xanthine are typical of xanthine oxidase substrates the name aldehyde oxidase implies a narrow and misleading specificity as aldehyde oxidation is much less significant than that of N-heteroaromatics. A more suitable term is that introduced by Bray (1975) to encompass both of these closely related 'Molybdenum Hydroxylases'. The role of these enzymes in metabolism and toxicity will be discussed and the reader is referred to recent comprehensive reviews covering biochemical and mechanistic aspects of the molybdenum hydroxylases (Bray 1975, Coughlan 1980, Rajagopalan 1980, Hille & Massey 1985, Beedham 1985, 1987, Parks & Granger 1986).

OXIDATION OF SUBSTRATES

The enzymes catalyse nucleophilic oxidation which can be represented as attack by hydroxyl ion (1).

$$RH + OH^- \longrightarrow ROH + 2e^- + H^+ \qquad (1)$$

Although molecular oxygen may be involved in the overall oxidation process the O atom incorporated into the product is ultimately derived from water. The following examples illustrate the above reaction and also highlight the differences between the oxidation products arising from it and microsomal Phase I metabolites.

Both oxidative functions may be seen in the same substrate: quinoline-6-aldehyde (1) is sequentially oxidised by aldehyde oxidase via the 2-quinolone to the corresponding carboxylic acid (Hijikata 1959).

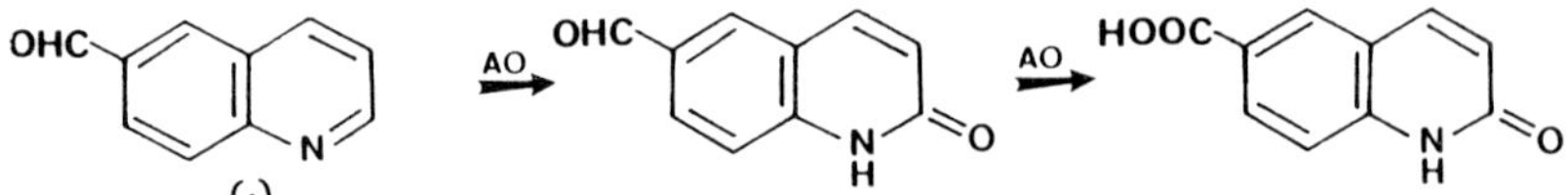

(1)

Heterocyclic compounds are generally better substrates than aldehydes for the molybdenum hydroxylases and thus ring oxidation precedes that of the aldehyde group. Aliphatic aldehydes have lower oxidation rates with xanthine oxidase than aldehyde oxidase although the affinity for both enzymes increase with an aromatic or heterocyclic substituent (Johns 1967, Morpeth 1983, Beedham 1987).

The most electropositive carbon in a heteroaromatic ring system is usually that adjacent to a ring N atom and this is the normal position of nucleophilic molybdenum hydroxylase attack. In contrast, microsomal oxidation would probably occur in the carbocyclic ring.

Uncharged carbocyclic compounds such as benzene and naphthalene are not substrates for the enzymes but as the number of N atoms in the molecules increase so does the affinity for the molybdenum hydroxylases. Thus, the tetra-N-substituted bases, purine (2) and pteridine (3), are oxidised exclusively by aldehyde oxidase and xanthine oxidase. This is a good example of the overlapping

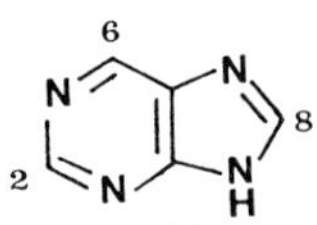

(2)

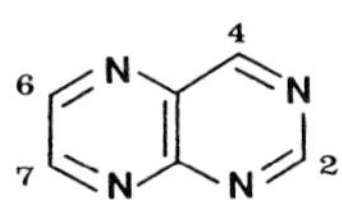

(3)

specificity of these enzymes and shows that although they both catalyse nucleophilic attack at an electron-deficient carbon, oxidation does not necessarily occur at the same position. Purine undergoes oxidation by xanthine oxidase sequentially at carbons 6,2 and 8 to give hypoxanthine, xanthine and uric acid respectively. Aldehyde oxidase can also catalyse the second step, the conversion of hypoxanthine, but it does not attack xanthine and purine is oxidised at carbon 8 (Krenitsky et al. 1972.) For aldehyde oxidase the overriding factor appears to be the electron density of the carbon undergoing oxidation - thus carbon 8 is the most electron deficient in purine (Nieman 1972). In contrast, the relative positions of the electronegative N atoms are thought to more important in binding and orientating the substrate within the active site of xanthine oxidase.

The final products of pteridine oxidation catalysed by xanthine oxidase and aldehyde oxidase are pteridin-2,4,7-trione and pteridin-2,4-dione respectively although the order of oxidation is not yet clearly defined (Hodnett et al 1976, Krenitsky et al 1972). Methotrexate, a pteridine analogue used as a cytotoxic drug (4), is oxidised by aldehyde oxidase to what is misleadingly called '7-hydroxy-methotrexate '(Johns 1967). However, the metabolite is not

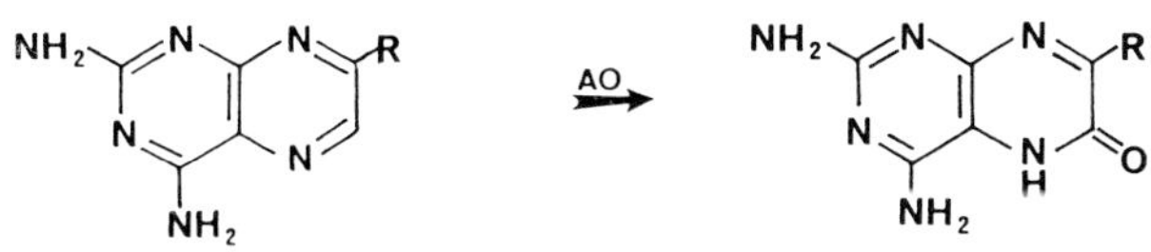

(4)

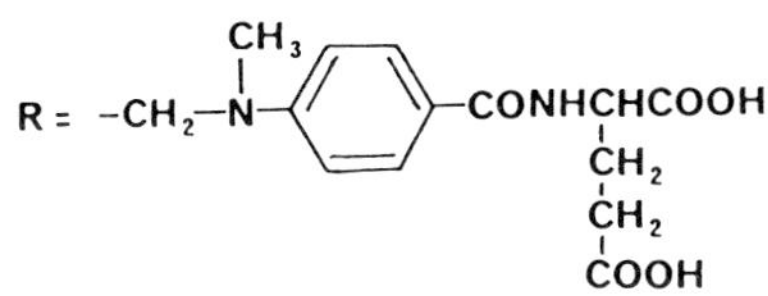

phenolic but exists as the lactam tautomer as do all molybdenum hydroxylase oxidation products. Thus, in contrast to microsomal oxidation products, these phase I metabolites do not form O-sulphates and glucuronides. In the case of methotrexate, plasma concentrations of the unchanged lactam, 7-hydroxymethotrexate, exceed that of the drug at the end of dosing (Chen 1982). Furthermore, there are also problems with the solubility of the lactams which are often less soluble than the parent compound: 7-hydroxy-methotrexate may cause nephrotoxicity because of its insolubility (Ertmann et al, 1985) and the purinone, uric acid, can crystallise out in the joints to cause the painful condition of gout.

Methylation of a ring N atom activates the α- and γ-carbons in an aromatic ring towards nucleophilic attack. The resulting heterocycles (cations) are generally good substrates of aldehyde oxidase but show only low oxidation rates with xanthine oxidase except at high pH values (Bunting et al 1980). We have shown that quinolinium salts (5) are simultaneously oxidised at carbons 2 and 4. The

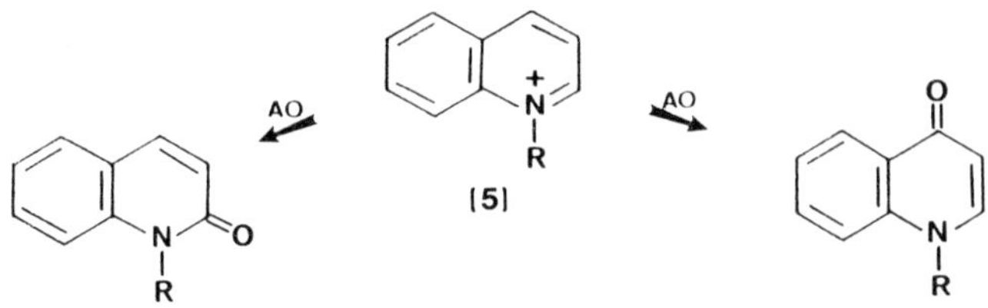

relative amounts of the two quinolones depend on the nature of the substituent and the species (Taylor et al 1984). Drugs may be methylated to form iminium ions in vivo but the intermediate (6) is often unstable and may be in equilibrium with the hydrated carbinolamine (7) and the ring-opened aldehyde (8).

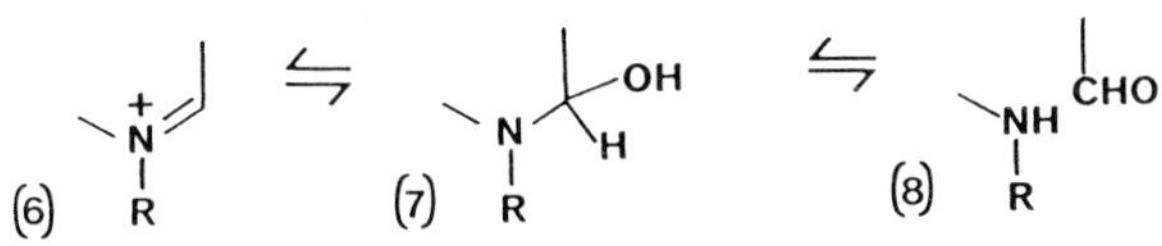

There are examples of both the iminium ion (nicotine and azapetine) and aldehyde (cyclophosphamide) intermediates undergoing aldehyde oxidase catalysed oxidation to the lactam and carboxylic acid metabolites respectively (Ruenitz et al 1979, Brandange & Lindblom 1979, Hill et al 1972). Oxidation of a hydrated carbinolamine to a lactam would appear to be a simple dehydrogenation reaction and not necessarily involve nucleophilic attack. However, we have shown that the analogous pseudobase, 3,4-dihydro-4-hydroxy-3-methyl-2-quinazolinone, is rapidly oxidised to the dione by aldehyde oxidase (Taylor 1984).

Finally, it has been thought until recently that there is a requirement for a heterocyclic N atom in substrates of the molybdenum hydroxylases. However, Banks and Barnett (1986) have shown that the carbocyclic tropylium cation (9) is

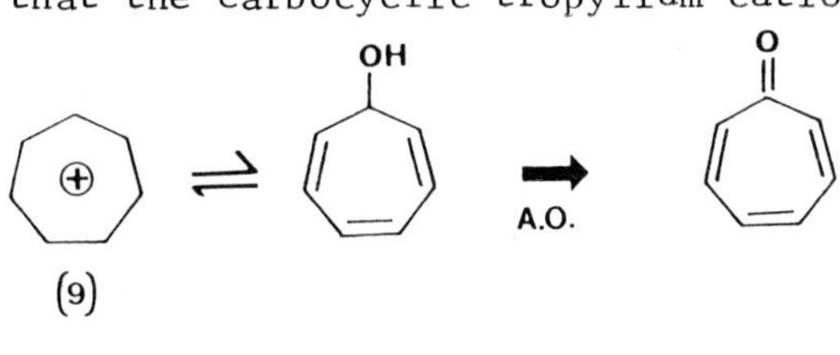

oxidised by aldehyde oxidase although no reaction was observed with xanthine oxidase.

DISTRIBUTION AND MOLECULAR PROPERTIES

In contrast to the microsomal system, the enzymes are found predominantly in the cytosol although there are recent reports of microsomal aldehyde oxidase activity (See Beedham 1987 for recent review). They are widely distributed throughout the animal kingdom from phylogenetically primitive species such as the sea anemone, crustaceans, insects, reptiles, birds and most mammals (Krenitsky et al 1974, Wurzinger & Hartentstein 1974) including man. Both aldehyde oxidase and xanthine oxidase are found in most tissues with highest levels in those tissues most often exposed to ingested foreign compounds; the former enzyme is most prevalent in the liver whereas the small intestine, milk and mammary gland contain the highest levels of xanthine oxidase (Beedham 1987).

The enzymes have a similar dimeric structure, each being composed of identical subunits containing molybdenum (1 atom Mo), flavin (1 mole FAD), and non-haem iron (2 Fe_2S_2 centres per subunit) (Coughlan 1980, Bray 1975). With the exception of NADH, reducing substrates such as purine interact at the Mo centre and the metal is reduced from Mo(VI) to Mo(IV). Bray (1984) has proposed that the substrate residue (R) reacts with an oxo ligand of the Mo and the released proton reduces a terminal sulphide of the Mo to the thiol with the concommitant reduction of the metal to give the complex below (10).

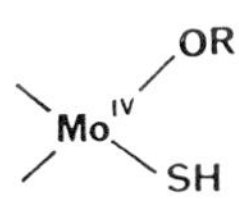

(10)

Hydrolysis of this complex releases the oxidised product and the Mo(IV) is reoxidised by intramolecular transfer of electrons to the other redox centres, Fe/SI, FE/SII and FAD.

Reoxidation of the reduced enzyme can occur at any of the redox groups but in vivo aldehyde oxidase and Type O xanthine oxidase react with oxygen and xanthine dehydrogenase and Type D xanthine oxidase reduce NAD+ (Scheme 1) (Coughlan & Ni Fhaolain 1979). 'Native' xanthine oxidase is thought mainly to exist as the D form but is readily converted to the O form during purification (Kaminski & Jezewska 1982, Kimm & Juhnn 1983).

Scheme 1. In vivo Reoxidation of Molybdenum Hydroxylases

$$\text{Enzyme-FADH}_2 \nearrow O_2 \xrightarrow{1e} O_2^- \quad (\text{AO, XO Type O})$$
$$\text{Enzyme-FADH}_2 \rightarrow O_2 \xrightarrow{2e} H_2O_2$$
$$\text{Enzyme-FADH}_2 \searrow NAD^+ \xrightarrow{1e} \text{NADH} \quad (\text{XO Type D})$$

Enzymic reduction of oxygen can proceed via a one-electron or two-electron process to yield either superoxide anion or hydrogen peroxide, the relative amounts of which depend on the reduction state of the enzyme (Coughlan & Ni Fhaolain, 1979, Porras et al 1981).

ROLE OF MOLYBDENUM HYDROXYLASES IN METABOLISM AND TOXICITY

Both enzymes react with endogenous substrates; xanthine oxidase is involved in the final stages of purine catabolism and aldehyde oxidase catalyses the oxidation of certain vitamins such as pyridoxal and N-methylnicotinamide. However, neither function appears to be vital to survival. On the other hand, they oxidise such a wide range of xenobiotics including aldehydes, uncharged bases, quaternary N-heterocycles and carbocycles that their role in the detoxication of these compounds can no longer be discounted. In addition, they may also be important in the production/ deactivation of toxic metabolites via reductive pathways. Thus aldehyde oxidase catalyses the reduction in vitro of aromatic nitro compounds, azo dyes, nitrosamines, N-oxides and sulphoxides (Sugihara & Tatsumi 1986). Xanthine oxidase has also been implicated in the activation of the pro-drug 6-deoxyacyclovir to acyclovir whereas aldehyde oxidase catalyses a competing deactivation pathway (Krenitsky et al 1984).

There are also a number of roles proposed for the active oxygen species, superoxide anion and hydrogen peroxide, arising from the oxidation of both endogenous and exogenous substrates. These include the organification of iodine (XO) and an antimicrobial function in the leucocytes (both molybdenum hydroxylases) (Fried et al 1973, Tubaro et al 1980, Beedham 1986). In contrast it has been suggested that tissue damage following ischaemia may be a result of the in vivo conversion of Type D $\rightarrow$ Type O xanthine oxidase and subsequent superoxide anion production (Adkinson et al 1986).

Finally, there is increasing evidence for the participation of xanthine oxidase in the storage and mobilisation of iron (Topham 1986) and it has been proposed that the high levels of maternal xanthine oxidase in colostrum and milk may be to effect maximum absorption of iron from the under-developed infant gut (Zikakis et al 1983).

REFERENCES

Adkinson, D., Hollwarth, M.E., Benoit, J.N., Parks, D.A. & Granger, D.N., 1986, Acta Physiologica Scandinavica, 126, Suppl. 548, 101.

Banks, R.B. & Barnett, B.D., 1986, Biochemical and Biophysical Research Communications, 140, 604.

Beedham, C., 1986, Journal of Pharmacy and Pharmacology, 38, 57.

Beedham, C., 1985, Drug Metabolism Reviews, 16, 119.

Beedham, C., 1987, Progress in Medicinal Chemistry, Vol. 24, edited by G.P. Ellis & G.B.West (Elsevier Science Publishers B.V.) (in the press).

Brandange, S.C. & Lindblom, L., 1979, Biochemical and Biophysical Research Communications, 91, 991.

Bray, R.C., 1975, The Enzymes, 3rd edn, Vol. 12, Part B, edited by P.D. Boyer (Academic Press, London & New York), p. 300.

Bray, R.C., 1984, Flavins and Flavoproteins, edited by R.C. Bray, P.C. Engel & S.G.Mayhew (Walter de Gruyter, Berlin-New York), p. 325.

Bunting, J.W., Laderoute, K.R. & Norris, D.J., 1980, Canadian Journal of Biochemistry, 58,49.

Chen, M.-L., 1982, Hplc assay and pharmacokinetics of methotrexate, Ph. D. thesis, University of Illinois.

Coughlan, M.P., 1980, Molybdenum and Molybdenum-Containing Enzymes, edited by M.P. Coughlan, (Pergamon Press, Oxford), p. 119.

Coughlan, M.P. & Ni Fhaolain, I., 1979, Proceedings of the Royal Irish Academy, 79B, 13.

Ertmann, R., Bielack, S. & Landbeck, G., 1985, Journal of Cancer Research and Clinical Oncology, 109, 86.

Fried, R., Fried, L.W. & Babin, D.R., 1973, European Journal of Biochemistry, 33, 439.

Hijikata, M., 1959, Nichidai Igaku Zasshi, 18, 1105.

Hill, D.L., Laster, W.R., & Struck, R.F., 1972, Cancer Research, 32 658.

Hille, R. & Massey, V., 1985, Molybdenum Enzymes, edited by T.P.Spiro (Academic Press, New York), p. 443.

Hodnett, C.M., McCormack, J.S. & Sabean, J.A., 1976 Journal of Pharmaceutical Sciences, 68, 1150.

Johns, D.G., 1967, Journal of Clinical Investigation, 46, 9.

Kaminski, Z.W. & Jezewska, M.M., 1982, Biochemical Journal,

207, 341.
Kimm, S.-W. & Juhnn, Y.-S., 1983, Korean Journal of Biochemistry, 15,71.
Krenitsky, T.A., Neil, S.M., Elion, G.B. & Hitchings, G.C., 1972, Archives of Biochemistry and Biophysics, 150, 585.
Krenitsky, T.A., Tuttle, J.V., Cattau, E.L. & Wang, P., 1974, Comparative Biochemistry and Physiology, 49B, 687.
Krenitsky, T.A., Hall, W.W., De Miranda, P., Beauchamp, L.M. M., Schaeffer, H.J. & Whiteman, P.D., 1984, Proceedings of the National Academy for Science, U.S.A., 81, 3209
Morpeth, F.F., 1983, Biochimica et Biophysica Acta, 744,328.
Nieman, Z., 1972, Israel Journal of Chemistry, 10, 819.
Parks, D.A. & Granger, D.N., 1986, Acta Physiologica Scandinavica, 548, 87.
Porras, A.G., Olsen, J.S. & Palmer, G., 1981, Journal of Biological Chemistry, 256, 9096.
Rajagopalan, K.V., 1980, Enzymatic Basis of Detoxication, Vol. 1, edited by W.B.Jakoby, (Academic Press, London and New York), p. 295.
Ruenitz, P.C., McLennon, T.P. & Sternson, L.A., 1979, Drug Metabolism and Disposition, 7, 204.
Sugihara, K. & Tatsumi, K., 1986, Archives of Biochemistry and Biophysics, 247, 289.
Taylor, S.M., 1984, Specificity of aldehyde oxidase towards N-heterocyclic cations, Ph.D thesis, University of Bradford.
Taylor, S.M., Stubley-Beedham, C. & Stell, J.G.P., 1984, Biochemical Journal,220, 67.
Topham, R.W., Jackson, M.R., Joslin, S.A. & Walker, M.C., 1986, Biochemical Journal, 235, 39.
Tubaro, E., Lotti, B., Santiangelli, C. & Cavallo, G., 1980, Biochemical Pharmacology, 29, 3018.
Wurzinger, K.H. & Hartenstein, R., 1974, Comparative Biochemistry and Physiology, 49B, 171.
Zikakis, Z.P., Dressel, M.A. & Silver, M.R., 1983, Instrumental Analysis of Foods, Vol. 2, edited by G. Charalambous & G. Inglett (Academic Press Inc.), p. 243.

THE FLAVIN-CONTAINING MONOOXYGENASE AS AN AMINE OXIDASE

L.A. DAMANI

Chelsea Department of Pharmacy,
King's College London (KQC),
Chelsea Campus, Manresa Road,
London SW3 6LX, U.K.

INTRODUCTION

The flavin-containing monooxygenase (FMO) is listed in Enzyme Nomenclature (Webb, 1984) as "Dimethylaniline monooxygenase (N-oxide forming, EC. 1.14.13.8)". This enzyme was first purified to homogeneity by Ziegler and his co-workers from pig liver microsomes (Ziegler & Mitchell, 1972), and later from rabbit liver (Hlavica & Hulsmann, 1979) rat liver (Kimura et al., 1983), and mouse liver (Levi & Hodgson, 1983; Sabourin et al., 1984). More recently, two other groups (Williams et al., 1984, and Tynes et al., 1985) have purified a FMO from rabbit lung that is catalytically and immunologically distinct from the liver enzyme. As in the case of cytochrome P-450 monooxygenases, it now seems likely that there may well be several microsomal flavin-containing monooxygenases with overlapping substrate specificities, and that the relative proportions of these isozymes may vary in different tissues within and between species.

The FMO and cytochrome P-450 are both located on the endoplasmic reticulum, and are the two main monooxygenases involved in the oxidative metabolism of xenobiotic amines (Gorrod, 1978; Ziegler, 1980; Damani, 1982; Gorrod & Damani, 1985 and references cited therein). Although the FMO was originally referred to as the microsomal mixed-function amine oxidase (Ziegler & Mitchell, 1972), it is now recognised that this enzyme can catalyse NADPH and O_2-dependent oxygenation at a variety of nucleophilic nitrogen, sulphur and phosphorus functionalities, but unlike cytochrome P-450 it cannot catalyse hydroxylation reactions at carbon. In view of this wider substrate specificity, it should no longer be referred to as an "amine oxidase", but more correctly as the "flavin-containing monooxygenase" or the "FAD-containing monooxygenase" (Poulsen & Ziegler, 1979).

Metabolic N-oxygenations represent important routes of metabolism for a large number of drugs and other foreign compounds. Therefore, there has been an interest in delineating the relative contributions of P-450 and FMO to such reactions. Any changes in the activity of enzymes involved in specific oxygenations, through environmental, physiological or genetic factors, would have an effect on drug disposition, and an effect ultimately on drug pharmacology and/or toxicology. Qualitative predictions as to which enzyme may be utilized for a specific N-oxygenation are possible, based on mechanistic and physicochemical considerations. In this brief review, the author examines the reaction mechanism and catalytic activity of the FMO towards primary, secondary and tertiary amines, and compares these with cytochrome P-450 mediated N-oxygenations. In addition, the status of both these monooxygenases in freshly prepared hepatocytes, and in hepatocyte monolayer cultures is described.

AMINE OXIDATION: RADICAL AND IONIC MECHANISMS

The consequence of enzymic amine oxidation may either be α -C-hydroxylation or N-oxygenation. This is dependent on the chemical environment of the nitrogen functionality and the reaction mechanism operative. The oxidation of amines by cytochrome P-450 probably occurs via a radical mechanism (White & Coon, 1980), whereas that of the FMO is by an ionic mechanism (Ziegler, 1980; 1984). The initial oxidative attack in the radical mechanism involves electron abstraction from nitrogen (Figure 1, a) to afford an amine cation radical. In

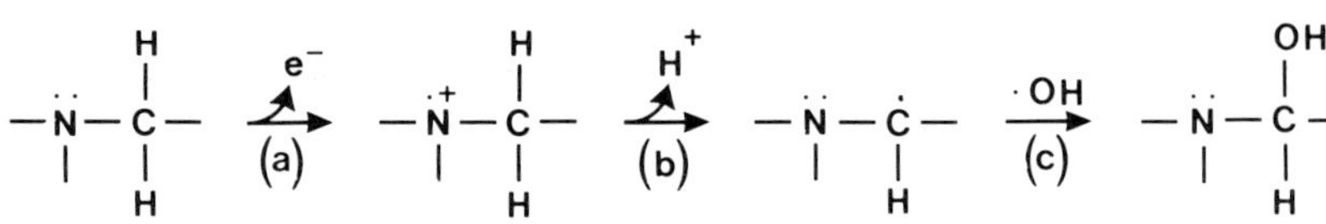

Figure 1. Cytochrome P-450 mediated amine oxidations (radical mechanism)

amines that have an available hydrogen on the carbon atom alpha to the nitrogen, there is rapid radical rearrangement (b) to the carbon radical followed by oxygenation (c) at this carbon centre. Consequently, cytochrome P-450 mediated amine oxidations, e.g. of N-alkylamines, afford intermediate carbinolamines, which rearrange to give N-dealkylated metabolites plus the corresponding aldehyde. Cytochrome P-450 catalysed N-oxidations (N-hydroxylations or N-oxide formation) are limited to compounds where radical rearrangement (Figure 1, b) is restricted for some reason, e.g. in amines that lack a hydrogen on the alpha carbon atom (e.g. phentermine). Nonetheless, cytochrome P-450 is involved in the N-oxygenation of several types of compounds e.g. primary arylamines (Uehleke, 1971), N-arylamides (Lotlikar, 1985), heteroaromatic amines (Gorrod & Damani, 1979), imines (Gorrod & Christou, 1985), and several other nitrogenous compounds (see Cho et al., 1984).

The catalytic cycle and mechanism of the flavin-containing monooxygenase is very different to that now well recognised for the P-450 isoenzymes. The FMO facilitates a direct two-electron oxidation of nucleophilic functional groups without formation of intermediate radicals (c.f. above for P-450 mediated amine oxidations). The mechanism for this enzyme has

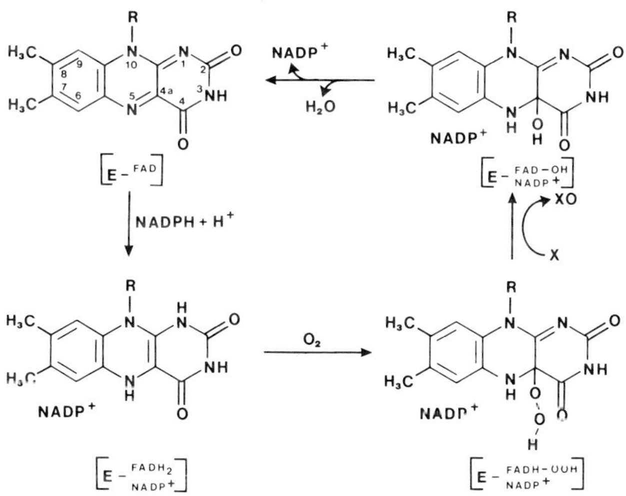

Figure 2. Catalytic cycle of the microsomal flavin-containing monooxygenase, illustrating changes in FAD-isoalloxazine ring system during N-, S- & P-oxygenations.

been described as ionic (Ziegler, 1980) and the essential features of the catalytic cycle are illustrated in Figure 2. Flavin reduction is achieved using NADPH as a source of reducing equivalents; oxygen binding is followed rapidly by internal electron transfer to oxygen to form the flavin 4a-hydroperoxide. The nucleophilic nitrogen (or sulphur or phosphorus) on the oxygenatable substrate then attacks the distal oxygen of the flavin 4a-hydroperoxide, affording the N-oxygenated metabolite and flavin 4a-hydroxide. Release of one molecule of water and finally the $NADP^+$ regenerates the oxidised enzyme (Bruice, 1984). Since the 4a-peroxide is a relatively strong oxidant species, it will oxidise any nucleophilic substrate that gains access to the enzyme active site; this is probably the most important limiting factor in oxygenation by this mechanism (see section below on substrate specificity).

AMINE N-OXYGENATION : SUBSTRATE SPECIFICITY OF THE FMO

Access to the reactive flavin 4a-hydroperoxide site on the enzyme is restricted to certain types of nucleophiles e.g. lipophilic non-ionic and mono-cationic amines. Nitrogenous compounds with two cationic groups at physiological pH, and those with an anionic group are not substrates and are thought to be excluded from the catalytic site. It has been suggested that this structural feature prevents the futile oxidation of normal cellular components, since most endogenous nucleophiles contain one or more negatively charged groups (Ziegler et al., 1980). Indeed, the only known physiological substrate for the FMO to date is the aminothiol cysteamine which is oxidised to the disulphide cystamine. Despite the limited accessibility of the enzyme active site, the substrate specificity of the FMO for xenobiotic amines is broad, amongst the better substrates being tertiary and secondary amines.

(a) $R_3N \longrightarrow R_3N^+{-}O^-$

(b) $RNHCH_2R' \longrightarrow RN(OH)CH_2R'$

(c) $RN(OH)CH_2R' \longrightarrow R\overset{+}{N}(O^-){=}CHR'$

(d) $RCH_2N(OH)CH_2R' \longrightarrow RCH_2\overset{+}{N}(O^-){=}CHR' + RCH{=}\overset{+}{N}(O^-)CH_2R'$

Figure 3: Xenobiotic amine substrates for the FMO

(a) Tertiary amines

Tertiary aliphatic, alicyclic and N,N-dialkylaryl amines are oxidised to amine N-oxides exclusively by the FMO (see Figure 3a). The reported N-oxygenation of N,N-dimethylaniline by rabbit liver cytochrome P-448 (Hlavica & Kehl, 1977) has been questioned (Ziegler, 1985), and to date there is no other convincing data that P-450 can mediate N-oxygenation of any of the above classes of tertiary amines. Indeed, incubation of N,N-dimethylaniline with a reconstituted system consisting of purified hepatic cytochrome P-450 or P-448 from rats was found to mediate N-demethylation but not N-oxidation (Houdi and Damani, 1985). The only tertiary amines N-oxidised by P-450 are the aromatic heterocyclic amines e.g. pyridine (Gorrod and Damani, 1979). The flavin 4a-hydroperoxide is apparently not a strong enough electrophile to N-oxidise pyridines or other amines where there is delocalisation of the nitrogen lone pair of electrons by conjugation with an aromatic system. The nitrogen in all FMO tertiary amine substrates has hybridised sp^3 orbitals; one of these contains the nonbonding electron lone pair, whereas the other three orbitals are used in σ-bond formation. Potentially chiral amines are not resolvable into their separate enantiomers because of rapid N-inversion. However, N-oxides of these amines do not undergo this inversion at nitrogen, and are resolvable into optically active forms. FMO mediated N-oxygenations of asymmetric tertiary amines are stereospecific, but only a limited amount of data is available in this respect with purified FMO. With many species, microsomal metabolism of (2'S)-(-)-nicotine leads to the preferential formation of (1'R; 2'S)-cis than (1'S; 2'S)-trans-N-oxide. With the unnatural (2'R)-(+)-isomer, the (1'R; 2'R) trans-N-oxide is the major product (Testa et al., 1976). The two enantiomers therefore appear to favour the formation of N-oxides with (1'R) configuration of the nitrogen atom. Our preliminary unpublished data (Damani, Pool & Crooks, 1987) on nicotine N-oxidation with purified pig liver FMO shows that the (2'S)-(-)-nicotine affords the cis- and trans- N-oxides in equal amounts, whereas the (2'R)-(+) isomer only affords the (1'R; 2'R) trans-N-oxide. In addition substrate stereoselectivity was also observed, the total N-oxide formed with the (2'S)-(-)-nicotine was half that formed from the (2'R) (+)-nicotine. Interestingly, a recent study (Lindeke et al., 1987) on the rat hepatic microsomal N-oxidation of the prochiral amine pargyline has revealed the complete absence of one of the pargyline N-oxide enantiomers. More detailed studies with the purified FMOs are required before any definitive statements can be made on substrate and product stereoselective amine N-oxygenations.

(b) Secondary amines

N,N-Disubstituted amines are initially oxygenated to hydroxylamines by the FMO (see Figure 3b). These N,N-disubstituted hydroxylamines almost invariably undergo further oxidation by the flavin enzyme. Hydroxylamines possessing at least one alkyl substituent with hydrogens on the α -carbon are probably transformed to highly unstable hydroxylamine N-oxides, which dehydrate to afford the nitrones (Figure 3c). When both substituents on nitrogen are aliphatic, further oxidation by FMO may afford two isomeric nitrones (Figure 3d). The ultimate products observed are dependent on the stability of the nitrone metabolites (see Coutts & Beckett, 1977); aliphatic nitrones are more susceptible to hydrolytic decomposition to aldehydes and primary hydroxylamines, but nitrones with an α -phenyl substituent are more stable. The principal catalyst for N-oxygenation of most acyclic and cyclic secondary aliphatic amines is the FMO (Ziegler, 1984). Whereas N-alkylarylamines (e.g. N-methylaniline, N-methyl-4-aminoazobenzene) are also substrates for the FMO (Ziegler, 1980; Kadlubar et al., 1976), there is some suggestion that cytochrome P-450 may also mediate the N-hydroxylation of certain substrates. For example, enzyme induction and inhibition studies indicated that microsomal N-oxidation of N-benzylaniline is catalysed predominantly by FMO, whereas N-oxidation of N-benzyl-4-chloroaniline is mediated by both the FMO and cytochrome P-450 (Gooderham & Gorrod, 1985). This tentative suggestion however needs confirmation with purified P-450 isozymes. Certain secondary hydroxylamines have also been reported to afford nitroxide radicals by microsomal FMO (Rauckman et al., 1979). Whereas secondary N-hydroxylamines and their further oxidation products (nitrones) have been detected *in vivo* with several medicinal secondary amines, the role of nitroxides in their metabolism and toxicity is as yet unresolved. At present there is no information available on the N-hydroxylation of N,N-diarylamines (e.g.

diphenylamine) and only one report on the N-hydroxylation of an aromatic heterocyclic secondary amine (2-phenylindole), which suggests that P-448 may be involved in this reaction (Jaccarini & Felice, 1978).

(c) Primary amines

The N-hydroxylation of virtually all primary arylamines (e.g. aniline) is mediated by cytochrome P-450. The only FMO arylamine substrates are compounds like 2-naphthylamine that readily form imine tautomers (Poulsen et al., 1976). N-Hydroxylation is also a route of metabolism for primary aliphatic amines (e.g. amphetamine, see Coutts & Beckett, 1977), but the pig liver FMO does not catalyse this reaction. Lipophilic primary aliphatic amines (e.g. *n*-octylamine) are not substrates for the pig liver FMO, but appear to interact with a regulatory site and stimulate two-fold the N-oxidation of tertiary amines (Ziegler et al., 1971). There is evidence for P-450 involvement in the N-oxidation of certain aliphatic amines. For example, N-hydroxylation of amphetamine and related primary amines was readily catalysed by purified reconstituted P-450 systems (Cho et al., 1984). N-Hydroxylation of phentermine was reported to be a P-450 reaction many years ago, and more recent work has demonstrated this with purified reconstituted P-450 systems (Duncan & Cho, 1982). There is an electronic basis for this P-450 substrate activity; phentermine has no available hydrogens on the α-C-atom and radical rearrangement is restricted (see section above on reaction mechanisms). However, there is no satisfactory electronic explanation as to why the FMO does not catalyse N-oxygenation of primary aliphatic amines (Ziegler, 1984). In this respect, recent reports that the mouse and rabbit lung FMOs both have the ability to N-oxidise *n*-octylamine (see Hodgson & Levi, this volume) are of interest. Detailed studies on the catalytic properties of these recently purified FMOs are not available, but it may be that other primary aliphatic amines are also substrates for these enzymes.

FMO ACTIVITY IN RAT HEPATOCYTE MONOLAYER CULTURES

In view of the importance of the FMO in the metabolism of numerous nitrogen and sulphur containing drugs, and in the production of toxic intermediates from some of these substrates, it is important to ascertain the status of this enzyme in any cellular system used as a model for mechanistic metabolic/toxicity studies. In contrast to studies on cytochrome P-450, the FMO has been less well studied in hepatocytes maintained in vitro. The normal hepatocyte preparation techniques do not appear to have any effect on the functional integrity of the enzyme. The rate of guanethidine N-oxidation in freshly prepared rat heptocytes was shown to be essentially equal to the rate predicted from measurements with isolated microsomes (McManus et al., 1983). We have recently examined the status of the FMO in rat hepatocytes maintained in primary monolayer culture (Damani & Sherratt, 1984; Sherratt & Damani, 1985; Sherratt, 1985). On the basis of previous studies with rat microsomes (Houdi & Damani, 1985), it was clear that N-oxidation of N,N-dimethylaniline was mediated exclusively via the FMO, whereas N-demethylation was by a phenobarbitone-inducible P-450. N,N-Dimethylaniline is therefore potentially an excellent single model compound for monitoring the activities of both these monooxygenases; an estimate of N-oxidase activity reflecting the status of the FMO, whereas N-demethylase activity would be a measure of the P-450 system. Optimal incubation conditions (incubation time, substrate concentration, cell number) were established for monitoring changes in the activities of these two monooxygenases in rat hepatocytes maintained in monolayer culture for various time periods (see Table 1)

Table 1. Changes in N,N-dimethylaniline "N-oxidase" and "N-demethylase" activities of rat hepatocytes maintained in monolayer culture.

Time in culture (hours)	% of initial activity "N-Oxidase"	"N-Demethylase"
2	100 (100)	100 (100)
8	70 (82)	57 (62)
24	84 (62)	22 (35)
48	103 (71)	15 (27)

Initial N-oxidase and N-demethylase activities were 300 ± 80 and 2240 ± 480 (n=3), respectively, in each case pmoles/mg protein/minute. (Data from Sherratt, 1985 and Sherratt and Damani, 1987, in preparation).

The N-oxidase and N-demethylase activities in 2 hour cultures were comparable to those in freshly isolated cells, indicating that the FMO and P-450 monooxygenases are stable during the 2 hour attachment period. These cultures exhibited a rapid decline in P-450, as seen by the lower N-demethylase activities over 48 hours (Table 1). This was validated by using a second model substrate, 7-ethoxycoumarin; the time decay profile of O-deethylase activity (data in parenthesis) was similar to that seen with N,N-dimethylaniline. These results are in agreement with other published data (e.g. Lake & Paine, 1982). In contrast, the FMO was relatively stable in rat hepatocytes cultured for 48 hours, as measured by N,N-dimethylaniline N-oxidase activity (Table 1), or by tetrahydrothiophene sulphoxidation (data in parenthesis); sulphoxidation of this cyclic sulphide is mediated exclusively by the FMO (Houdi & Damani, 1984). The stability of the flavin monooxygenase on short-term culture makes this model particularly suitable for examining this enzyme at the cellular level. In this respect, more detailed studies with hepatocytes from different species are required, since the P-450 instability seen in rat hepatocytes is not always seen with other species, e.g. rabbit and man (Poole et al., 1982; Strom et al., 1982).

CONCLUSIONS

The FMO is found in almost all mammalian tissues, but the highest concentration is in the liver, with significant amounts in the lungs and kidneys of some species. The activity of FMO in pig and human liver is very high, but lesser amounts are also present in livers from rodents and other small animals. The broad substrate specificity coupled with the wide tissue distribution of the enzyme suggests that the FMO plays a major role in the metabolism and excretion of numerous nitrogenous, sulphur and phosphorus drugs and other xenobiotics. The FMO is clearly a very effective 'amine oxidase', but it is probably an even better 'S- and P-oxidase'. With certain sulphur and phosphorus xenobiotics, an S- or P-oxygenated metabolite may be produced by both P-450 and FMO (see Hodgson & Levi, this volume). However, to date there is no convincing data that an N-oxygenated metabolite is produced by both these monooxygenases. Although certain amines may be substrates for both the P-450 and the FMO, the products with each enzyme are invariably different.

REFERENCES

Bruice, T.C., 1984, In "Flavins and Flavoproteins", edited by R.C. Bray, P.C. Engel & S.G. Mayhew, W. de Gruyter, Berlin. pp 45-55.

Cho, A.K., Duncan, J.D., Fukuto, J.M. & Lindeke, B., 1984, The metabolic disposition of organonitrogen compounds. In "Foreign Compound Metabolism", edited by J. Caldwell & G.D. Paulson, Taylor & Francis, London. pp 79-89.

Coutts, R.T. & Beckett, A.H., 1977, Drug Metabolism Reviews, 6, 51.

Damani, L.A., 1982, Oxidation at nitrogen centers. In "Metabolic Basis of Detoxication", edited by W.B. Jakoby, J.R. Bend & J. Caldwell, Academic Press, New York. pp 127-149.

Damani, L.A., Pool, W.F., & Crooks, P.A., 1987, University of Kentucky, Unpublished observations.

Damani, L.A. & Sherratt, A.J., 1984, Journal of Pharmacy and Pharmacology, 36 (supplement), 31P.

Duncan, J.D. & Cho, A.K., 1982, Molecular Pharmacology, 22, 235.

Gooderham, N.J. & Gorrod, J.W., 1985, Microsomal N-oxidation of secondary aromatic amines. In "Biological Oxidation of Nitrogen in Organic Molecules", edited by J.W. Gorrod & L.A. Damani, Ellis Horwood, Chichester. pp 81-95.

Gorrod, J.W., 1978, On the multiplicity of microsomal N-oxidase systems. In "Mechanisms of Oxidizing Enzymes" edited by T.P. Singer & R.N. Ondarza, Elsevier, New York. pp 189-197.

Gorrod, J.W. & Christou, M., 1985, Metabolic N-hydroxylation of acetophenone imines. In "Biological Oxidation of Nitrogen in Organic Molecules", edited by J.W. Gorrod & L.A. Damani, Ellis Horwood, Chichester. pp 278-289.

Gorrod, J.W. & Damani, L.A., 1979, Xenobiotica, 9, 219.

Gorrod, J.W. & Damani, L.A., 1985, editors "Biological Oxidation of Nitrogen in Organic Molecules" Ellis Horwood, Chichester.

Hlavica, P. & Kehl, M., 1977, Biochemical Journal, 164, 487.

Hlavica, P. & Hulsmann, S., 1979, Biochemical Journal, 182, 109.

Houdi, A.A. & Damani, L.A., 1984, Journal of Pharmacy and Pharmacology, 36 (supplement), 62P.

Houdi, A.A. & Damani, L.A., 1985, N-Demethylation and N-oxidation of N,N-dimethylaniline by rat liver microsomes. In "Biological Oxidation of Nitrogen in Organic Molecules", Ellis Horwood, Chichester. pp 96-100.

Jaccarini, A. & Felice, M.A., 1978, The metabolism of pyrroles and indoles: Ring nitrogen oxidation. In "Biological Oxidation of Nitrogen", edited by J.W. Gorrod, Elsevier, Amsterdam. pp 169-176.

Kadlubar, F.F., Miller, J.A. & Miller, E.C., 1976, Cancer Research, 36, 1196.

Kimura, T., Kodama, M. & Nagata, C., 1983, Biochemical Biophysical Research Communications, 110, 640.

Lake, B.G. & Paine, A.J., 1982, Biochemical Pharmacology, 31, 2141.

Levi, P. & Hodgson, E., 1983, International Journal of Biochemistry, 15, 349.

Lindeke, B., Weli, A.M. & Hermansson, J., 1987, University of Uppsala, unpublished data.

Lotlikar, P.D., 1985, Enzymatic N-hydroxylation of aromatic amides. In "Biological Oxidation of Nitrogen in Organic Molecules", edited by J.W. Gorrod & L.A. Damani, Ellis Horwood, Chichester. pp 163-174.

McManus, M.E., Grantham, P.H., Cone, J.L., Roller, P.P., Wirth, P.J. & Thorgeirsson, S.S., 1983, Biochemical Biophysical Research Communications, 112, 437.

Poole, A., Chasseaud, L.F. & Bridges, J.W., 1982, Toxicology, 24, 141.

Poulsen, L.L., Masters, B.S.S. & Ziegler, D.M., 1976, Xenobiotica, 6, 481.

Poulsen, L.L. & Ziegler, D.M., 1979, The Journal of Biological Chemistry, 254 6449.

Rauckman, E.J., Rosen, G.M. & Kitchell, B.B., 1979, Molecular Pharmacology, 15, 131.

Sabourin, P., Symser, B. & Hodgson, E., 1984, International Journal of Biochemistry, 16, 713.

Sherratt, A.J., 1985, Ph.D. Thesis, University of Manchester, U.K.

Sherratt, A.J. & Damani, L.A., 1985, The metabolism of N,N-dimethylaniline by rat hepatocytes. In "Biological Oxidation of Nitrogen in Organic Molecules", edited by J.W. Gorrod & L.A. Damani, Ellis Horwood, Chichester. pp 101-106.

Strom, S.C., Jirtle, R.L., Jones, R.S., Novicki, D.L.,

Rosenberg, M.R., Novotny, A., Irons, G., McLain, J.R. & Michalopoulos, G., 1982, Journal of the National Cancer Institute, 68, 771.

Testa, B., Jenner, P., Beckett, A.H., & Gorrod, J.W., 1976, Xenobiotica, 6, 553.

Tynes, R., Sabourin, P. & Hodgson, E., 1985, Biochemical Biophysical Research Communications, 126, 1069.

Uehleke, H., 1971, Xenobiotica, 1, 327.

Webb, E.C., 1984, editor, "Enzyme Nomenclature", published for the International Union of Biochemistry by Academic Press, Inc., Florida, (U.S.A.) p 125.

White, R.E. & Coon, M.J., 1980, Annual Reviews in Biochemistry, 49, 315.

Williams, D., Ziegler, D.M., Hardin, D., Hale, S., & Masters, B., 1984, Biochemical Biophysical Research Communications, 125, 116.

Ziegler, D.M., 1980, Microsomal Flavin-containing monooxygenase: Oxygenation of nucleophilic nitrogen and sulphur compounds. In "Enzymatic Basis of Detoxication", Vol. 1, edited by W.B. Jakoby, Academic Press, New York. pp 201-227.

Ziegler, D.M., 1984, Metabolic oxygenation of organic nitrogen and sulphur compounds. In "Drug Metabolism and Drug Toxicity", edited by J.R. Mitchell and M.G. Horning, Raven Press, New York. pp 33-53.

Ziegler, D.M., 1985, Molecular basis for N-oxygenation of sec- and tert- amines. In, "Biological Oxidation of Nitrogen in Organic Molecules", edited by J.W. Gorrod & L.A. Damani, Ellis Horwood, Chichester. pp 43-52.

Ziegler, D.M. & Mitchell, C.H. (1972), Archives Biochemistry Biophysics, 150, 116.

Ziegler, D.M., Poulsen, L.L. & Duffel, M.W., 1980, Kinetic studies on mechanism and substrate specificity of the microsomal flavin-containing monooxygenase. In, "Microsomes, Drug Oxidations, and Chemical Carcinogenesis", edited by M.J. Coon, A.H. Conney, R.W. Estabrook, H.V. Gelboin, J.R. Gillette & P.J. O'Brien, Vol. II, Academic Press, New York, pp. 637-645.

Ziegler, D.M., Poulsen, L.L. & McKee, E.M., 1971, Xenobiotica, 1, 523.

FLAVIN OXYGENASES - GENERAL ASPECTS
ACTIVATION OF MOLECULAR OXYGEN BY FLAVIN

Sandro Ghisla
Fakultät Biologie der Universität,
D-7750 Konstanz, RFG

Introduction

Flavins are one of the few catalysts used by living cells which have the capacity to activate molecular oxygen. Flavin enzymes having such a function are widespread, and can be subdivided roughly into two categories: The oxidases, which use O_2 as terminal acceptor, and the monooxygenases, which additionally catalyze the insertion of one atom of oxygen into a substrate. In order to understand the mechanisms by which these enzymes work (cf. below), the basic aspects of the activation of O_2 by flavins will be discussed briefly.

a) Mode of activation of O_2 by the flavin

This activation is carried out by either the fully reduced form, $Fl_{red}H_2$ (or $Fl_{red}H^-$), or, under certain circumstances, by the radical form, $FlH^\cdot$ (or $Fl^{\cdot -}$) of the flavin itself. Since the flavin is normally in the oxidized form (Fl_{ox}) under aerobic conditions, this implies, that a reduction (eq. 1) must precede oxygen activation. The reducing equivalents required for this can originate from a variety of sources. With the "oxidases" it will be the substrate which is dehydrogenated by the flavin. With the "external monooxygenases" reduction is provided by NAD(P)H. In the case of the "internal monooxygenases" the reducing equivalents arise from dehydrogenation of the same substrate which subsequently will become oxygenated:

$$Fl_{ox} + 2\ e + H^+ \rightleftharpoons Fl_{red}H^- \qquad (1)$$

The mechanism of the activation of oxygen has been unraveled only recently [cf. several articles in "Flavins and Flavoproteins", 1984, Eberlein and Bruice, 1982]. This essentially involves the inversion of the spin of one electron of paramagnetic oxygen (↑O-O↑), and is envisaged as starting by a (thermodynamically unfavourable, although feasible [Kemal et al., 1977]) step in which one electron is transferred from the reduced flavin to dioxygen to form the (caged) complex of neutral flavin radical and superoxide anion (2):

$$Fl_{red}H^- + \uparrow O_2 \uparrow \rightleftharpoons [FlH^{\cdot}\uparrow\uparrow O_2^{\cdot -}] \quad (2)$$

Note that in this complex the spins of the two unpaired electrons still have the same orientation. This complex might now dissociate into the components according to (3a);

$$[FlH^{\cdot}\uparrow\uparrow O_2^{\cdot -}] \longrightarrow FlH^{\cdot} + O_2^{\cdot -} \quad (3a)$$

or, a further electron can be transferred from the flavin radical to superoxide to yield oxidized flavin and hydroperoxide anion (3b):

$$[FlH^{\cdot}\uparrow\uparrow O_2^{\cdot -}] \longrightarrow Fl_{Ox} + HO_2^- \quad (3b)$$

The production of superoxide by the flavin enzymes xanthine oxidase and by the superoxide generating system of neutrophiles might be best represented by the sequences (2) + (3a).

On the other hand, most recent results from the groups of Massey and Anderson [Anderson et al., 1987], involving rapid reaction techniques and pulse radiolysis indicate that the sequences represented by equations (1) and (3b) best explain the observations made during the reoxidation of glucose oxidase, a typical flavin oxidase.

The second important alternative consists in a spin inversion which occurs inside the above complex leading to a species which is simply a different representation of a covalent bond between the flavin and oxygen (4):

$$[FlH^{\cdot}\uparrow\uparrow O_2^{\cdot -}] \longrightarrow [FlH^{\cdot}\downarrow\uparrow O_2^{\cdot -}] \longrightarrow FlH\text{-}OOH \quad (4)$$

This would represent the mode of activation of oxygen in all those cases, in which oxygen is "further used", e.g. for monooxygenation reactions. The structure of the flavin hydroperoxide formed in the reaction sequence (4) is of great importance, and has long been the object of dispute and controversy [Bruice, 1980]. This species was first observed spectrophotometrically during single turnover reactions of phenolic hydroxylases in Massey's group [Spector & Massey, 1972, Strickland & Massey 1973, Entsch et al. 1976], and was isolated as a metastable intermediate from the reaction of luciferase-bound reduced FMN with O_2 at low temperature [Hastings et al., 1973]. It has the structure of a 4a,5-dihydro-4a-hydroperoxy-flavin as shown on Scheme 1. This structure has since been confirmed by ^{13}C-NMR spectroscopy using FMN selectively enriched at the C(4a)-position [Ghisla et al., 1978, Vervoort et al., 1986]. In the free system it will not be stable since it decays to form oxidized flavin and H_2 (Scheme 1). Its spectrum has been observed in pulse radiolysis studies and its rate of decay estimated as ~300 s^{-1} [Anderson, 1982]. Flavin-4a-hydroperoxides, on the other hand, are stable when the position N(5) is blocked, e.g. by alkylation. Thus Bruice and coworkers were able to isolate an N(5)alkylated-lumiflavin-4a-hydroperoxide and study its properties. Its UV absorption spectrum is clearly similar to that of the corresponding flavin-4a-hydroxide (a product obtained upon reaction of the hydroperoxide, cf. below), and to that of the enzymatically observed species.

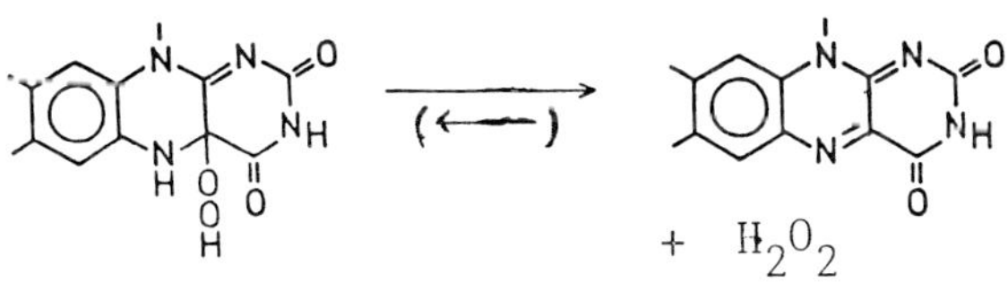

Scheme 1: Structure of the flavin-hydroperoxide (4a,5-dihydroflavin-4a-hydroperoxide), and dissociation to form free HOOH and oxidized flavin.

Stabilisation of the hydroperoxide by the enzyme is equivalent to the prevention of the elimination of H_2O_2. Earlier proposals [Entsch et al., 1976, Kurfürst et al., 1982] invoke for this a strong hydrogen bridge between N(5)-H and a protein base. Recent NMR investigations carried out with reduced (1,5-dihydro) flavin bound to bacterial luciferase indicate that the environment around N(5)-C(4a) in reduced (1,5-dihydro) flavin is very hydrophobic and that accessibility of solvent to this part of the molecule might be restricted [Verwoort et al., 1986]. These effects might result in impeding the elimination of H_2O_2 (i.e. of H^+, and HOO^-). Regardless of the details of the mechanism, the stability of enzyme bound flavin-hydroperoxide can be remarkable, and reach the order of hours at low temperature in the cases of bacterial luciferase [Tu, 1979] or N,S-monooxygenase [Beaty & Ballou, 1981].

b) Flavoprotein Oxidases

Due to their dual function, these proteins should be better named "dehydrogenase-oxidases". They catalyze the transfer of two-electron equivalents from an organic substrate to molecular oxygen, the latter being reduced to H_2O_2 [Massey & Ghisla, 1983]:

$$SH_2 + O_2 \text{ ----(Oxidase)-----> } S + H_2O_2$$

In general, with oxidases stabilization of the flavin-4a-hydroperoxide has not been observed. It is thus likely, that the reaction with O_2 proceeds via steps (2) + (3). A characteristic of oxidases is the accessibility of positions N(5) and C(4a) to the solvent, other regions being rather shielded, and the presence of a protein positive charge in the vicinity of N(1), C(2)=O, which is assumed to serve in stabilization of the reduced flavin anion [Massey & Ghisla, 1983]. The reactivity of anionic reduced flavin is indeed greater compared to that of the neutral species [Bruice, 1984].

c) Flavoprotein Monooxygenases

Typical for this class is that in most cases so far studied the reactive intermediate is the flavin-4a-hydroperoxide, which can exhibit different degrees of stability. This class can also be subdivided according to two criteria: Either according to the mechanism of "oxidation" of the substrate, or according to the source of reducing equivalents required for the reduction of the flavin (cf. reaction (1) above). Thus, depending on whether the flavin is reduced by NAD(P)H, or by substrate, according to the second criterion, enzymes have been named "internal" as opposed to "external" monooxygenases. For a detailed discussion of the criteria applied to this or other classifications we refer to Massey & Hemmerich, [1980].

If on the other hand mechanistic criteria are applied, then three different classes emerge:

i) Flavin enzymes involved in "hydroxylation" of activated aromatic compounds (note that, in contrast to P-450-dependent enzymes, flavin monooxygenases cannot process alkanes or aromatic compounds not activated by e.g. a hydroxyl function, such as phenols).

ii) Monooxygenations involving direct nucleophilic or electrophilic attack of the hydroperoxide to the substrate.

iii) Monooxygenations proceeding possibly via a radical type mechanism.

i) The class of the so called "hydroxylases" such as p-OH-benzoate hydroxylase or phenol hydroxylase are among the best studied, and mechanistically most intriguing flavin enzymes. In spite of this, the mechanism of insertion of "O" into the aromatic substrate is still elusive. Extensive studies mainly from the group of Massey have demonstrated that the primarily formed flavin-4a-hydroperoxide, which is characterized by a single-banded absorption in the near UV (λ_{max} ~ 375 nm), is converted in the presence of substrate to a species having a high extinction maximal around 390-410 nm, which has an apparent pK ~7.8 [Wessiak et al., 1984]. Subsequently the latter species is converted to the flavin-4a-hydroxide, and this in turn splits off water to reform oxidized flavin [Entsch et al., 1976, Wessiak et al., 1984].

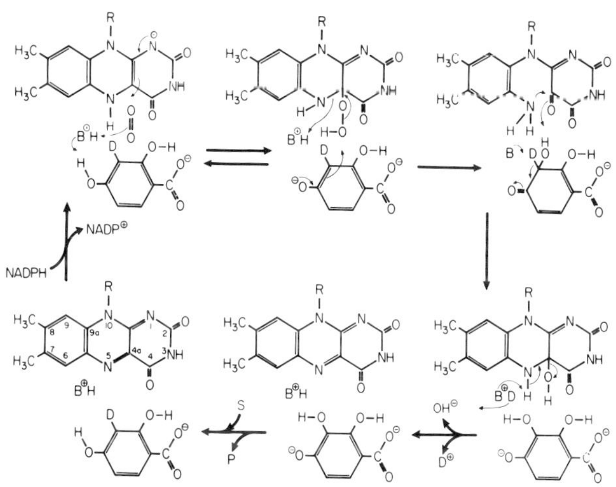

Scheme 2: Reaction sequence proposed by Massey's group to rationalize the reactions occurring during catalytic hydroxylation of phenols, and the accompanying spectral changes (adapted from Massey & Ghisla, 1983).

Current studies on this subject focus on the chemical structure of the high extinction intermediate, which has been proposed to result from intermediate opening of the central ring of the isoalloxazine system.
Synthesis of model compounds having an "opened" structure did not provide conclusive evidence whether a ring opening

occurs or not during hydroxylation [Wessiak et al.,1984]. While several possible intermediates, which have been suggested by various chemists without reference to actual experimental findings have been ruled out (see Wessiak et al., 1984) the definite nature of the high extinction intemediate has remained unsolved.

ii) The nucleophilic reaction of the flavin-4a-hydroperoxide to form an adduct which will then decay by a Baeyer-Villiger type mechanism is the sequence now generally accepted for the reaction of cyclohexanone monooxygenase [Branchaud & Walsh, 1985]:

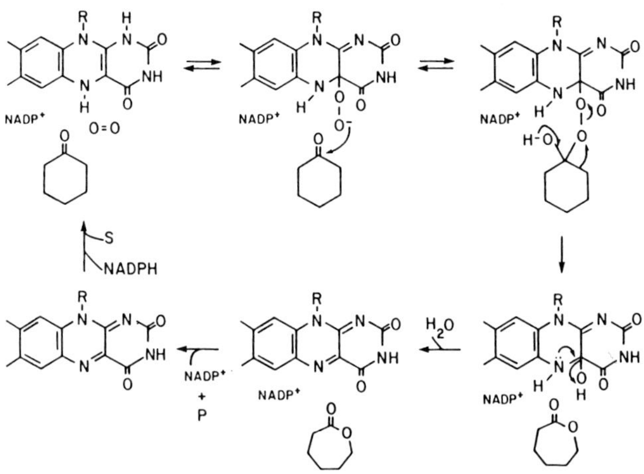

Scheme 3: Mechanism proposed by Walsh's group for the monooxygenation of cyclohexanone by cyclohexanone monooxygenase (adapted from Massey & Ghisla, 1983).

In the case of L-lactate monooxygenase [Lockridge et al., 1972] and lysine monooxygenase [Flashner & Massey, 1974] hydrogen peroxide is formed either via sequence (3b) or decay of the flavin-4a-hydroperoxide; it then reacts nucleophilically with the α-carbonyl function of substrate at the enzyme active site and induces decarboxylative fragmentation as shown on Scheme 4:

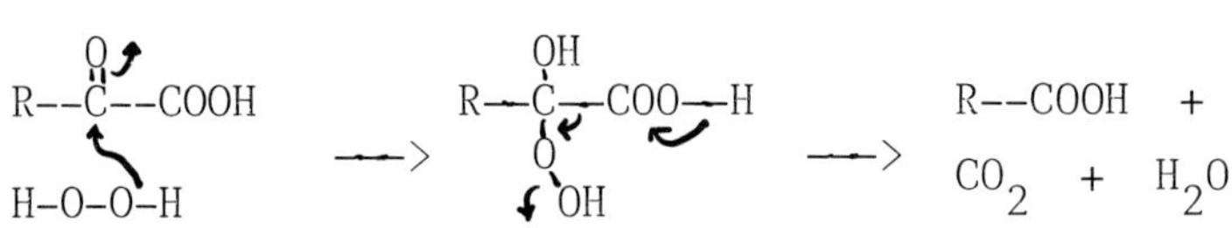

The mechanism proposed for the microsomal flavin mixed function oxidase involves the attack of the nucleophile to be oxidized at the distal oxygen of the flavin-4a-hydroperoxide [Bruice, 1984]. In this case the flavin-4a-hydroxide is formed directly, no intermediates (e.g. such as those observed during the reactions of the hydroxylases) have been observed in the reaction [Beaty and Ballou 1981]:

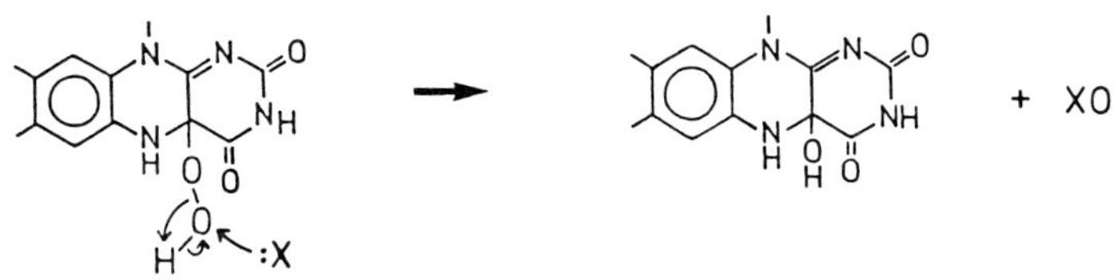

Scheme 4: Mode of oxidation of nucleophilic substrates by enzyme bound flavin-hydroperoxide in N,S-monooxygenase Substrate X = -N-, -S- or I^-.

It should be pointed out, however, that the information available to date cannot exclude for the mixed function oxidase a kinetic mechanism involving rapid sequences of single electron transfer.

iii) The case of bacterial luciferase appears to be a very particular one. This enzyme forms a flavin-4a-hydroperoxide, which then oxidizes long chain aldehydes to the corresponding carboxylic acids (Scheme 5). During the process an excited state is produced, which emits light maximal at ~ 485 nm [Ziegler & Baldwin, 1981] Until recently the assumption was accepted, that also in this case a Baeyer-Villiger type mechanism was operative, as originally proposed by Eberhard & Hastings [1972]. This mechanism in its original formulation, however, does not permit the conversion of chemical energy into light. In order to circumvent this problem mechanisms and experiments have been designed, which suggest, that the reaction of the peroxide with the aldehyde is initiated by an electron transfer [Macheroux & Ghisla, 1985]. The excited state would thus be generated via a so called CIEEL-mechanism (Chemically Induced Electron Exchange Mechanism), which was originally put forward by Schuster [1979].

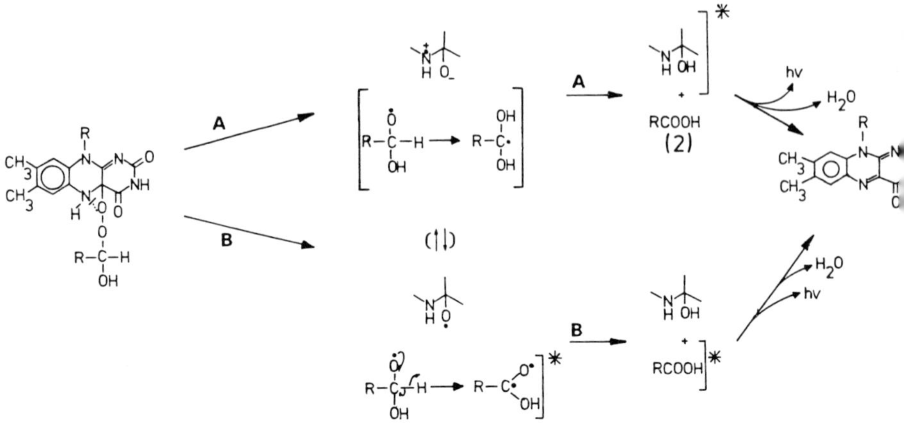

Scheme 5: Reaction sequence proposed for the processes catalyzed by bacterial luciferase. Note that the reduced (1,4-dihydro) flavin N(5) atom acts as a donor to generate the radical pairs shown, either by pathways A or B. In the first case the flavin-4a-hydroxide will be to be generated in the excited state. Alternatively (pathway B), the excited carboxylate might be an intermediate (adapted from Macheroux & Ghisla, 1985)

Conclusions

Whether a (reduced) flavin enzyme will react with dioxygen appears to be governed by the accessibility of the latter from the solvent. Shielding of the N(5)-C(4a) loci might be of particular importance. The pattern of O_2 reactivity resulting in formation of the flavin-4a-hydroperoxide, of H_2O_2 or of $O_2^{\cdot -}$ depends on the relative rates of steps (2-4), which in turn will clearly be governed by the protein interactions. In addition, the stabilization of the peroxide requires a specific interaction, probably a strong hydrogen bridge towards N(5)-H. With respect to the steering of the modes of reaction of the peroxide itself no clear cut pattern is yet apparent. Depending on the type of substrate a "hydroxylation", a nucleophilic attack or a radical reaction might be induced, this again requiring steering by interactions with the protein. The flavin thus seems to provide the basic capability to activate oxygen, the modes of reaction of active intermediates being governed by the features of the enzyme active center.

REFERENCES

Anderson, R.F., 1982, in "Flavins and Flavoproteins", proceedings of the 7th intern. symposium (Massey, V., and Williams, Ch.H., eds) Elsevier North Holland, Amsterdam, pp. 278-283.

Anderson, R.F., Schopfer, L.M., & Massey, V. (1987) unpublished result

Beaty, N.B., & Ballou, D.P., 1981, J. Biol. Chem. 256, 4619-4625

Branchaud, G.P., & Walsh, C.T., 1985, J. Am. Chem. Soc. 107, 2153-2161

Bruice, T.C., 1980, in "Advances in Chemistry Series", No. 191, Biomimetic Chemistry (Dolphin, D., McKenna, C., Murakami, Y., & Tabushi, I., eds), Amer. Chem. Soc., pp. 89-118

Bruice, T.C., 1984, in "Flavins and Flavoproteins", proceedings of the 8th intern. symposium (Bray, R.C., Engel, P.C., & Mayhew, S.G. eds) W.de Gruyter, Berlin, New York, pp. 45-55.

Eberhard, A., & Hastings, J.W., 1972, Biochem. Biophys. Res. Commun. 47, 2444-2449

Eberlein, G., & Bruice, T.C., 1982, J. Amer. Chem. Soc. 104, 1449-1452 Flavins and Flavoproteins, proceedings of the 8th intern. symposium (Bray,R.C., Engel, P.C., & Mayhew, S.G., eds) W de Gruyter, Berlin, New York.

Flashner, M.I.S., & Massey, V., 1974, J. Biol. Chem. 249, 2579-2586

Entsch, B., Ballou, D.P., Massey, V., 1976, J. Biol. Chem. 251, 2550-2563

Ghisla, S., Hastings, J.W., Favaudon, V., Lhoste, J.M., 1978, Proc. Nat. Acad. Sci. USA, 75, 5860-5863.

Hastings, J.W., Balny, C., Le Peuch, C., Douzou, P. 1973, Proc. Natl. Acad. Sci. USA 70, 3468-3472

Kemal, C., Chan, T.W., & Bruice, T.C., 1977, J. Amer. Chem. Soc. 99, 7272-7286

Kurfürst, M., Ghisla, S., Presswood, R., & Hastings, J.W., 1982, Eur. J. Biochem. 123, 355-361.

Lockridge, O., Massey, V. & Sullivan P.A., 1972, J. Biol. Chem. 247, 8097-8106

Macheroux, P., & Ghisla, S., 1985, Nachr. Chem. Tech. Lab. 33, 785-790

Massey, V., & Ghisla, S., 1983, in "Biological Oxidations", 34. Mosbach Colloquium (Sund, H., & Ullrich, V., eds) Springer, Berlin, Heidelberg, pp. 114-139.

Massey, V., & Hemmerich, P., 1980, Biochem. Soc. Transactions 8, 246-257.

Schuster, G.B., 1979, Acc. Chem. Res. 12, 366-373
Spector, T., & Massey, V., 1972, J. Biol. Chem. 247, 5632-5636.
Strickland, S., & Massey, V., 1973, J. Biol. Chem. 248, 2953-2962.
Tu, S.C. 1979, Biochemistry, 18, 5940-5945.
Vervoort, J., Müller, F., Lee, J., W.A.M. van den Berg, C.T.W., Moonen, 1986, Biochemistry, 25, 8062-8067.
Vervoort, J., Müller, F., O'Kane, D., Lee, J., Bacher, A., 1986, Biochemistry 25, 8067-8075
Wessiak, A., Schopfer, L.M., & Massey, V. 1984, J. Biol. Chem. 259, 12547-12556
Wessiak, A., Schopfer, L.M., Yuan, L.C., Bruice, T.C., & Massey, 1984, Proc. Natl. Acad. Sci. USA, 81, 4246-4249
Ziegler, M.M., & Baldwin, T.O., 1981 Current topics in Bioenergetics, 12, 65-113

THE FLAVIN-CONTAINING MONOOXYGENASE AS A SULFUR OXIDASE

E. Hodgson & P. E. Levi

Toxicology Program, North Carolina State University, Raleigh, North Carolina 27695 USA

INTRODUCTION

The flavin-containing monooxygenase (FMO), formerly known as N,N-dimethylamine N-oxidase, EC 1.14.13.8 and originally described as an amine oxidase, is an enzyme located in the endoplasmic reticulum. This enzyme and the cytochrome P-450-dependent monooxygenase system (P-450), also located in microsomes, are the major enzymes catalyzing the oxidation of lipophilic foreign compounds. Their products have increased water solubility and serve as substrates for conjugation reactions forming glucuronides, glycosides, and sulfates which are readily excretable.

Purification of pig liver FMO was accomplished some time ago and the capability of this solubilized enzyme to catalyze the oxidation of a wide variety of nucleophilic nitrogen- and sulfur-containing compounds has been well established (Ziegler 1980; Poulsen 1981). The physiological substrate for this enzyme is thought to be cysteamine, which is oxidized to cystamine providing a thiol oxidant for the synthesis of peptide disulfides (Ziegler & Poulsen 1977). The pioneering studies of Ziegler and his co-worker on pig liver FMO provided the basis for the recent expansion of knowledge concerning this enzyme.

Hajjar & Hodgson (1980, 1982a) reported that pig liver FMO could form sulfoxides from thioether-containing organophosphate and carbamate pesticides and moreover that this enzyme could catalyze the oxidative desulfuration of fonofos to form fonofos oxon (Hajjar & Hodgson 1982b). The formation of oxons is an activation reaction resulting in more potent cholinesterase inhibitors.

It is important that the FMO specifically oxidizes sulfides to (R)-(+)-sulfoxide enantiomers, while P 450 oxidations yield predominantly sulfoxides in the S(-) configuration as shown with tolyl ethyl sulfide (Light et al., 1982; Waxman et al., 1982). Similarly, although both P-450 and the FMO are able to catalyze the oxidative desulfuration of fonofos, the two enzymes are thought to form the opposite oxon isomers (Hajjar & Hodgson 1982b). The two isomers of fonofos have different toxicities in mammals and insects (Lee et al., 1976, 1978a,b). Thus, the potential exists that selective monooxygenation to toxic or less toxic chiral products could be involved in selective toxicity.

Since oxidative metabolism can be carried out by both the FMO and P-450, the relative involvement of the two monooxygenases toward the overall metabolism of a particular substrate is of importance. The distribution of the FMO in non-hepatic tissues and its contribution to complex metabolic pathways is also of importance. In this brief review we will document the reactions in which the FMO is known to oxidize sulfur and summarize our own studies on the relative importance in liver and in extrahepatic tissues of the FMO and P-450 in the oxidation of substrates common to both enzymes. Finally, we will illustrate the role of the FMO as a phosphorus oxidase.

SULFUR OXIDATIONS

In general these reactions have been characterized by Ziegler and co-workers (Ziegler 1980, Poulsen 1981) using purified pig liver FMO and are summarized below:

<u>Sulfides & Sulfoxides</u>

RSR-- NADPH, O_2 --> RS(O)R-- FMO, NADPH, O_2 --> RS(O_2)R

egs. Phorate, Methylphenylsulfide

<u>Thiols, Sulfenic Acids, Disulfides</u>

RSH-- NADPH, O_2 --> RSOH -->RSSR

RSSR-- NADPH, O_2 --> RSS(O)R-->

egs. Cysteamine, 1-Butanethiol

<u>Thioamides</u>

RC(S)NH_2 -- NADPH, O_2 --> RC(SO)NH_2

egs. Thioacetamide, Thiobenzamide

Thiocarbamides

$RNHC(S)NH_2$ -- NADPH, O_2 --> $RNCH(SO)NH_2$

egs. Thiourea, Methimazole, Phenylthiourea

Several points about these reactions should be noted. First, there is a wide variation in Km among the many substrates. For example, sulfides are readily oxidized to sulfoxides but, because the Km for sulfoxides is usually several orders of magnitude higher than that for the corresponding sulfide, the second step is not usually seen. Second, many of the initial products are sequentially oxidized by the FMO to further products and last, many of these products are highly reactive and undergo additional reactions with endogenous compounds such as glutathione. Some of the results of our studies of FMO activity in mouse, rat, rabbit, and pig liver microsomes are shown in Table 1.

Table 1. Oxidation of sulfur-containing compounds by hepatic microsomes.

Substrate	Activity[a]			
	Mouse[b]	Rat[b]	Rabbit[b]	Pig[c]
Thiourea	18.9	7.8	12.3	12.9 (31.4)
Phenylthiourea	9.0	4.4	7.7	9.3 (26.1)
α-Naphthylthiourea	7.3	4.0	6.6	7.9 (21.6)
Methimazole	17.4	7.2	10.2	14.3 (30.4)
2-Mercaptobenzimidazole	6.1	2.9	6.1	8.3 (18.8)
Ethylene sulfide	16.6	6.7	11.0	11.3 (21.7)
Methylphenylsulfide	10.2	4.7	7.1	9.9 (25.6)
Thioacetamide	18.6	7.5	11.6	13.4 (31.0)
Cysteamine	17.8	8.1	11.6	13.6 (30.9)
1-Butanethiol	9.2	4.1	7.2	7.8 (20.7)
trans-o-Dithiane-4,5-diol	4.8	2.5	6.9	7.3 (10.9)

[a]Activity:nmol NADPH/min/mg microsomal protein. [b]Incubation included 5 mg antireductase IgG/mg microsomal protein. [c]Incubations contained 3.0 mM metyrapone to inhibit P-450; values in parenthesis determined in presence of n-octylamine.

Source: modified from Tynes & Hodgson, Archives of Biochemistry & Biophysics 1985. 240, 77.

PURIFICATION AND CHARACTERIZATION

Because of the need to study the relative roles of the FMO and P-450 isozymes, it was necessary to purify the FMO and P-450 isozymes from the same species. Becaue of our extensive use of the mouse for P-450 studies, both enzyme systems were purified from mouse liver (Sabourin et al., 1984, Levi & Hodgson 1983).

Subsequently our group (Tynes et al., 1985, 1986) as well as Williams et al., (1984) purified the FMO from rabbit lung, demonstrating that it is immunologically and catalytically distinct from that of the liver. The mouse and rabbit lung FMOs have a unique ability for N-oxidation of the primary aliphatic amine, n-octylamine, commonly included in microsomal incubations to inhibit P-450. In the mouse lung, this compound not only serves as a substrate but is also a positive effector of metabolism. The mouse and rabbit lung enzymes have a higher pH optimum, near 9.8, compared to the liver enzymes which have peaks near pH 8.8. Using antibodies raised in goats, Ouchterlony immunodiffusion analysis indicated that the liver and lung proteins are immunochemically dissimilar (Tynes & Hodgson 1985).

RELATIVE IMPORTANCE OF FMO AND CYTOCHROME P-450 IN MICROSOMAL PREPARATIONS

In order to study the relative importance of these two enzymes in microsomal membranes we developed methods to measure each separately in the same preparation. The most useful of these techniques consisted of inhibition of P-450 activity by using an antibody to the NADPH cytochrome P-450 reductase thus permitting measurement of FMO activity alone. A second procedure was heat treatment of microsomal preparations (50°C for 1 minute) to inactivate the FMO, thus permitting determination of P-450 activity, which was unchanged by the heat treatment (Tynes & Hodgson 1983).

The relative contributions of the two enzyme systems with thiobenzamide as a substrate are summarized in Table 2. Note the higher FMO activity in female than in male mouse liver as well the difference in relative contribution in lung and liver for the mouse but not the rat. Similar studies have been carried out using the insecticide, phorate (Table 3) (Kinsler et al., in preparation).

COMPLEX METABOLIC PATHWAYS

The microsomal oxidation of the insecticide, phorate (O, O-diethyl S-(ethylthio) methylphosphorodithioate was utilized as a model system for the investigaton of FMO contribution to a complex oxidative pathway (Levi & Hodgson, in the press).

Table 2. Relative contribution of the FMO & P-450 to the oxidation of thiobenzamide

Species	Sex	Tissue	Treatment	Relative Activity	
				P-450	FMO
Mouse	M	Liver	--	50	50
Mouse	M	Liver	Phenobarbital	65	35
Mouse	F	Liver	--	25	75
Mouse	M	Lung	--	20	80
Rat	M	Liver	--	35	65
Rat	M	Lung	--	40	60

Source: modified from Tynes & Hodgson 1983. Biochemical Pharmacology, 32, 3419.

Table 3. Relative contributions of the FMO & P-450 to the oxidation of phorate by mouse microsomes

Tissue	Sex	Relative Activity	
		P-450	FMO
Liver	M	80	20
	F	75	25
Lung	M	40	60
	F	45	55
Kidney	M	30	70
	F	10	90

Source: Kinsler, Levi & Hodgson (unpublished results)

Both P-450 and the FMO catalyze the initial sulfoxidation of thioether-containing organophosphate insecticides such as phorate and disulfoton. The stereospecificity of the oxidation of phorate to phorate sulfoxide as well as the further oxidations of phorate sulfoxide to the sulfone, the oxon sulfoxide, and the oxon sulfone were examined, using purified FMO and purified P-450 isozymes isolated from mouse liver microsomes.

The FMO catalyzed the formation of (-)-phorate sulfoxide, while two P-450 isozymes (P-450-B2, a constitutive form, and P-450-PB, the principal form induced by phenobarbital) produced (+)-phorate sulfoxide. The other three constitutive P-450 isozymes examined yielded racemic mixtures.

The FMO had the lowest Km for the sulfoxidation reaction, 32 µm, while the Km values for the P-450 isozymes ranged from 67 µm to 250 µm (Table 4). No additional oxidation of phorate sulfoxide by the FMO was detected using either (+)-phorate sulfoxide or (-)-phorate sulfoxide as substrates. By contrast, all five P-450 isozymes tested formed additional oxidation products with both (+) and (-) phorate sulfoxide; (+)-phorate sulfoxide was the preferred substrate for all P-450 forms.

The final oxidation product, phorate oxon sulfone, was derived by desulfuration of phorate sulfone, with the formation of the oxon sulfoxide being a terminal pathway.

Table 4. Oxidation of phorate to optically active phorate sulfoxides by P-450 isozymes and FMO

Enzyme	Optical Activity	Km (µm)[a]	Vmax[b]
P-450 A1	None	111	31
P-450 B1	None	125	50
P-450 B2	(+)	100	111
P-450 B3	None	250-333	50
P-450 PB	(+)	67	91
FMO	(-)	32	80

[a]Km values were determined using substrate concentrations from 5-125 µm. [b]nmol p. sulfoxide formed/min/nmol enzyme.
Source: Levi & Hodgson, 1987 (in the press).

FMO AS A PHOSPHOROUS OXIDASE

Oxidative desulfuration, previously considered to be entirely due to P-450, is with some substrates also an FMO reaction. Desulfuration of phosphonate insecticides, such as fonofos (S-phenyl ethyl ethylphosphonodithioate) and its analogs, is catalyzed by pig liver microsomal FMO although desulfuration of phosphorodithioates, such as parathion, is not. (Hajjar & Hodgson 1982). Trivalent phosphorus-containing compounds are also excellent substrates for the enzyme. Diethylphenylphosphine has a K_m value lower than 2.5µM. Stoichiometry studies with diethylphenylphosphine and its sulfide showed that O_2 and NADPH consumption were approximately equal to the substrate consumed. Diethylphenylphosphonite also appears to be an excellent substrate but its rapid nonenzymatic hydrolysis and/or oxidation precludes accurate K_m determinations. The major metabolite of both diethylphenylphosphine and its sulfide was the phosphine oxide (Smyser & Hodgson 1985).

Subsequent studies have shown that phosphines are also excellent substrates for the FMO from mouse, rat and rabbit liver. They are not, however, particularly good substrates for P-450 isozymes although they do bind to P-450 giving rise to spectrally observable complexes and will inhibit the oxidation of other substrates such as p-nitroanisole (Smyser et al., 1986).

CONCLUSIONS

The FMO of mammalian microsomes from both hepatic and extrahepatic tissues is a versatile sulfur oxidase, frequently contributing more than cytochrome P-450 to the oxidation of common substrates.

Its role in oxidative metabolism and complex metabolic pathways has been determined in part but further resolution is required. Of more critical importance, perhaps, is the further definition of tissue-specific forms of the enzyme and the molecular biology of their expression.

REFERENCES

Hajjar, N. & Hodgson, E., 1980, Science, 209, 1134.

Hajjar, N. & Hodgson, E., 1982, Biochemical Pharmacology, 31, 745.

Hajjar, N. & Hodgson, E., 1982b the microsomal FAD-dependent monooxygenase as an activating enzyme:fonofos metabolism. In Biological Reactive Intermediates II, Part 1, edited by R. Snyder, D. Parke, J. Kocsis, D. Jollow, C. Gibson, & C. Witmer (Plenum Publishing Co.), p. 1245.

Lee, P., Allahyari, R. & Fukuto, T., 1976, Biochemical Pharmacology, 25, 2671,

Lee, P., Allahyari, R. & Fukuto, T., 1978a, Pesticide Biochemistry and Physiology, 8, 158.

Lee, P., Allahyari, R. & Fukuto, T., 1978b, Pesticide Biochemistry and Physiology, 8, 146.

Levi, P. & Hodgson, E., 1983, International Journal of Biochemistry, 15, 349.

Light, D., Waxman, D. & Walsh, C., 1982, Biochemistry, 21, 2490.

Poulsen, L., 1981, Reviews in Biochemical Toxicology, 3, 33.

Sabourin, P., Symser, B. & Hodgson, E., 1984, The International Journal of Biochemistry, 16, 713.

Smyser, B. & Hodgson, E., 1985, Biochemical Pharmacology, 34, 1145.

Smyser, B., Levi, P. & Hodgson, E., 1986, Biochemical Pharmacology, 35, 1719.

Tynes, R. & Hodgson, E., 1985, Archives of Biochemistry and Biophysics, 240, 77.

Tynes, R., Sabourin, P. & Hodgson, E., 1985, Biochemical Biophysical Research Communications, 126, 1069.

Tynes, R. & Hodgson, E., 1983, Biochemical Pharmaccology, 32, 3419.

Waxman, D., Light D. & Walsh, C., 1982, Biochemistry, 21, 2499.

Williams, D., Ziegler, D., Hardin, D., Hale, S., & Masters B., 1984, Biochemical Biophysical Research Communications, 125, 116.

Ziegler, D. microsomal flavin-containing monooxygenase: oxygenation of nucleophilic nitrogen and sulfur compounds. In Enzymatic Basis of Detoxication, Vol. 1, edited by W. Jakoby (Academic Press), 1980.

Ziegler, D. & Poulsen, L., 1977, Trends in Biochemical Sciences, 2, 79.

3. Metabolism of anticancer drugs

Metabolism of Anticancer Drugs

H. OELSCHLÄGER

Institut für Pharmazeutische Chemie
der Johann Wolfgang Goethe-Universität
Georg-Voigt-Str. 14
6000 Frankfurt am Main 11, FRG

Introduction

Tumours are one of the most frequent causes of mortality. Of the population, 20-25% in industrialized countries die of malignant tumours. About 35% of cancer patients will be cured by surgical methods or radiotherapy, while chemotherapy accounts for a further 14% of definitive cures.

During the last 20 years decisive changes have occurred in the way of thinking about and the interpretation of the tumour problem. New horizons concerning the possibilities of therapy are emerging. In this respect, I would like to point out the discovery of the;

1. Restriction enzymes by Arber and Smith (1971)
2. Reverse transcriptase by Baltimore (1975)
3. First oncogenes by Duesberg (1975) and
4. Tumour necrosis factor by Lloyd Old (1975).

We now know with more certainty that the development of malignomas is an extremely complex and dynamic process. The critical question is why do tumour cells escape body-specific immunology?

In the chemotherapy of tumours the following groups of compounds have proved successful:

1. National products, e.g. vinca alkaloids inhibiting mitosis
2. Alkylating agents, which may cause cross-

linking between two nucleic acid chains
3. Antimetabolites
4. Antibiotics, especially anthracycline types
5. Hormones and their antagonists
6. Miscellaneous agents, e.g. hydroxyurea.

Vincristin, cyclophosphamide and methotrexate are the most frequently administered drugs in this country. The lack of success with antineoplastic agents is probably due to cell-cycle kinetics (Fig.1).

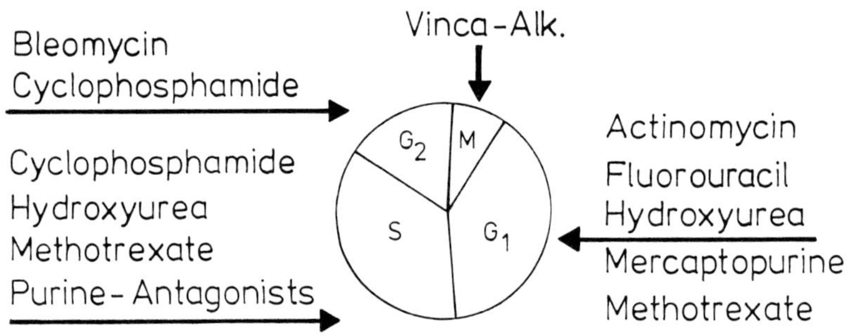

Fig.1: Cell-Cycle Kinetics and Action of Antineoplastic Agents

Although differences in the duration of the cell cycle occur between cells of various types all cells display a similar pattern during the division process. This may be characterized as follows: (1) there is a presynthetic phase (G_1); (2) the synthesis if DNA occurs (S); (3) an interval follows the termination of DNA synthesis, the post-synthetic phase (G_2); and (4) mitosis (M) ensues - the G_2 cell, containing a double complement of DNA, divides into two daughter G_1 cells. Each of these may immediately re-enter the cell cycle or pass into a non-proliferative stage, referred to as G_0. The cells of certain specialized tissues may differentiate into functional cells that are no longer capable of division. On the other hand, many cells, especially those in slow growing tumours, may remain in the G_0 state for prolonged periods, only to be recruited into the division cycle again at a much later time. Most antineoplastic agents act specifically on processes such as DNA synthesis, transcription, or the function of the mitotic splindle and, therefore, are regarded as cell-cycle specific. It is obvious that further understanding of the cell cycle and of the factors that regulate the recruitment of G_0 cells into the cycle should prove of great value in future attempts to develop chemotheraprutic measures for slow-growing tumours. Human malignancies that are currently most susceptible to chemotherapeutic measures are those with a large growth fraction, i.e. a high percentage of cells in the process of division. On the other hand, slow-growing tumours with a small growth fraction, e.g. carcinomas of the colon or lung, are often unresponsive to cytotoxic drugs.

It must be taken into account that normal tissues which proliferate rapidly (bone marrow, hair follicle and intestinal epithelium) are often subject to damage by some of these potent antineoplastic drugs and such toxicity often limits drug utility.

The cytotoxic effect of these chemotherapeutic agents often depends on their biotransformation. Cyclophosphamide, cisplatin or fosfestrol are prodrugs which will be transformed into the active species in the body, mostly by unspecific enzymes. Furthermore, 5-fluorouracil will be converted enzymatically to F-UMP- i.e. fluoro-desoxyuridine - monophosphate. The degradation of the antineoplastic agents occurs predominantly in the liver, the kidney, the lung and the GI-tract. This implies that the risk of injury to these organs must be considered before administration of these drugs.

Our investigations on the behaviour of fosfestrol (Fig.2) in human beings indicate the necessity of very sensitive and specific analytical methods for the determination of the parent substance and its metabolites in biological fluids. Fosfestrol has been on the market as Honvan® for more than 30 years and represents a useful therapeutic agent against pro-static carcinoma. It is an inactive form of transport of the lipophilic diethylstilbestrol (E-DES) with good aqueous solubility. DES suppresses the level of testosterone plasma down to castration level.

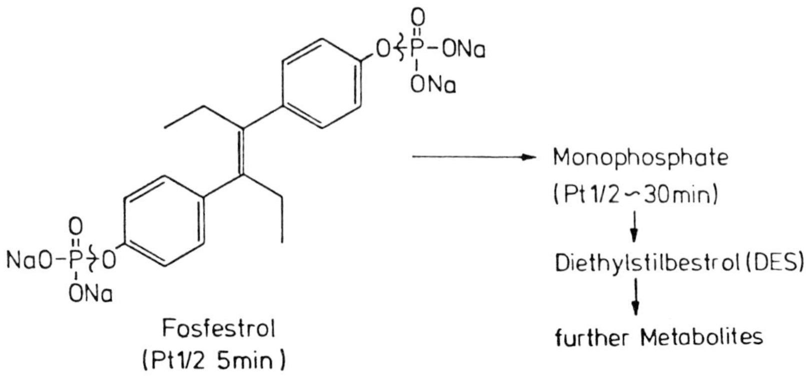

Fig.2: Enzymatic Cleavage of Fosfestrol

All investigators have accepted the theory up till now that fosfestrol accumulates in the tumour tissue where it is cleaved at its ester groups by the high concentration of acid phosphatase present. But until now nobody has been able to simultaneously determine fosfestrol and its metabolites in plasma and in tumour tissues and to prove this hypothesis. However, we have developed a new technique for measuring fosfestrol and its metabolites in plasma and tissues. The steps are illustrated in Fig.3.

The basis of this method utilizes the so-called homogeneous ion pair extraction using tetrabutylammoniumphosphate which forms ion pairs with the anions of the phenolic compounds. After partitioning by HPLC the detection occurs by UV-spectroscopy and, in the case of the free phenols, by an electro-chemical detector (ECD) equipped with 3 electrodes. The phenols are oxidised at +1 V at the working electrode consisting of pressed carbon paste (Fig.4).

Fig.5 and Fig.6 show the results of plasma investigations of a patient who was treated daily over a period of 10 days with 1500 mg fosfestrol intravenously. No accumulation of fosfestrol and its main metabolites (2, 3 and 4) could be observed. After oral administration of 360 mg fosfestrol neither fosfestrol nor its DES-

Measurement of Plasma Levels of Fosfestrol and its Metabolites

1. Centrifugation of the heparinised blood sample
2. Addition of 0,5 ml tetrabutylammoniumphosphate (0,03 mol) to 1 ml plasma
3. Slow precipitation of plasma proteins by addition of methanol and subsequent centrifugation
4. Decanting of the supernatant aqueous methanolic solution
5. Extraction of the remaining residue with 2 ml methanol
6. Pooling of the methanolic phases
7. Filtration and HPLC assay of 100 µl (UV detection 236 nm)

Fig.3: Steps of the Analytical Technique

Reaction at the Electrode

(carbon paste anode constructed in this laboratory)

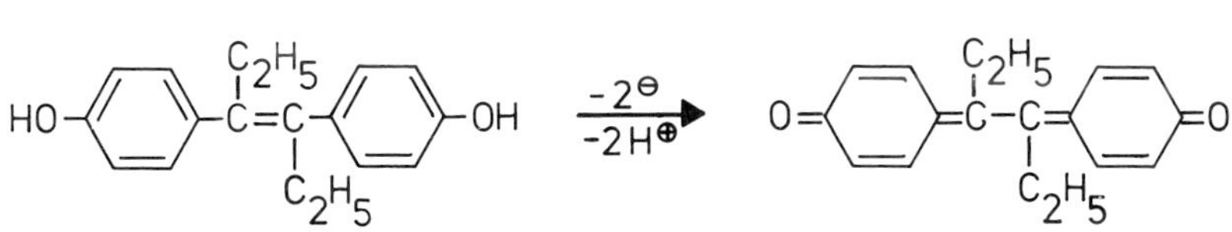

Fig.4: Electrochemical Determination of E-DES

monophosphate could be detected in plasma, due to the hydrolysis by the enzymes of the gut-wall mucosa. In this case we have only estimated certain amounts of DES and its conjugates. The latter are involved in enterohepatic recycling.

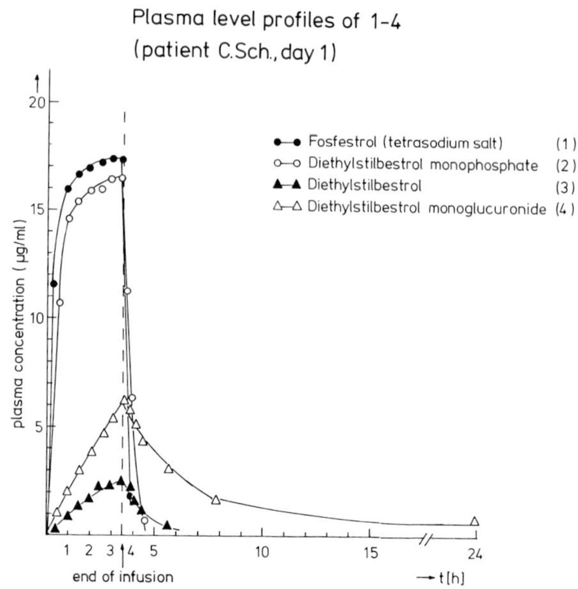

Fig.5: Plasma Level Profiles of Fosfestrol and its Main Metabolites (day 1)

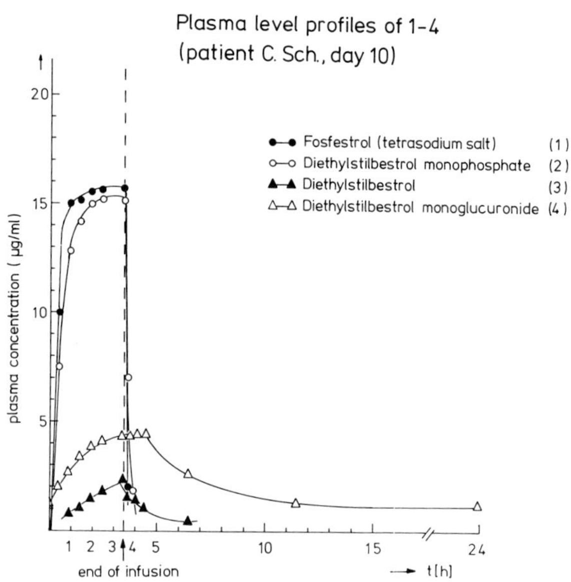

Fig.6: Plasma Level Profiles of Fosfestrol and its Main Metabolites (day 10)

The central question is: do we have a chance to solve the tumour problem and to defeat this cruel disease?

Little hope is to be found in the synthesis and clinical trials of new anticancer drugs from the aforementioned types of anti-proliferative agents. Nevertheless, a major breakthrough lies in the consequent development of monoclonal antibodies in the area of diagnosis and for the therapy of malignancies. Monoclonal antibodies are used routinely today for early diagnosis of tumours; their application in therapy is at present in its early stage. The general realization of this principle has shown little progress, because specific tumour antigens of all tumours could not be detected and therefore the required tumour-specific antibodies have not been available in all cases.

A selective destruction of tumour cells ought to be achieved by monoclonal antibodies carrying cytotoxic compounds, e.g. alkylating agents, which react specifically with those proteins produced by the tumour nucleic acid. In this case, the normal tissues may be protected against the attack of the antiproliferative compounds.

REFERENCES

Oelschläger, H., 1984, Krebschemotherapeutika aus pharmakokinetischer Sicht. In *Schriftenreihe der Bundesapothekerkammer zur wissenschaftlichen Fortbildung*, Bd. XII/Gelbe Reihe, p.41.

Oelschläger, H., 1984, Fosfestrol: Pharmakokinetische Untersuchungen. In *Pharmazeutische Zeitung*, 129, 2271.

Oelschläger, H. et al., 1984, Plasmaspiegel von Fosfestrol und seinem Monophosphat, von Diethylstilbestrol und seinem Monoglucuronid nach intravenöser Gabe bei Patienten mit metastasierendem Prostatakarzinom. In *Arzneimittelforschung/Drug Research*, 34, 1333.

Oelschläger, H. et al., 1986, Direkte Bestimmung von Diethylstilbestrol und seinen Monokonjugaten im Plasma. In *Arzneimittel-Forschung/Drug Research*, 36, 759.

Oelschläger, H. et al., 1986, Plasmakonzentrationen von Fosfestrol sowie von Diethylstilbestrol und seinen Konjugaten nach intravenöser Gabe an Prostatakarzinom-Patienten. In *Arzneimittelforschung/Drug Research*, 36, 1284

Rothley, D. & Oelschläger, H., 1986, Direkte Approximation von Plasma-Konzentrations-Zeit-Kurven des E-Diethylstilbestrol-Monoglucuronids nach oraler und i.v. Gabe von Fosfestrol. In *Pharmazie*, 41, 862.

Alkylating Agents
Metabolism and Anticancer Selectivity

H.J. HOHORST, G. VOELCKER and L. BIELICKI

University of Frankfurt/Main
Zentrum der Biologischen Chemie, Abtlg.Zellchemie
Theodor-Stern-Kai 7, D-6000 Frankfurt/Main 70

The main problem associated with using alkylating agents as anticancer drugs is essentially the same as for nearly all other drugs used in cancer chemotherapy - namely the lack of specificity and the low therapeutic index. Metabolism and bioactivation of latent prodrugs cannot improve this principal shortcoming since the activated metabolites resulting from oxidation or reductive biotransformation do not react by themselves with the target molecule but through spontaneous and therefore highly unspecific release of reactive species. Specificity may be expected only from those metabolic processes in which the ultimate cytotoxic agent will be released at that specific site which is critical for (cancer) cell proliferation or DNA replication. Theroetically highest specificity may be expected from drugs which are enzyme mechanism-based suicide inactivators of DNA polymerase α-holoenzyme. According to Hubscher (1983) this enzyme is the replicator for chromosomal DNA in eukaryotic cells (Fig.1).

DNA polymerase α holoenzyme offers several points for attack by suicide inactivators. Besides the DNA polymerase activity it contains at least six subunits which according to Ottiger and Hubscher (1984) contribute to the complex DNA replication on both the leading and lagging strand. One of the subunits is 3'-5'exonuclease which Brudlag and Byrnes demonstrated to confer "proof reading" activity to the DNA polymerase α holoenzyme. Studying the toxicogenation of acti-

Fig.1. Bioactivation and cytotoxic specificity of anticancer drugs.

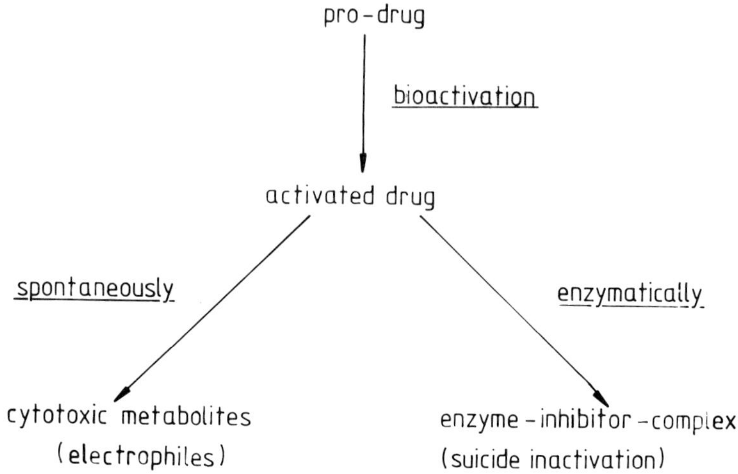

vated cyclophosphamide (4-OH-CP) Hohorst et al. (1986) demonstrated that spontaneous β-elimination of acrolein from 4-OH-CP to yield phosphoramide mustard (PAM) as the ultimate alkylating product does not work in vivo (Fig.2). Moreover an enzymatic mechanism with hydrolytic attack by phosphodiesterases on the phosphorester bound in 4-OH-CP was observed. By comparing the toxicogenating activity of various phosphodiesterases and exonucleases with 4-OH-CP as substrate, Bielicki et al.(1983) showed that only those exonucleases which are capable of hydrolysing phosphodiester bonds on the 3'-OH-terminal of monostranded DNA or polynucleotides (thus operating in the 3'-5'direction) could also hydrolyse activated CP.

Most interesting was the observation that 3'-5'exonucleases firmly associated with DNA polymerases like the Kornberg enzyme, DNA E.coli polymerase I or DNA polymerase δ which was first isolated from rabbit bone marrow by Byrnes, showed the highest specific activities for toxicogenation of 4-OH-CO. Furthermore, Bielicki et al. (1984) demonstrated that toxicogenation of 4-OH-CP by he 3'-5'exonuclease subsite of DNA polymerase I led to an irreversible inactivation of the DNA polymerase core enzyme by alkylation

Fig.2. Metabolism of cyclophosphamide.

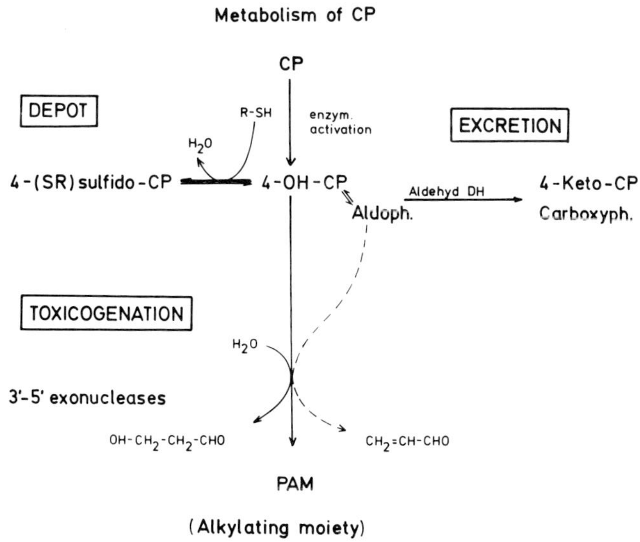

with PAM. This means that 4-OH-CP acts on these key enzymes of DNA replication as an enzyme-mechanism-based suicide inactivator. Hohorst et al. (1986) postulated that cytotoxic specificity of 4-OH-CP depends on this property. In addition a site-specific alkylation of DNA might also occur.

In any case the ultimate alkylation on the replication machinery must be very specific and must be restricted to active replicating sites of the chromatin (replication forks).

However in the case of activated CP the high cytotoxic specificity is overlapped by nonspecific toxicities resulting from the high reactivity of the hemiaminal group on C4 of the oxazaphosphorine ring and by toxicogenation of activated CP by free exonucleases that are not linked to DNA polymerase (Fig.3). This explains why cyclophosphamide, despite its high cytoxic specificity, is far from being an ideal anticancer agent and is still limited in its curative possibilities by toxicity especially on bone marrow and the urinary and gastrointestinal tracts.

Attempts are in progress to design suicide inactivators of DNA polymerase holoenzyme in which those toxic unspecificities are eliminated.

Fig.3. Doses of phosphoramide-ester NSC 612567 D and range of toxicities.

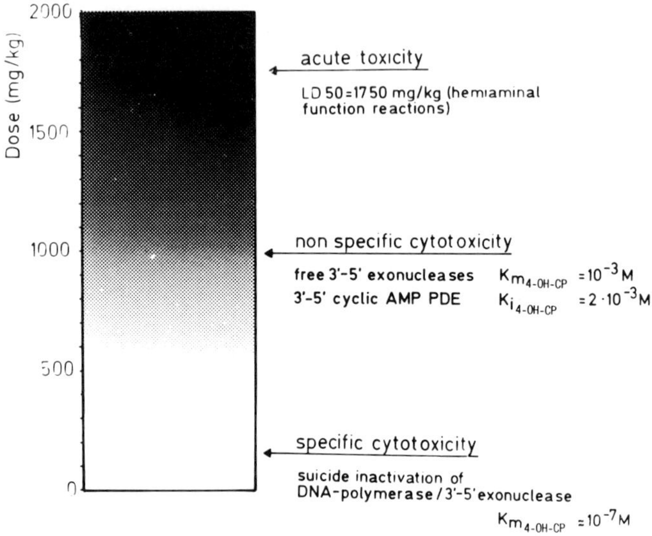

Single i.p. injection of drug with BDF_1 mice + with P815 Mastocytoma ascites.

Following these attempts we aim to develop alkylating anticancer drugs with high efficacy and low toxicity.

REFERENCES

Bielicki, L., Voelcker, G. & Hohorst, H.-J., 1983, *Journal of Cancer Research and Clinical Oncology*, 105, 27.

Bielicki, L., Voelcker, G. & Hohorst, H.-J., 1984, *Journal of Cancer Research and Clinical Oncology*, 107, 195.

Brudlag, D. & Kornberg, A., 1972, *Journal of Biological Chemistry*, 247, 241.

Byrnes, J.J., Downey, K.M., Black, V.L. & So, A.G., 1976, *Biochemistry*, 5, 2817.

Hohost, H.-J., Bielicki, L. & Voelcker, G., 1986, The enzymatic basis of cyclophosphamide specificity. In *Advances in Enzyme Regulation*, Vol. 25, edited by George Weber (Pergamon Press), p.99.
Hübscher, U., 1983, *Experientia*, 39, 1.
Ottiger, H.P. & Hübscher, U., 1984, *Proceedings of the National Academy of Science of the U.S.A.*, 81, 3993.

METABOLISM OF PLATINUM COMPOUNDS*

G. Ehninger, C. Haag, G. Vossler, and H.D. Waller

Medizinische Universitätsklinik, Otfried-Müller-Str., 7400 Tübingen, FRG

Introduction

The unexpected and interesting biologic acitivity of platinum complexes was first noted in the laboratories of B. Rosenberg (1965, 1985). In a study that was designed to test the influence of electric fields on growing cells, cell division was inhibited by an electrolysis product of the platinum electrode formed in the presence of the ammonium chloride in the nutrient medium. Further analysis showed that this chemical was the classic Peyrone's chloride, cis-dichlorodiammineplatinum (II).

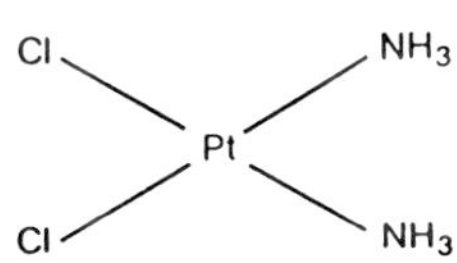

Figure 1. Structure of cisplatin

Platinum is in the oxidation state +2 and has four bonds that point to the corners of a square. The high stability of these isomer implies an energy barrier to exchange between ligands. Platinum II complexes are accessible to attack from above and below the plane where additional two platinum orbitals can be directed for bond formation. Although

* Dedicated to Prof. Dr. G.W. Lohr on the occasion of his 65 th birthday.

complexes of platinum II and platinum in oxidation state +4 have antitumor activity, the activity of platinum IV complexes may be due to conversion of the +2 state in the cell. Combined or intermediate states of oxidation occur in the platinum pyrimidine blue complexes, which are potenially interesting new antitumor agents (Arrizabalga 1984).

In 1968, some platinum complexes were tested for anticancer activity in a mouse-tumor model system. Cisplatin (drug generic name of c-DDP) completely inhibited the development of the solid Sarcoma-180 tumor (Hill 1972). In further clinical trials cisplatin showed considerable activity against several tumors, although clinical use was limited by a considerable toxicity, particularly nephrotoxicity. Other side effects include nausea and vomiting, myelosuppression, ototoxicity, peripheral neuropathy, electrolyte disturbances, seizures, and allergic reactions.

A significant breakthrough occurred when Hayes and associates (1977) dicovered that the simple trick of hydrating the patient markedly diminished the nephrotoxicity without loss of anticancer activity. Since that time cisplatin is used successfully in a wide range of tumours e.g. testicular cancer, ovarian cancer, non small cell lung cancer and sarcomas.

Measurement of Pt complexes in biologic samples

Pharmacokinetic studies are most often done by use of flameless atomic absorption spectroscopy (FAAS). Samples are atomized at 2700°C and absorbance is measured at 265.9 nm. The major disadvantages of flameless atomic absorption spectroscopy are the expense and complexity of the apparatus, matrix effects in clinical samples and the lack of specificity due to the measurement of the total Pt content. Free Pt can be separated from protein-bound Pt in plasma by centrifuge ultrafiltration.

Pharmacokinetics of cisplatin

In our pharmacokinetic studies cisplatin was administered as iv infusion over 8 hours at a dose of 50 mg/m^2 to 75 mg/m^2 (Ehninger 1984). Figure 2 shows a typical concentration-time curve of platinum in serum in treatment cycle two 5 weeks after the first treatment course. The terminal half-life was 87.3 h $\pm$ 37 h (N=23). The non-protein bound cisplatin

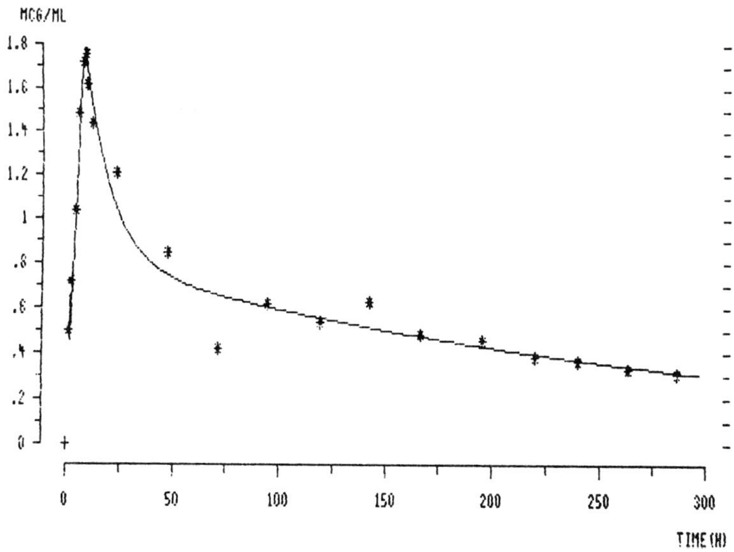

Figure 2. Total serum platinum concentration

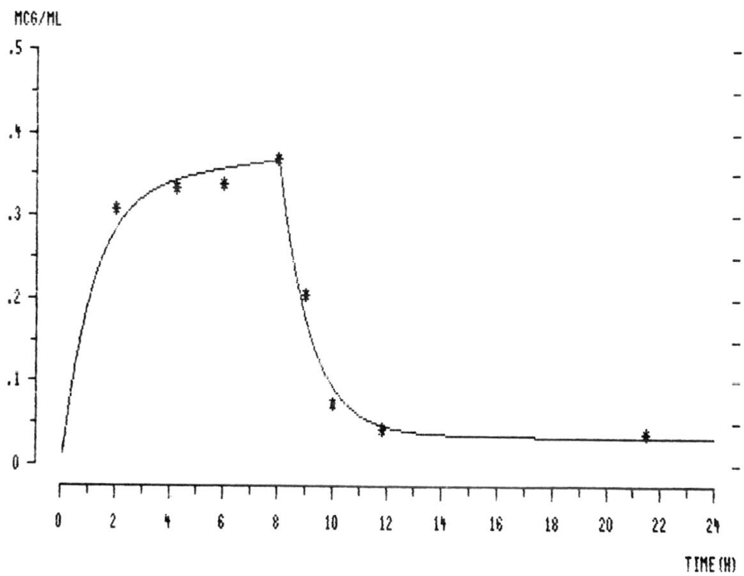

Figure 3. Non-protein-bound platinum concentration

concentration was measured by flamless atomic absorption spectroscopy after ultrafiltration. At the end of the 8-h-infusion, the concentration rapidly declined with a half-life of $0.4\ h \pm 0.3\ h$ (N=11). At the end of the infusion 50 % was protein bound, and four hours after infusion more than 90 per cent was protein bound (Figure 3).
The protein-bound fraction is not cytotoxic. Therefore the most important pharmacologic parameter is the plasma concentration of unbound Pt as a function of time.

Mean cumulative urinary excretion at 24 hours was $34.5\ \% \pm 12.9\ \%$ (N=24). The excreted amount per day was much lower on the following days, and after 5 days 51.3 ± 14.8 % of the administered amount are excreted in urine.

Reaction of cisplatin with water

The biologically most important reactions involve the replacement of one ligand by another. The reactions of cisplatin with water are summarized in Figure 4 (Zwelling 1982). Although the Pt-water bond is weaker than the Pt-Cl bond, the overwhelming concentration of water molecules can override the difference in bond stability.
This can occur only when the Cl^- concentration is very low, since Cl^- will shift the equilibrium away

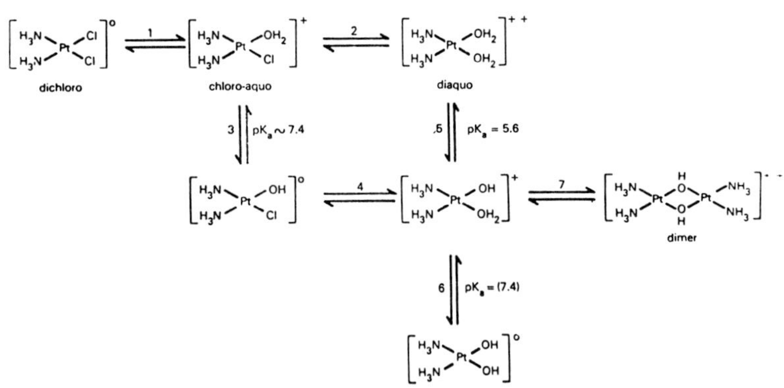

Figure 4. Reactions of cisplatin with water (from Zwelling 1982)

from the aquo forms. The chlorides of cisplatin can be replaced by water molecules in a sequence of two steps: reactions 1 and 2 in Figure 3. Each of the bound water molecules can dissociate a proton, with acid dissociation constants. In addition, two Pt complexes can combine to form dimers and higher polymers. The Pt species connected by this network of reactions would be expected to differ in their pharmacokinetic behaviour and in their reactivity with biomolecules.

Pharmacokinetic studies with ^{13}N labelled cisplatin did not provide any evidence that ammonia was released from cisplatin in vivo. (Haber 1984)

Protein binding

The Cl^- concentration of plasma should prevent the aquation reaction and therefore maintain the drug in the relatively unreactive dichloro form. The process of progressive binding of Pt to plasma proteins must therefore be a result of covalent binding with sulfhydryl-groups. In dialysis experiments, we could demonstrate that the binding of cisplatin was irreversible (Ehninger 1984). After binding to plasma proteins, the drug is no longer cytotoxic to cells in culture systems (Takahashi 1985). Cisplatin binds to a variety of plasma proteins (Gullo 1980), and cisplatin would remain in the plasma as long the protein molecule to which it is bound.

The percentage of the drug in the reactive chloro-aquo form would be about 1 per cent as estimated from the equilibrium constants.

Reactions of cisplatin in plasma

However, the investigations of Daley-Yates and Mc Brien (1984) were controversial in some respects.

Cisplatin and metabolite species and unchanged cisplatin present in samples of protein-free plasma were separated by HPLC. The fractions of the column effluent were analysed for platinum using flameless atomic absorption spectroscopy. Seven different species could be detected in protein-free plasma of rats obtained 2 hr after injection of cisplatin.

The authors measured the concentrations of these compunds over three hours after injection. The concentration of free platinum falls rapidly, reflecting both an increase in the binding to protein and the removal of soluble platinum species by the kidney.

By 3 hr following dosing the concentration of unchanged cisplatin remaining in the plasma was very low or undetectable. Two principal metabolite species were detected, designated C and F. Fifteen minutes after injection C is the most abundant metabolite and accounts for approximately 10% of the total ultrafiltrable plasma platinum. At 3 hr post injection, when almost no unchanged cisplatin remains in the plasma and the total platinum content of the plasma is much lower, species F is the most abundant metabolite and C and F are approximately 15 % and 50 % of the ultrafiltrable plasma platinum respectively.

When cisplatin is incubated in vitro with whole plasma or protein free plasma, species can be recognized which have the same retention times as those formed in vivo, although they are present in different proportions. These differences are explained by differential excretion and differences in the availability of substituting ligands. The authors were not able to produce metabolite species sufficiently pure and in the quantities required for unambiguous analysis. However, several data indicate that species F is a hydrolysis product and cochromatographs with diaquodiammine platinum. It is very surprising that these species are produced in the presence of chloride concentrations of 100 mM as present in plasma. It is therefore mandatory that in plasma an agent is present which can catalyse this hydrolysis reaction.

The authors demonstrated that two other species C and D are methionine complexes with cisplatin (McAuliffe 1972). Further experiments showed that mixed metabolites and hydrolysis products are more nephrotoxic than cisplatin, although the cisplatin-methionin complex was not nephrotoxic. The mixed metabolites do have some antitumour effect, but are less effective than the parent compound.

Reactions of cisplatin inside cells

Segal and Le Pecq (1985) investigated the reactions of cisplatin inside cells where it reacts with many different molecules e.g. proteins and nucleic acids. The formation of DNA adducts is thought to be the main cause of cytotoxicity. In medium containing no anions other than Cl^-, the monoaqua and diaqua species are the only reactive derivatives. In medium containing other ions such as acetate, phosphate, and pyrophosphate these anions were able to exchange with chloride to form aceto, phosphato, or pyrophosphato complexes. Ap_4A, a signal nucleotide possibly involved in the control of DNA replication initiation, also reacts with cisplatin, but the biological significance of this reaction is not fully elucidated.

Binding of cisplatin to DNA

A clear indication of the biologic role of DNA damage in cisplatin-treated bacteria was the finding that mutants defective in DNA excision or recombination repair have increased sensitivity to the drug. The DNA site of greatest intrinsic reactivity with cisplatin is the guanine-N_7 position and some recent data indicate that cisplatin binds to the N_7 and O_6 positions of the same guanine base (Eapen 1985, Johnson 1985, Miller 1985, Pinto 1985, Raudaschl-Sieber 1985, Sherman 1985). Three types of Pt cosslinks involving DNA have been identified: interstrand, intrastrand, and DNA-protein crosslinks (Zwelling 1979).

Cisplatin analogs

The clinical efficacy and the severity of side effects of cisplatin have led to the development of several hundred analogs. The principle of the second generation platinum coordination complexes is the replacement of the two chlorides by more stable ligands or, in additon, the substitution of the ammonia ligands. JM-9 (CHIP, Iproplatin), an octahedral platinum (IV) compound and carboplatin (CBDCA) are compounds of great clinical interest. These compounds showed antitumor affects as good as those of cisplatin in some experimental tumors and in man, but had decreased toxicity. The key pharmacological differences of these cisplatin derivatives are the formation of less degradation products, a longer half-life of free non-protein-bound fractions, and a higher urinary excretion of unchanged parent compound (Lee 1983, Pendyala 1983, Momburg 1985, Laznichova 1986, van der Vijgh 1986).

In chloride-free phosphate buffer, cisplatin had a half-life of 2.4 h in contrast to a half-life of 268 h for carboplatin (Knox 1986). By use of a ^{14}C labelled ligand, carboplatin was shown to bind monofunctionally to DNA after monoaquation. The CBDCA ligand now becomes a more labile group which results in a difunctional binding to DNA. This work has shown that once bound to DNA in equal amounts both cisplatin and carboplatin cause equal difunctional lesions, interstrand crosslinks, and cytotoxicity. A enzymatic activation of carboplatin does not occur.

The pharmacokinetics of iproplatin were investigated by Creaven (1986). The plasma decay of the unchanged drug is rapid. In vitro studies demonstrated that iproplatin itself does not bind to plasma protein. Total platinum decays with a biexponential decay, and the non-protein bound platinum fraction shows the same pattern. Thus, iproplatin is metabolized to protein bound and non-protein bound metabolites. The chemical structure of these compounds is unknown.

Summary

The conversion of cisplatin probably involves simple chemical reactions and possibly some enzymatic reactions. The details of these mechanisms and the extent of their contribution to the overall changes have not been elucidated.

The chlorides of cisplatin are replaced by water molecules, the aquo-complexes, which are reactive compounds.

Additional complexing with methionine was observed.

Cisplatin reacts via sulfhydryl groups directly with proteins. The protein-bound fraction is inactive and is irreversibly bound. A ligand exchange is also possible with acetate, phosphate and pyrophosphate.

Cisplatin derivatives are more stable than cisplatin itself. Carboplatin also reacts with DNA via the exchange of ligands.

REFERENCES

Arrizabalaga, P., Castan, P., Laurent, J.-P., Cros, S., Francois, G., 1984, European Journal of Medical Chemistry, 19, 501.

Creaven, P.J., Pendyala, L., Madajewicz, S., 1986, Drugs under Expermental and Clinical Research, 12, 287.

Daley-Yates, P.T., McBrien, D.C.H., 1984, Biochemical Pharmacology, 33, 3063.

Eapen, S., Green, M., Ismail, I.M., 1985, Journal of Inorganic Biochemistry, 24, 233.

Ehninger, G., Haag, C., Wilms, K., 1984, Tumordiagnostik und Therapie, 5, 147.

Gullo, J.J., Litterst, C.L., Maguire, P.J., Sikic, B.I., Hoth, D.F., Woolley, P.V., 1980, Cancer Chemotherapy and Pharmacology, 5, 21.

Haber, M.T., Cooper, A.J.L., Rosenspire, K.C., Ginos, J.Z., Rottenberg, D.A., 1985, Journal of Labelled Compounds and Radiopharmaceuticals, 22, 509.

Johnson, N.P., Mazard, A.M., Escalier, J., Macquet, J.P., 1985, Journal of the American Chemical Society, 107, 6376.
Knox, R.J., Friedlos, F., Lydall, D.A., Roberts, J.J., 1986, Cancer Research, 46, 1972.
Laznickova, A., Laznicek, M., Kvetina, J., Drobnik, J., 1986, Cancer Chemotherapy and Pharmacology, 17, 133.
Lee, F.H., Canetta, R., Issell, B.F., Lenaz, L., 1983, Cancer Treatment Reviews, 10, 39.
McAuliffe, C.A., Murray, S.G., 1972, Inorganica Chimica Acta Reviews, 103, 121.
Momburg, R., Bourdeaux, M., Sarrazin, M., Roux, F., Briand, C., 1985, European Journal of Drug Metabolism and Pharmacokinetics, 10, 77.
Pendyala, L., Greco, W., Cowens, J.W., Madajewicz, S., Creaven, P.J., 1983, Cancer Chemotherapy and Pharmacology, 11, 23.
Pinto, A.L., Lippard, S.J., 1985, Biochimica et Biophysica Acta, 780, 167.
Rosenberg, B., 1985, Cancer, 55, 2303.
Sherman, S.E., Gibson, D., Wang, A.H.-J., Lippard, S.J., 1985, Science, 230, 412.
Segal, E., Le Pecq, J.-B., 1985, Cancer Research, 45, 492.
Takahashi, K., Seki, T., Nishikawa, K., Minamide, S., Iwabuchi, M., Ono, M., Nagamine, S., Horinishi, H., 1985, Japanese Journal of Cancer Research, 76, 68.
Van der Vijgh, W.J.F., Klein, I., 1986, Cancer Chemotherapy and Pharmacology, 18, 129.
Zwelling, L.A., Kohn, K.W., 1979, Cancer Treatment Reports, 63, 1439.
Zwelling, L.A. Kohn K.W., 1982, Platinum complexes. In Pharmacologic Principles of Cancer Treatment, edited by B. Chabner (Saunders, Philadelphia), p. 309.

ANTITUMOR ANTHRACYCLINES

Federico Arcamone

Farmitalia Carlo Erba, Milan, Italy

INTRODUCTION

Daunorubicin (I) and doxorubicin (adriamycin, II) are antitumor antibiotics produced by *Streptomyces peucetius* that have considerable importance in the medical treatment of different types of human cancer (Arcamone 1981). Doxorubicin is endowed with a wide spectrum of activity against solid tumors and is currently used mainly in drug combinations. More than fifteen years after its introduction in therapy new clinical applications are still studied. These include new disease targets, dose-schedule alterations, special routes of administration and combined modality therapies (Praga et al., 1982). However, the presence of dose limiting toxic side effects, together with the low, if any, responsiveness of important diseases such as non small cell lung cancer, colorectal cancer, pancreatic adenocarcinoma, prostatic cancer, renal cancer and malignant melanoma, have stimulated the development of analogs aimed at improved efficacy and tolerability or at a wider spectrum of activity.

Most available experimental evidence indicates nuclear DNA as the main biological target of the antitumor anthracyclines, possibly through multiple mechanisms (Capranico et al., 1986). However, other cellular targets, e.g. plasma membrane redox systems, might be of relevance (Sun et al., 1984). The metabolism of I and II has been studied by Takanashi & Bachur (1976). The constitutive enzyme daunorubicin-reductase catalyzes efficiently the conversion of I and less extensively of II into the corresponding 13-dihydroderivatives that still exhibit bioactivity comparable to the parent cpmpounds. A second metabolic reaction, whose pharmacological relevance is still to be established, is the reductive deglycosidation to the biologically inert 7-deoxyaglycones. The latter compounds may also be eliminated in conjugated form after 4-demethylation.

It now appears that metabolism of anthracycline glycosides in the body is a main factor influencing their pharmacological behavior. Work carried out in the author's laboratory on the new clinically useful analogs of the biosynthetic antitumor anthracyclines is presented here. These studies relate to the clinically important second generation anthracyclines epirubicin (III) and idarubicin (IV). The former is a better tolerated analog of doxorubicin showing a similar spectrum of activity in solid tumors, and differs from the parent compound in the orientation of the 4'-hydroxyl group. The second is a totally synthetic analog of I, lacking the methoxyl group at C-4, and endowed with potent antileukaemic activity. Another important aspect of anthracycline metabolism is represented by the redox reactions involving the quinone system. Both the structural requirements of these reactions and their relevance to the bioactivity of the anthracyclines are subjects of current interest in this area.

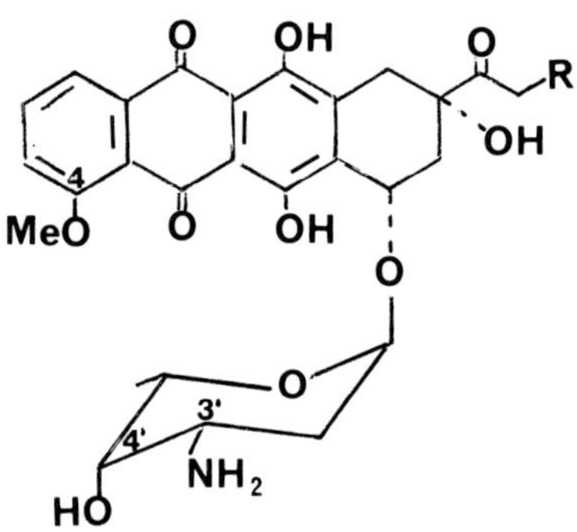

I : R = H
II : R = OH

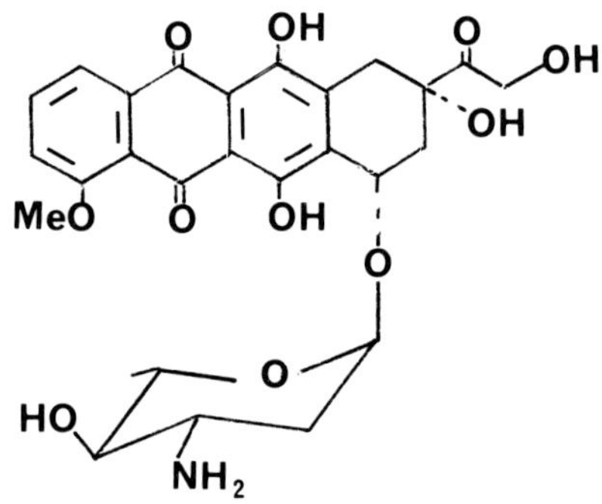

III

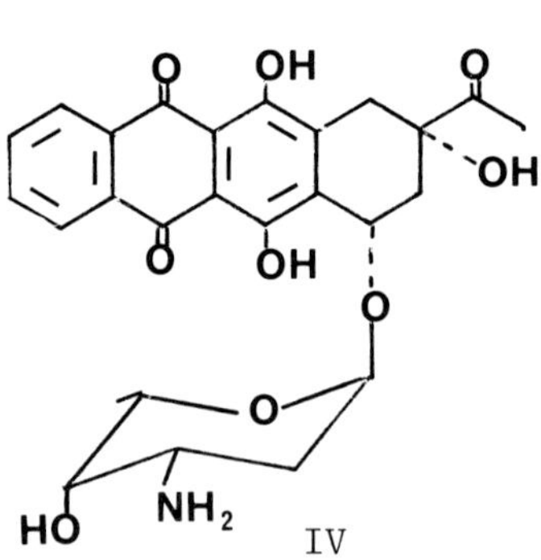

IV

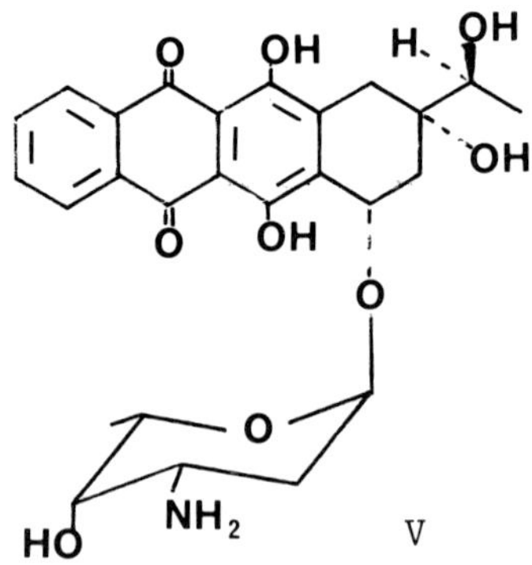

V

EPIRUBICIN

The synthesis of [14-^{14}C]epirubicin was performed starting from epirubicin itself according to a general procedure developed in our laboratory (Arcamone et al., 1984). The labelled compound was used in the rat studies showing that III gives lower blood levels and generally higher tissue concentrations of radioactivity in the first day after iv treatment when compared with II. This behavior was confirmed in the patient studies. However, the new analog was found to follow, in the human body, a different fate as the main metabolite was found to be the 4'-O-β-D-glucuronide of III, accompanied by a lower amount of the same conjugate of the 13-dihydroderivative. This conjugation is unique among the clinically useful anthracyclines and most likely is the cause of the different clinical toxicity of epirubicin when compared with doxorubicin. On the other hand III exhibits response rates in different solid tumors of the same order of magnitude as those exhibited by II at comparable dosage (Hurtelup & Ganzina 1986).

IDARUBICIN

The metabolism of IV was established both on the basis of the analysis of human metabolites and of radioisotopic studies. Also in this case transformations that take place in the body play a relevant role. In fact IV is extensively converted to the 13-dihydro metabolite V, a compound exhibiting a relatively slow biliary elimination rate (Penco et al., 1985; Zini et al., 1986). The extent of the said conversion is consistent with the absence of the hydroxyl at C-14 because it is known that the enzyme daunorubicin reductase, reduces much more efficiently the C-13 carboxyl group in I than in II (Felsted et al., 1977). The intrinsic antitumor activity and elevated concentrations of V in the plasma of the patients is apparently responsible for the clinical efficacy of the drug (Hurtelup & Ganzina 1986). Further metabolism in laboratory animals includes the formation of conjugated forms of the 7-deoxy-13-dihydroaglycone (Zini et al., 1986).

REDOX REACTIONS

In the presence of a suitable redox enzyme the anthracyclines may undergo either an one or a two electron reduction. In aerobic conditions the reduced form promptly passes the electrons to oxygen with the formation of radical species (Bachur et al., 1982). In the absence of oxygen deglycosidation with production of a quinone methide takes place. The latter reacts with a proton to give the corresponding 7-

deoxyquinone (Kleyer & Koch 1984). However, the intermediate quinone methide may also react as an electrophile in selected situations (Ramakrishnan & Fisher 1986).

Intermediate formation of semiquinone radical species seems not to be the case when a typical anthracycline such as I is incubated with rat liver microsomes and NADPH in anaerobic conditions and at concentrations lower than 10^{-3}M. On the other hand a small amount of a radical species is formed in the same conditions from 6-deoxy-carminomycin (VI) probably arising by a disproportionation process. A major difference is however represented by the deglycosidation reaction that occurs promptly with I whereas the reduced form of VI does not undergo the fission of the C7-O7 bond. This diverse reactivity does not influence the bioactivity as both I and II are endowed with antitumor and cardiotoxic properties. On the other hand it has been found that L-xylo aminoglycoside VII, showing a relatively low affinity for native calf-thymus DNA, is clearly much less cytotoxic than "isodoxorubicin" VIII that has an affinity for DNA of the same order of magnitude as the isomeric I. Both compounds VII and VIII are reductively deglycosidated in anaerobic conditions with the enzyme preparation. It can be concluded that the ability to form reactive quinone-methide intermediates does not imply the expression of cytotoxic properties.

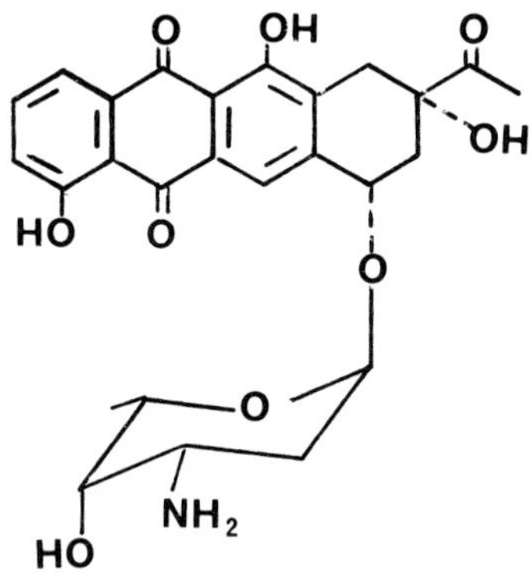

VI

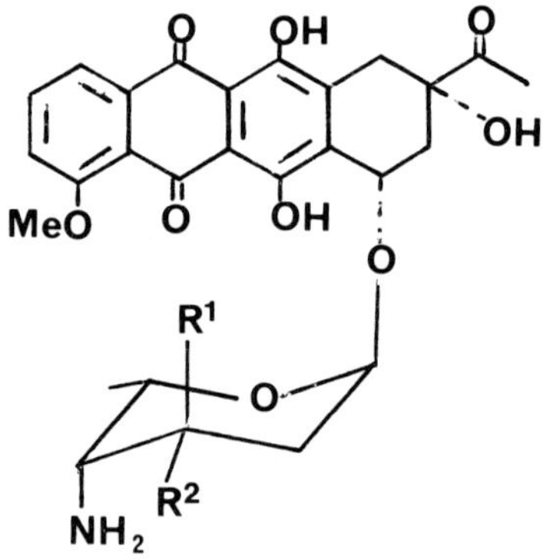

VII : R^1 = OH, R^2 = H

VIII : R^1 = H, R^2 = OH

REFERENCES

Arcamone, F., 1981, Doxorubicin, Anticancer Antibiotics, Vol. 17, edited by G. deStevens (Medicinal Chemistry Series) (Academic Press).

Arcamone, F., Lazzati, M., Vicario, G.P. & Zini, G., 1984, Cancer Chemotherapy and Pharmacology, 12, 157.

Bachur, N.R., Gee, M.V. & Friedman, R.D., 1982, Cancer Research, 42, 1078.

Capranico , G., Soranzo, C. & Zunino, F., 1986, Cancer Research, 46, 5499.

Felsted, R.L., Pichter, D.R. & Bachur, N.R., 1977, Biochemical Pharmacology, 26, 1117.

Hurtelup, P. & Ganzina, F., 1986, Drugs. In Experimental Clinical Research, 12, 233.

Kleyer, D.L. & Koch, T.H., 1984, Journal of the American Chemical Society, 106, 2380.

Penco, S., Cassinelli, G., Vigevani, A., Zini, P., Rivola, G. & Arcamone, F., 1985, Gazzetta Chimica Italiana, 115, 195.

Praga, C., Beretta, G., Bawa, O., Tabanelli, D. & Zanon, P., 1982. In Anthracycline Antibiotic in Cancer Therapy, edited by F.M. Muggia, C.W. Young & S.K. Karter (Developments in Oncology) (Martinus Nijhoff Publishers), p. 384.

Ramakrishnan, K. & Fisher, J., 1986, Journal of Medicinal Chemistry, 29, 1215.

Sun, I.L., Crane, F.L., Löw, H. & Grebing, C., 1984, Journal of Biogenetics and Biomembranes, 16, 209.

Takanashi, S. & Bachur, N.R., 1976, Drug Metabolism and Disposition, 4, 79.

Zini, G., Vicario, G.P., Lazzati, M. & Arcamone, F., 1986, Cancer Chemotherapy and Pharmacology, 16, 107.

ANTIHORMONES IN THE TREATMENT OF CANCER

Rolf Geiger

Hoechst AG, D-6230 Frankfurt/Main-80

INTRODUCTION

The treatment of cancer with antihormones presupposes that hormone receptors exist on cancer cells and that cell-growth and -proliferation depend on the respective hormone.

In a narrower sense, we understand a true antihormone to be a substance which competes with the hormone at its receptor. In practice, however, suppression of hormonal activity can be accomplished at several stages, biosynthesis, receptor interaction or inhibition of a post-receptor event.

A special but important case is overstimulation, if it results in a negative feedback which blocks a step in a hormonal reaction sequence. This principle works e.g. in the hypothalamic-hypophyseal-gonadal axis.

ANTIGLUCOCORTICOIDS

In Cushing's syndrome, caused by adrenal hyperplasia or tumors, but also by high levels of ACTH which may stem from ectopic ACTH-producing tumors, excessive amounts of corticosteroids are released from the cortex of the adrenal gland.

The adverse anabolic effect of androgens, e.g. testosterone, on glucocorticoid-induced catabolism antagonizes the action of cortisol on tissues but also inhibits the effect of ACTH on the adrenal gland. This stimulated the search for other steroidal antihormones (Sakiz 1986 I). An 11-substituted synthetic norandrostane derivative though, RU 38 486, has been characterized as a potent glucocorticoid antagonist and has been shown to be clinically active in Cushing's syndrome (Nieman et al.,1984). This compound however, is also a strong antiprogestin (Sakiz 1986 II).

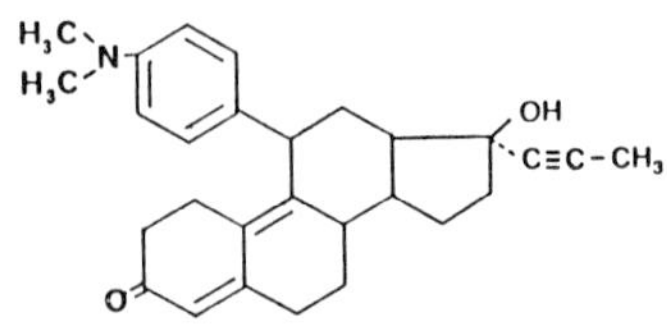

RU 38 486

ANTIHORMONES IN THE REPRODUCTIVE SYSTEM

The most prominent cases for antihormonal treatment of cancer are tumors of the reproductive system. They are intimately related with the endocrine system and are subject of its delicate control mechanisms. Some of them are structurally and functionally similar to their tissue of origin and respond to hormonal treatment.

Figure 1: Female hormone regulation

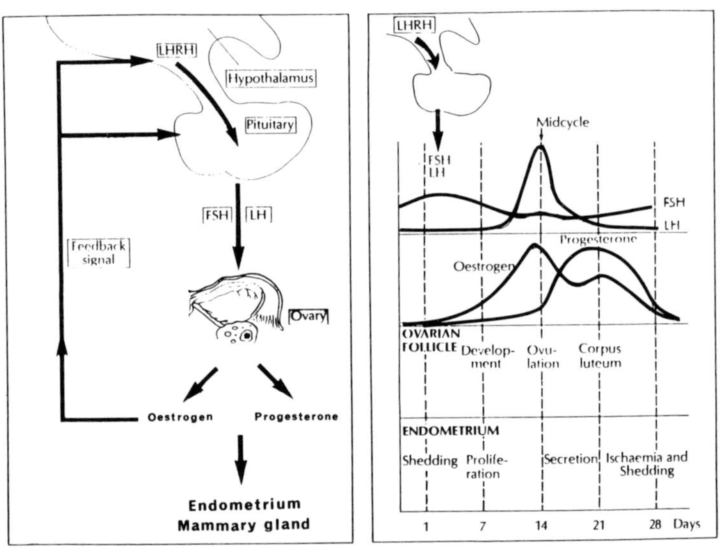

Figure 1 gives a picture of the mechanisms which regulate the hypothalamic-hypophyseal-gonadal axis in the female.

The hypothalamic hormone LHRH (Matsuo et al.,1971),

```
pGlu-His-Trp-Ser-Tyr-Gly-Leu-Arg-Pro-Gly-NH
  1   2   3   4   5   6   7   8   9   10
                 LHRH
```

stimulates the production of the hypophyseal hormones FSH and LH. These sex-independent glycoproteins, for their part, regulate synthesis and release of the steroidal sex hormone in the ovaries and testes.

A complicated feedback system adjusts and controls the equilibrium between these hormones. Figure 1 also demonstrates the rhythmic pattern in the release of FSH and LH in the female as a consequence of signals from the central nervous system, mediated by LHRH. This chronobiological rhythm causes the different pattern of oestrogen and gestagen release which results in effects seen in the menstrual cycle.

Tumors which derive from glandular or endometrial tissues often possess the same hormonal stimulation mechanisms as the parent ones, i.e. they bear hormone receptors. Consequently, deprivation of hormones or their displacement from the receptors may provide an effective therapeutic principle.

PROSTATIC CANCER

In prostatic cancer, orchectomy removes the source of the male hormone testosterone which provides about 90% of the circulating androgens. The rest comes from the adrenals which continue to produce androgenic steroids under the influence of the hypophyseal hormone ACTH.

Another way to block testosterone production is the oral administration of oestrogens which inhibit pituitary production of LH and subsequently testosterone. Oestrogens, however, increase the incidence of cardiovascular complications and places the patient at risk of severe cardiovascular accidents (Geller et al., 1976).

A true antihormonal approach is the application of antiandrogens, possessing receptor-blocking properties and antigonadotropic effects.

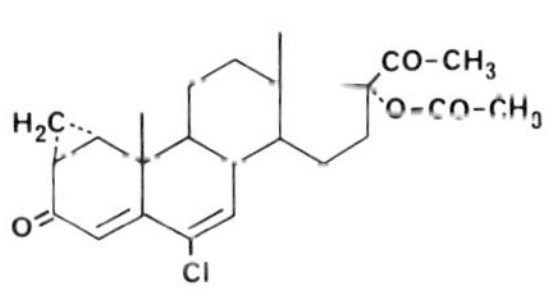

Cyproterone acetate

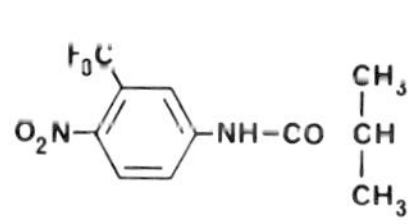

Flutamide

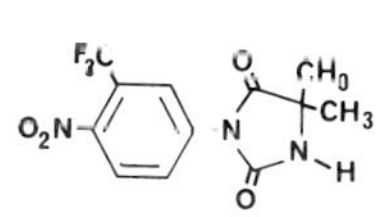

Anandron

The steroidal antiandrogen cyproterone acetate rapidly decreases plasma testosterone (Jacobi et al., 1980). Surprisingly, a non-steroidal compound, flutamide, strongly and selectively binds to and blocks androgen receptors (Koch 1984). Cyclization of flutamide results in the analogue anandron which is more resistent to metabolic attack. Antiandrogens, however, turned out to be less active than oestrogens and frequently caused an "escape phenomenon" of testosterone (Di Silverio & Sciarra 1986).

The most recent development in the treatment of prostatic carcinoma has been the replacement of surgical castration by medical castration following the administration of so-called super-agonistic analogues of LHRH. These highly potent compounds desensitize FSH and LH producing pituitary cells by down-regulation of their LHRH receptors. The synthesis of FSH and LH stops and after initial stimulation, plasma testosterone is reduced to castration levels (Labrie et al., 1980, 1985).

The discovery of these potent agonists was the result of extensive structure-activity relationship studies (Geiger 1984, Karten & Rivier 1986). In a first step, 10-glycin-amide could be replaced by ethylamide yielding a 3 to 5-fold increase in biological activity. The systematic substitution of alanine for each amino acid showed a remarkable decrease in hormonal potency, teaching the importance of side-chain interactions with the receptor. Another series of analogues, however, in which every amino acid was replaced by D-alanine, resulted in the surprising finding that D-alanine in position 6 enhances the hormonal potency about sevenfold. Combination of both substitutions gave a thirtyfold increase.

Table 1: Biological activity of LHRH analogues, modified in positions 6 and 10

Side-chain of D-amino acids in position 6	Residue in position 10	Approximate biol. activity in vivo (LH-RH = 1)
$-H$	$-NH-C_2H_5$	4
$-CH_3$	$-Gly-NH_2$	7
$-CH_3$	$-NH-C_2H_5$	30
$-CH_2-CH(CH_3)_2$	$-NH-C_2H_5$	80
$-CH_2-O-C(CH_3)_2-CH_3$	$-NH-C_2H_5$	140

Finally, a 140-fold increase was observed with buserelin (last compound in Table 1), the strongest agonist within a series of D-amino acids with aliphatic side-chains.

In contrast to agonistic analogues of LH-RH, where most favourable substitutions had been found within a relatively short time, the development of strong antagonists took about a decade. On the other hand, the search was unique as regards the result - a several thousandfold increase in binding, compared to that which had been shown by the first antagonistic compounds. In the most active analogues, 50% of the amino acids are replaced by (mostly non-natural) D-amino acids (Table 2; Karten & Rivier 1986).

Table 2: Antagonistic analogues of LHRH

		Replacement in positions 1	2	3	6	10	Inhibitory dose (µg/rat)
1	1972	pGlu		Trp	Gly	Gly-NH_2	
2	1974	pGlu	D-Phe	Trp	Gly	Gly-NH_2	
3	1976	pGlu	D-Phe	D-Trp	D-Phe	Gly-NH_2	1000
4	1978	Ac-Pro	D-Phe	D-Trp	D-Trp	Gly-NH_2	200
5	1979	Ac-D-Phe	D-(pCl)Phe	D-Trp	D-Trp	Gly-NH_2	30
6	1981	Ac-Δ^3Pro	D-(pF)Phe	D Trp	D-Trp	Gly-NH_2	5
7	1982	Ac-D-(pCl)Phe	D-(pCl)Phe	D-Trp	D-Arg	D-Ala-NH_2	1
8	1983	Ac-D-Nal(2)	D-(pCl)Phe	D-Trp	D-hArg$(Et)_2$	D-Ala-NH_2	0,5

Despite the outstanding success in the design of LH-RH antagonists, these compounds are not yet being considered for use as antihormones. Still, the amount required for a sufficient blockade of the gonads is too high. Furthermore, the antagonists cause a release of histamine which cannot be tolerated. Thus, the so-called super-agonists remain the compounds of choice in the treatment of hormone-dependent cancer or cell proliferation. They are able to bring the serum concentration of sex hormones to castration levels, and only in the beginning stimulatory phase is the application of e.g. an antiandrogen recommended in the treatment of prostate carcinoma.

More recently, however, combinations of a highly active LH-RH agonist such as buserelin with the antiandrogene flutamide or anandron have been desribed in the continuous treatment of prostate carcinoma. LH-RH agonists cannot stop the synthesis of steroid hormones with androgenic potency in the adrenals which provide about 10% of androgen supply. Only an antiandrogen is able to suppress this activity by blocking androgen receptors on the cancer cells. The reported results are promising (Labrie et al., 1986)

BREAST CANCER

In the breast cancer, radical mastectomy was for a long time considered the best treatment regardless of stage. Today, this opinion is undergoing extensive reevaluation.

The response rate to antihormonal therapy depends on the receptor status as shown in Table 3 (Williams 1981).

Table 3: Response Rates to Endocrine Therapy as a Function of Steroid Hormone Receptor Status in Metastatic Breast Cancer

ER Status	PgR-Status	Approximate Response
positive	positive	80 %
positive	negative	30 %
negative	positive	not established
negative	negative	5 %

ER = oestrogen receptor
PgR = progesterone receptor

Oestradiol itself which promotes cell growth at low doses, is inhibitory at high doses. Again, however, oestrogens are inadequate for therapy because of their cardiovascular side-effects. The antioestrogen Tamoxifen is used for palliative treatment and can inhibit even oestrogen receptor-negative cell-lines (Chouvet & Saez 1985). Treatment with high doses of androgens have been effective for a limited time but virilising effects and hypercalcaemia limit this therapy.

Down-regulation of the pituitary by LHRH analogues such as Buserelin may therefore be the method of choice in the endocrine treatment of hormone dependent mammary carcinoma, alone or in combination with an anti-oestrogen. There are still many open questions with regard to correct dosage and optimal chronobiological pattern of treatment. It is to be hoped, however, that the resolution of these questions may open the door to an alternative therapy for late-stage breast cancer patients.

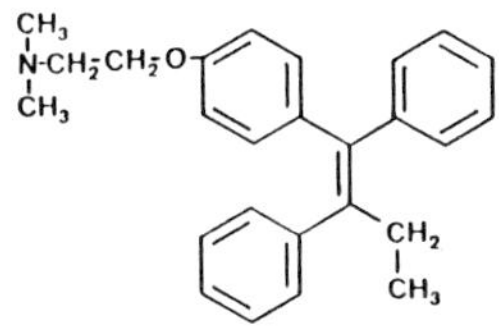

Tamoxifen

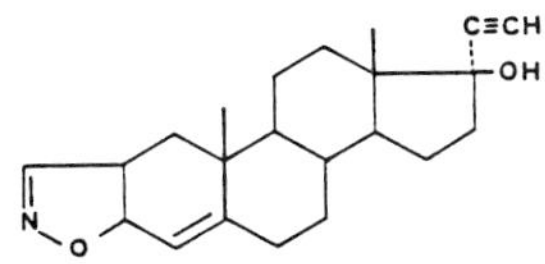

Danazol

ENDOMETRIOSIS

Buserelin has proved to be highly effective in the treatment of endometriosis, a benign proliferation of endometrial tissue outside its normal site. It may therefore replace the synthetic androgen Danazol whose application is associated with many side-effects including its androgenic and anabolic properties.

CONCLUSION

Considering the experience gathered so far, we must admit that treatment of cancer with true antihormones is restricted to few cases within the field of malignancy in the endocrine system. The indirect way by depriving hormone-dependent tumors of their hormonal growth factors seems presently to be a most effective and tolerable approach in the treatment of those tumors.

REFERENCES

Chouvet, D. & Saez, S., 1985 OH-Tam activity in mammary cell lines devoid of estrogen receptor. In Abstr.76th Meeting of the American Association for Cancer Research No. 752

Geiger, R., 1984 design and synthesis of LHRH agonists and antagonists. In LHRH and its analogues, edited by F. Labrie, A. Bélanger & A. Dupont (Excerpta medica international congress series 656, p. 36)

Jacobi, G.H., Altwein, J.E., Kurth, K.H., Basting, R. & Hohenfellner, R., 1980 British Journal of Urology, 52, 208

Karten, M.J. & Rivier, J.E., 1986 Endocrine Reviews, 7, 44

Koch, H., 1984 Drugs Today, 20, 561

Labrie, F., Bélanger, A., Cusan, L., Séguin, C., Pelletier, G., Kelley, P.A., Lefèvre, F.A., Lemay, A. & Raynaud, J.P. 1980 Journal of Andrology, 1, 209

Labrie, F., Dupont A., Bélanger, A., Lachance, R. & Giguère, M., 1985 British Journal of Medicine, 291, 369

Labrie, F., Dupont, A., Giguère, M., Borsanyi, J.P., Bélanger, A., Lacourcière, Y., Emond, J. & Monfette, G., 1986 Journal of Steroid Biochemistry, 25, 877

Matsuo, H., Baba, Y., Nair, R.M.G., Arimura, A. & Schally, A.V., 1971 Biochemical Biophysical Research Communications 43, 1334

Momany, F.A., 1976 Journal of the American Chemical Society, 98, 2996

Nieman, L.K., Chrousos, G.P., Spitz, I. et al. 1984 Clinical Research, 32, 271 A

Raynaud, J.P., Moguilewsky, M., Tournemine, V., Coussedière, D., Salmon, J., Husson, J.M., Bertagna, C., Tremblay, D., Pendyala, L., Brisset, J.M., Vallancien, G., Serment, G., Navratil, H., Dupont, A. & Labrie, F., 1985 Pharmacology and clinical studies with Anandron. In EORTC Genitourinary Group Monograph 2 Part A. Therapeutic Principles in Metastatic Prostatic Cancer, edited by F.H. Schöder & B. Richards (Alan R. Liss, New York), p. 99

Sakiz, E., 1986 I Survey on Antiglucocorticoids. In Pharmacology and clinical uses of inhibitors of hormone setion and action, edited by B.J.A. Furr & A.E. Wakeling (Baillière Tindall), p. 212

Sakiz, E., 1986 II Mifepristone (RU 486): A New Antiprogestin. ibid., p. 170

Di Silverio, F. & Sciarra, F., 1986 Journal of Steroid Biochemistry, 25, 773

Williams, R.H., 1981 Textbook of Endocrinology, 6th Edition (B.W. Saunders & Co., Philadelphia)

Figures have been taken from Geiger (1984) and from Busereline (Programme of the Hormone Group ZPM, Hoechst AG) 1984

THE METABOLISM OF SOME NOVEL ANTICANCER DRUGS

Andreas Gescher

Cancer Research Campaign Experimental
Chemotherapy Group, Pharmaceutical Sciences Institute,
Aston University, Birmingham, U.K.

INTRODUCTION

The "NCI Investigational Drugs Pharmaceutical Data" compendium published by the National Cancer Institute in 1986 lists more than 70 drug products which are currently or shortly undergoing either phase 1 clinical evaluation or toxicological testing as a prelude to trials. These products are novel compounds or investigational drug formulations. In view of this large number the selection of a few of these drugs to illustrate the importance of metabolism in therapy with novel agents is bound to be arbitrary. In the case of the eleven drugs discussed here, metabolism is important either as (i) an activation mechanism, (ii) a route of deactivation, (iii) a mode of toxification or (iv) a pivotal step in drug discovery.

DRUGS WHICH ARE METABOLICALLY ACTIVATED

Tiazofurin (I, Fig. 1) is a thiazole-C-nucleoside which is structurally related to the antiviral agent ribavirin. Tiazofurin is excreted predominantly unchanged and to a minor extent as its 5'-phosphate (Arnold et al., 1984). Anabolism to tiazofurin adenine dinucleotide (TAD) in the target cell appears to be vital for its antitumour activity. TAD inhibits inosine monophosphate dehydrogenase, which is the rate-limiting enzyme involved in guanosine nucleotide synthesis (Lui et al., 1984).

The aziridinylbenzoquinone drug diaziquone (II, Fig. 1) was synthesised with the rationale to obtain a cytotoxin with sufficient lipophilicity to penetrate the central nervous system. The drug is metabolised in *vivo* and in vitro (Spiegel et al., 1982). To date it has not been possible to isolate its metabolites and therefore their chemistry is unknown. Tumour cells are capable of reducing II to its free radical anion (Gutierrez et al., 1985). This biotransformation depends upon the presence of the intact aziridine moieties in the quinone molecule. Probably the radical produced by one-electron reduction is the ultimate cytotoxic species. Alternatively, it might generate cytotoxic radicals derived from oxygen.

FIG. 1. Structures of tiazofurin (I) and diaziquone (II).

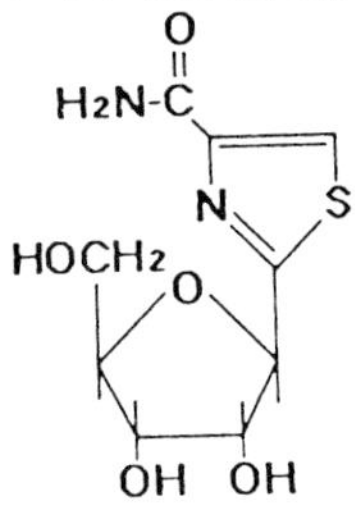

I

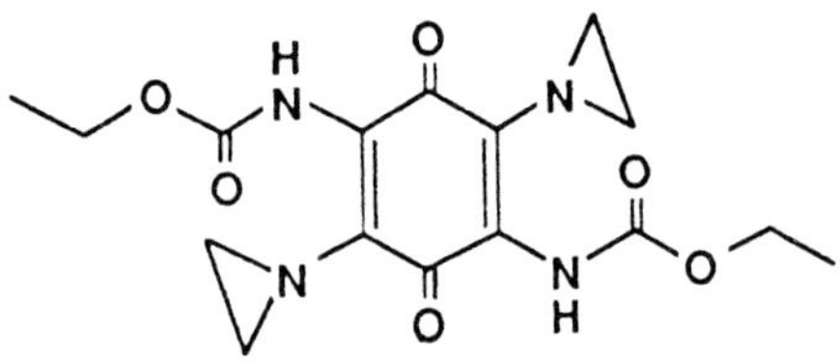

II

DRUGS WHICH ARE METABOLICALLY DEACTIVATED

The epipodophyllotoxin etoposide (III, Fig. 2) and its congener teniposide have been among the very few therapeutically successful novel drug entities introduced into the oncologist's drug armamentarium in recent years. Etoposide is cytotoxic because it is capable of causing DNA breakage either by interaction with DNA topoisomerase II or by generation of free radical intermediates (O'Dwyer et al., 1985). The metabolites of III which have been found to date are the hydroxy acid formed by hydrolysis of the lactone ring and the cis-lactone which are only weakly cytotoxic (Evans et al., 1982; D'Incalci et al, 1985). The antineoplastic potential of etoposide glucuronides (Colombo et al, 1985) remains to be characterised.

Pyridoglutethimide (IV, Fig. 2) has been developed as a potential successor to aminoglutethimide (AG), a drug effective in the treatment of mammary carcinoma in postmenopausal women. AG is thought to act by inhibition of aromatase, an enzyme complex involved in oestrogen synthesis. Pyridoglutethimide is a more selective aromatase inhibitor than AG. Whereas the AG molecule undergoes metabolism at four different molecular sites (Foster et al., 1984), IV is biotransformed only to the corresponding pyridine-N-oxide (Seago et al., 1986). The metabolites of AG or IV, do not inhibit aromatase. Human interferons (HIfns) are endogenous proteins with a molecular weight of between 15000 and 25000 which possess antiviral properties. Their potential use in cancer chemotherapy has elicited considerable attention in the lay press, but the clinical trials conducted thus far have not fulfilled the exaggerated hopes which were raised by their discovery. HIfns are rapidly catabolised by proteolytic enzymes in the liver and kidneys (Mannering & Deloria, 1986). There are dramatic differences in the distribution, rate and locus of catabolism and rate of elimination between the different HIfns (Pelleroni & Bohoslawec, 1984). This finding renders it feasible that recombinant interferons will soon be biosynthetically tailored to seek out target organs with some selectivity.

FIG. 2: Structures of etoposide (III) and pyridoglutethimide (IV).

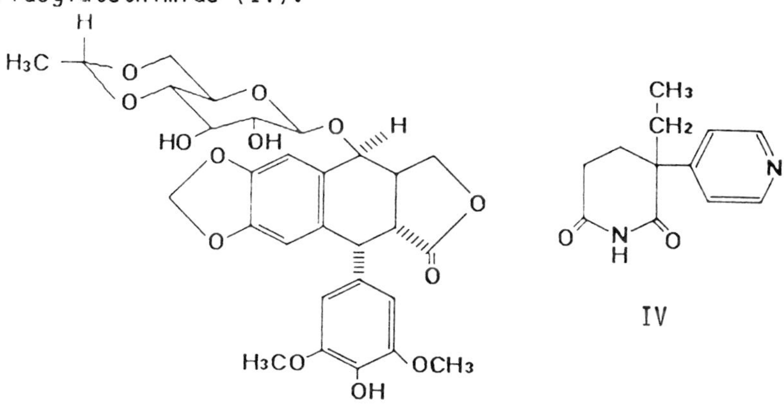

III

IV

DRUGS WHICH ARE METABOLICALLY TOXIFIED

Lack of cytotoxic selectivity remains the major drawback of the treatment of malignancies with drugs. A case in point is the nitrosourea semustine (V, Fig. 3) which has been under investigation for many years as it possesses excellent activity against a wide spectrum of murine tumours. In patients repeated administration of V can cause a delayed, irreversible and often fatal nephrotoxicity. There is now good evidence that the nephrotoxic species is a product of the hepatic metabolism of V (Kramer et al., 1986). Semustine undergoes rapid non-enzymic degradation and enzymatic hydroxylation in the liver, and both processes together yield a plethora of highly reactive carbamoylating and alkylating intermediates.

Certain protein growth factors and small molecular weight compounds can induce differentiation in a number of leukaemia cell lines, probably by altering the expression of specific genes. Once differentiated the cells cease to proliferate. Conceptually, these agents represent a novel non-toxic approach to the chemotherapy of neoplasias. Hexamethylene bisacetamide (VI, Fig. 3) and N-methylformamide (VII, Fig. 3) are examples of such inducers of differentiation. However, whether they cause their anti-neoplastic activities against murine tumours *in vivo* by this mechanism remains exceedingly doubtful. In patients VI undergoes metabolic deacetylation and oxidation to acetamidohexanoic acid (VIII, Fig. 3) which might be responsible for the metabolic acidosis and neurotoxicity associated with high doses of VI (Callery et al., 1986).

The major toxicities of N-methylformamide (VII) in patients are general malaise and liver damage (McVie et al., 1984). The drug has been shown to be metabolised mainly to carbon dioxide, methylamine (Kestell et al., 1985) and N-acetyl-S-(N-methylcarbamoyl)cysteine (IX, Fig. 3) (Kestell et al., 1986). The pathway which leads to the formation of the thiocarbamate (IX) involves oxidation of the N-formyl group and subsequent conjugation with glutathione. It appears likely that the hepatotoxin derived from VII is a reactive species formed as intermediate along this pathway.

FIG. 3: Structures of semustine (V) and of hexamethylene bisacetamide (VI), its major metabolite acetamidohexanoic acid (VIII), N-methylformamide (VII) its major metabolite N-acetyl-S-(N-methylcarbamoyl)cysteine (IX).

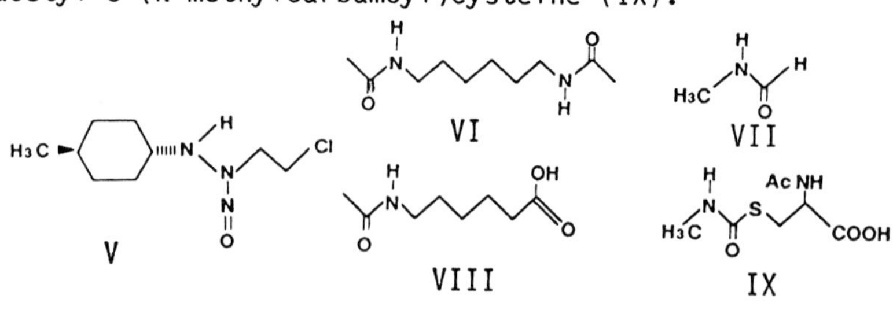

METABOLISM AND ANTICANCER DRUG DISCOVERY

Trimelamol (X, Fig. 4) is an investigational drug which was developed as the logical extension of studies of the metabolism of hexamethylmelamine (HMM) (Gescher et al., 1980) and pentamethylmelamine (PMM) (Rutty et al., 1982). Both HMM and PMM require metabolic activation to N-hydroxymethyl compounds. In patients the rate of their metabolism is slow compared to that in mice, which is reflected in the marked differences in treatment responses between man and mouse (Rutty et al., 1982). Trimelamol which does not require metabolic activation seems to be effective in patients and is also much less neurotoxic than PMM (Rutty et al., 1985).

The diethylaminoethyl ester (XI, Fig. 4) of flavone acetic acid is an interesting agent as it is completely devoid of activity against the murine tumour models which have been used traditionally as part of the NCI screen for novel anti-cancer drugs. However, XI inhibited the growth of a colon carcinoma model which is exceedingly refractory to most anticancer drugs (Plowman et al., 1986). During preliminary investigations XI was found to be much more active when given by the intraperitoneal route compared to intravenous administration. Not surprisingly XI is hydrolysed rapidly in human plasma to the very active flavone acetic acid (XII, Fig. 4) which lacks the cardio-vascular toxicity of XI (Kerr et al., 1986). Therefore XII has now replaced XI in clinical investigations. Structure-activity studies on a series of imidazotetra-zinones related to mitozolomide (XIII, Fig. 4) have shown the need for the presence of N-H in the 8-carboxamido moiety for optimum activity. Dimethylmitozolomide (XIV) is much less cytotoxic towards mouse lymphoma cells than XIII, but in vivo both are almost equiactive (Horspool, Gescher and Stevens, unpublished). This unexpected activity of XIV in vivo has been shown to be due to its metabolism. Dimethylmitozolomide is rapidly N-demethylated by mouse hepatic microsomes to yield XV and possibly XIII (Horspool, Gescher & Stevens, unpublished).

FIG. 4: Structures of trimelamol (X), flavone acetic acid (XII), its diethylaminoethyl ester (XI), mitozolomide (XIII) and its methyl (XV) and dimethyl derivatives (XIV).

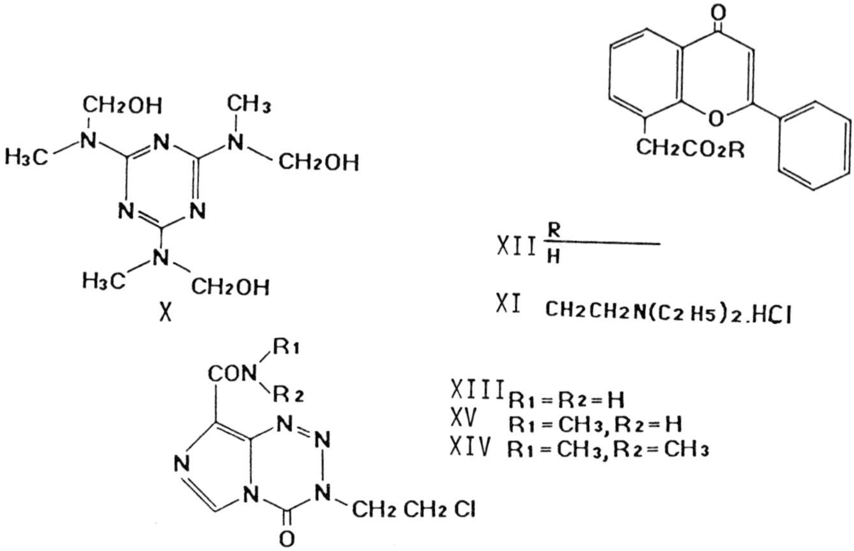

CONCLUSION

The examples described above illustrate that metabolism plays a pivotal role in the wanted or unwanted effects of many new antineoplastic agents. But attempts to design novel drugs which target their antiproliferative potential selectively towards tumour cells by exploiting e.g. differences in metabolism between host and tumour have hitherto not been very successful. Progress in cancer chemotherapy depends more than ever before on the collaboration between biochemists, cell biologists, pharmacologists, medicinal chemists and clinical oncologists. Such collaboration might eventually yield better, i.e. more selective, anticancer drug molecules as a consequence of the progress currently made in the molecular biology and the cellular physiology of normal and neoplastic cells.

REFERENCES

Arnold, S.T., Jayaram, H.N., Harper, G.R., Litterst, C.L., Malspeis, L., Desouza, J.J.V., Staubus, A.E., Ahluwalia, G.S., Wilson, Y.A., Cooney, D.A. & Johns, D.G., 1984, Drug Metabolism and Disposition, 12, 165.

Callery, P.S., Egorin, M.J., Geelhaar, L.A. & Nayar, M.S.B., 1986, Cancer Research, 46, 4900.

Colombo, T., D'Incalci, M., Donelli, M.G., Bartosek, I., Benfenati, E., Farina, P. & Guaitani, A., 1985, Xenobiotica, 15, 343.

D'Incalci, M., Sessa, C., Rossi, C., Roviaro, G. & Mangioni, C., 1985, Cancer Treatment Reports, 69, 69

Evans, W.E., Sinkula, J.A., Crom, W.R., Dow, L., Look, A.T. & Rivera, G., 1982, Cancer Chemotherapy and Pharmacology, 7, 147.

Foster, A.B., Griggs, L.J., Howe, I., Jarman, M., Leung, C.S., Manson, D. & Rowlands, M.G., 1984, Drug Metabolism and Disposition, 12, 511.

Gescher, A., D'Incalci, M., Farina, P. & Fanelli, R., 1980, Life Sciences, 26, 147.

Guttierez, P.L., Egorin, M.J. & Fox, B.M., 1985, Biochemical Pharmacology, 34, 1449.

Kestell, P., Gescher, A. & Slack, J.A., 1985, Drug Metabolism and Disposition, 13, 587.

Kestell, P., Gledhill, A.G., Threadgill, M.D. & Gescher, A., 1986, Biochemical Pharmacology, 35, 2283.

Kerr, D.J., Kaye, S.B., Graham, J., Cassidy, J., Harding, M., Setanoians, A., McGrath, J.C., Vezin, W.R., Cunningham, D., Forrest, G. & Soukop, M., 1986, Cancer Research, 46, 3142.

Kramer, R.A., McMenamin, M.G. & Boyd, M.R., 1986, Toxicology and Applied Pharmacology, 85, 221.

Lui, M.S., Faderan, M.S., Liepuieks, J.J., Natsumeda, Y., Olah, E., Jayaram, H.N. & Weber, G., 1984, Journal of Biological Chemistry, 259, 5078.

Mannering, G.J. & Deloria, L.B., 1986, Annual Review of Pharmacology and Toxicology, 26, 455.

McVie, J.G., Ten Bokkel Huinink, W.W., Simonetti, G. & Dubbelman, R., 1984, Cancer Treatment Reports, 68, 607.

O'Dwyer, P.J., Leyland-Jones, B., Alonso, M.T., Marsoni, S. & Wittes, R.E., 1985, New England Journal of Medicine, 312, 692,

Palleroni, A.V. & Bohoslawec, O., 1984, Journal of Interferon Research, 4, 493.

Plowman, J., Narayanan, V.L., Dykes, D., Szarvasi, E., Briet, P., Yoder, O.C. & Paul, K.D., 1986, Cancer Treatment Reports, 70, 631.

Rutty, C.J., Judson, I.R., Abel, G., Graham, M.A., Calvert, A.H., & Harrap, K.R., 1985, British Journal of Cancer, 52, 466.

Rutty, C.J., Newell, D.R., Muindi, J.R.F. & Harrap, K.R., 1982, Cancer Chemotherapy and Pharmacology, 8, 105.

Seago, A., Goss, P.E., Griggs, L.J. & Jarman, M., 1986 Biochemical Pharmacology, 35, 2911.

Spiegel, J.F., Egorin, M.J., Collins, J.M., Lerner, B.D. & Bachur, N.R., 1982, Drug Metabolism and Disposition, 11, 41.

4. Developments in analytical techniques in xenobiotic research

Introduction: Importance and Impact of Analytical Techniques in Xenobiotic Research

WOLFGANG RITTER

Bayer AG, Institute of Clinical Pharmacology, Wuppertal, FRG

The progress in foreign compound metabolism and disposition from its very beginning in the 19th century up to now was always based on an idea, or a hypothesis, and on the experimental realisation to prove that idea or hypothesis - in most cases something which can be called, in a broad sense, an analytical method. However, since there have always been more ideas than have been realized or proven by an experiment (because an appropriate technique was not available) it can be stated simply that progress in xenobiotic research is based almost entirely on the advances in analytical methodology.

For illustration of this I have chosen three examples, each one from the past and the present and one pointing to the future.

THE NITROFURANS

For more than 20 years from about 1950, the nitrofurans were of great importance as antibacterial agents. The chemical structure of most of the derivatives can be described by the general formula of an azomethine of 5-nitrofuraldehyde (Miura & Reckendorf, 1967).

Beginning with the discovery of the antibacterial activity of nitrofurazone, more than 7000 papers have been published on the nitrofurans (Burger, 1970) and it can be assumed that a few hundred of them were devoted to their disposition, metabolism, and biochemistry. Most of the collected data, however, remained obscure mainly because reliable and specific analytical methods for the nitrofurans were not available in the 1950's and 60's.

It was only in 1977 that a specific assay by HPLC was described for one of the most important drugs of the nitrofuran family, nitrofurantoin (Aufrère et al., 1977). Two years later, an improved procedure with a detection limit of 20 ng/ml was published by Vree et al. (1979). In the same paper, Vree also presented for the first time reliable data on the plasma levels of nitrofurantoin in man - about 25 years after its introduction for the treatment of urinary tract infections.

The first real pharmacokinetic study was published only a few years ago (Niazi and Vishnupad, 1983), stating that "no plasma level study has been reported on nitrofurantoin ... due mainly to the lack of availability of a sensitive analytic methodology".

A similar situation can be observed looking at the metabolism of the nitrofurans, again because appropriate methods were not available at that time. Several metabolites including the hydroxylamine were already found or proposed 20 to 30 years ago, based on UV and infrared spectroscopy and in part elemental analysis of isolated products from in vitro and in vivo experiments (Miura and Reckendorf, 1967).

It was only in 1978 that Aufrère et al. gave clear evidence of the main metabolites of nitrofurantoin using HPLC and mass spectrometry (MS). Ionen et al. (1980) identified a hitherto unknown type of metabolite, the 4-hydroxy derivative of nitrofurantoin, obtained from the urine of rats pretreated with 3-methylcholanthrene. The metabolites of another once important nitrofuran derivative, furazolidone, now primarily used as a feedgrain additive for antibacterial prophylaxis in livestock-breeding, were published only in 1984 (Abraham et al.).

Thus, the advent of specific assay methods and modern instrumental technology finally gave the answers to the many questions which were open 20 years earlier when the nitrofurans belonged to the armamentarium of antibacterial treatment.

GLYCERYL TRINITRATE

Glyceryl trinitrate, better known perhaps as "nitroglycerin", is one of the old but still important drugs, used for the treatment of angina pectoris since 1879.

The therapeutic plasma levels are about 1 ng/ml and even lower. It is not surprising, therefore, that nearly 100 years passed until a determination of the plasma levels in man was possible (Rosseel and Bogaert, 1973). But even today, this assay procedure by gas chromatography (GC) with electron capture detection is not entirely sufficient, mainly due to the low plasma levels which rapidly decline with a plasma half-life of only a few minutes.

In 1983 (Settlage et al.), plasma level data were reported obtained by GC linked to negative ion chemical ionisation MS.

Because of the limited sensitivity of the detectors, HPLC could not be applied until the thermal energy analyser (TEA) was introduced (Spanggord and Keck, 1980). Detection is based on the chemiluminescence of nitrogen dioxide radicals produced by pyrolysis of the organic nitrate.

However, the TEA seems not to be suitable for routine drug monitoring, hence Bogaert (1987) in his very recent review on glyceryl trinitrate characterized the situation briefly by stating that "the assay in plasma remains difficult" and "assay problems ... are probably responsible for some of the discrepancies between published results". Taylor et al. (1987) have recently reviewed the analytical methods and pharmacokinetics for organic nitrate drugs.

THE PROSTAGLANDINS

As a third example to illustrate the importance of appropriate methods I have chosen a group of compounds which are a real challenge for the xenobioanalyst at present and for the future: the prostaglandins and their specific assay in the pg/ml range. Synthetic prostaglandins are now under investigation world-wide and various methods are used for determination of parent compound and metabolites in blood plasma.

Apart from one unique example, arbaprostil, which after derivatisation can be determined by HPLC with fluorescence detection with an outstanding sensitivity of 10 pg/ml (Pullen & Cox, 1985), all of the published assays are based on GC/MS.

The first specific assay of prostaglandins by GC linked to electron impact MS was described already in 1971 (Axen et al.). Morita et al. (1978) tried GC with positive ion chemical ionisation MS but this procedure, despite several advantages, is hampered by its low sensitivity. GC with negative ion chemical ionisation MS was first published for the analysis of a prostaglandin E_2 analogue (Min et al., 1980). This procedure was subsequently used by several other groups and seems to be the method of choice at present for the assay of prostaglandins.

However, even this analytical technique is very likely to be too insensitive for determination of a prostaglandin E_1 analogue with plasma levels expected in the range between 1 and 10 pg/ml after a dose of 50 µg/man. The author is at present working on this problem.

In conclusion, the three examples chosen illustrate that the progress in xenobiotic research was always, and still is, dependent nearly exclusively on the analytical techniques available.

Today, with stable isotopes combined with modern separation techniques it would not take 20 to 30 years to elucidate the fate of the nitrofurans in the organism.

Disposition of glyceryl trinitrate in man is now well established, but drug monitoring in patients is still a problem due to the low plasma levels. It is not unlikely that the recent developments in HPLC with new types of detectors now on the horizon will finally solve the dilemma of glyceryl trinitrate assay.

Finally, determination of the prostaglandins with physico-chemical methods will remain a challenge for the future years. Perhaps HPLC linked to MS will be the answer because a large amount of substance can be separated under less extreme conditions conditions than in gas chromatography.

REFERENCES

Abraham, R.T., Knapp, J.E., Minnigh, M.B., Wong L.K., Zemaitis, M.A., & Alvin, J.D., 1984, Drug Metabolism and Disposition, 12, 732.

Aufrère, M.B., Hoener, B., & Vore, M.E., 1977, Clinical Chemistry, 23, 2207.

Aufrère, M.B., Hoener, B., & Vore, M., 1978, Drug Metabolism and Disposition, 6, 403.

Axen, U., Grêen, K., Hörlin, D., & Samuelsson, B., 1971, Biochemical and Biophysical Research Communications, 45, 519.

Bogaert, M.G., 1987, Clinical Pharmacokinetics, 12, 1.

Burger, A., 1970, Medicinal Chemistry, Third Edition, Part 1 (Wiley, New York) p. 645.

Ionen, H.G., Oesch, F., & Platt, K.L., 1980, Drug Metabolism and Disposition, 8, 446.

Min, B.H., Pao, J., Garland, W.A., de Silva, J.A.F., & Parsonnet, M., 1980, Journal of Chromatography, 183, 411.

Miura, K., & Reckendorf, H.K., 1967, Progress in Medicinal Chemistry 5, edited by G.P. Ellis and G.B. West (Butterworths, London), p. 320.

Morita, I., Murota, S., Suzuki, M., Ariga, T., & Miyatake, T., 1978, Journal of Chromatography, 154, 285.

Niazi, S., & Vishnupad, K.S., 1983, Biopharmaceutics & Drug Disposition, 4, 213.

Pullen, R.H., & Cox, J.W., 1985, Journal of Chromatography, 343, 271.

Rosseel, M.T., & Bogaert, M.G., 1973, Journal of Pharmaceutical Sciences, 69, 754.

Spanggord, R.J., & Keck, R.G., 1980, Journal of Pharmaceutical Sciences, 69, 444.

Settlage, J.A., Gielsdorf, W., & Jaeger, H., 1983, Journal of High Resolution Chromatography & Chromatography Communications, 6, 68.

Taylor, T., Taylor, I.W., Chasseaud, L.F. & Bonn, R., 1987, Progress in Drug Metabolism, Vol. 10, edited by J.W. Bridges, L.F. Chasseaud and G.G. Gibson (Taylor & Francis, London) p. 207.

Vree, T.B., Hekster, Y.A., Baars, A.M., Damsma, J.E., & Van der Kleijn, E., 1979, Journal of Chromatography, 162, 110.

THE UTILIZATION OF STABLE ISOTOPES IN DRUG METABOLISM STUDIES

H. R. Sullivan and R. B. Franklin
Lilly Research Laboratories
Indianapolis, Indiana 46285, USA

The utilization of stable isotope labelling as a technique in biomedical research has increased dramatically in the last ten years. This has been particularly true in studies of the *in vitro* and *in vivo* metabolic transformation and pharmacokinetic studies of drugs and metabolites. In combination with the high resolving capabilities of GC and HPLC, and with the specificity and sensitivity of quantitative MS, stable isotope labelling has provided a unique method of analysis, certainly not available by other methods. One of the first and most fundamental applications of this technique has been the study of the mechanisms and stereochemistry involved in the *in vitro* and *in vivo* biotransformation of drugs. Examples of *in vitro* studies using this technique are the isotopic, stereochemical and induction studies of the hepatic hydroxylation of ethyl benzene to methylphenyl carbinol (MPC).

IN VITRO HYDROXYLATION OF ETHYL BENZENE

The *in vitro* enzymic hydroxylation of ethyl benzene (EB) using the 15000 g rat liver supernatant fraction has been shown to be under stereochemical control producing 80% R(+)- and 20% S(-)-MPC (McMahon *et al.*, 1966). In order to study the mechanism by which hydroxylation occurred, the reaction was carried out in an atmosphere of ^{18}O (68 atom %) and the ^{18}O content of the resulting MPC was found to be 62%. Thus, the hydroxylation of EB was the result of a mixed-function oxidase reaction employing molecular oxygen rather than oxygen from water. That hydrogen from water was not involved in the reaction was demonstrated by conducting the reaction using deuterium oxide. No isotopic hydrogen appeared in the resulting MPC.

Next, the primary isotope effect on the hydroxylation of α,α-d_2-EB was investigated. The rate of formation of MPC from the deuterated substrate was substantially slower than the non-deuterated compound due to the deuterium isotope effect, kH/kD=1.8. As expected from a true mixed-function oxidase reaction, the MPC formed retained one of the deuterium atoms. Subsequent oxidation of the MPC-d_1 with CrO_2 yielded acetophenone containing no deuterium, thereby showing that no shift of a deuterium atom (such as was seen in aromatic hydroxylation reactions by Guroff *et al*. 1967), occurred during the formation of MPC. The optical purity of the MPC-d_1 was comparable to that of the MPC from EB, i.e., 81% R(+).

From the results described above it was apparent that the hydroxylation of EB proceeded by the direct displacement of one of its alkyl α-hydrogen atoms by oxygen. To elucidate whether this displacement occurred by backside displacement (inversion) or by frontside displacement (retention), S(+)-α-d-EB (see Fig. 1) was synthesized and its hydroxylation by the rat hepatic 15000g supernantant system was studied. The MPC formed retained 86% of the deuterium present in the optically active EB. In addition, the MPC had an $(\alpha)_D$ of 37.3° equivalent to 91.7% R (+)-α-d-MPC. These results demonstrated that the hydroxylation of EB occurred with retention of configuration; i.e., oxygenation proceeded by a front side displacement or "insertion" reaction as shown below.

Figure 1. *In vitro* hydroxylation of S(+)-α-d-ethyl benzene.

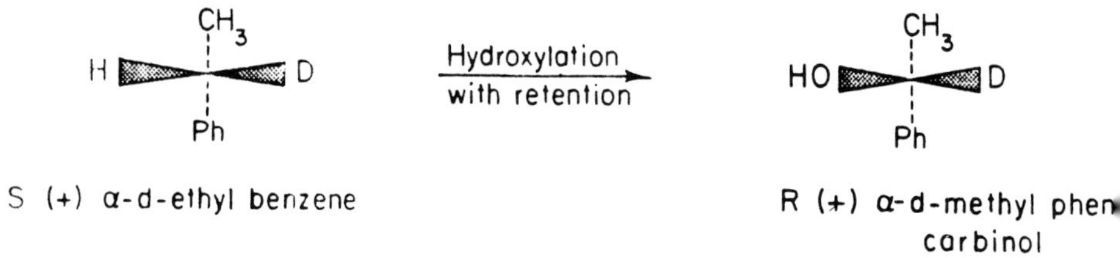

The effect of three inducing agents on the stereochemical nature of this hydroxylation of EB was also investigated. Results showed that chemical induction of the enzymes by phenobarbital, *m*-bromophenobarbital or chlorcyclizine substantially diminished the stereoselectivity of the reaction. Results obtained from a similar study using α,α-d_2-EB as the substrate confirmed these results and were important since α-d-MPC, unlike MPC, was not significantly dehydrogenated to acetophenone. Thus, the stereochemistry of this reaction cannot be based upon differential further reaction of the MPC isomers. The effect of induction on the stereospecificity may be the result of differential induction of the various isozymes of P_{450}.

IN VIVO METABOLISM STUDIES OF NABILONE, A 9-KETOCANNABINOID

Another important application of stable isotopes and GC/MS is the quantitative determination of concentrations of drugs and metabolites in biological media. This is particularly true when the experimental drug is very potent and total doses given are in the 1 mg range. It is usually the only available method that possesses both sufficient sensitivity and specificity to be applicable. Nabilone, a 9-ketocannabinoid, is an orally-effective anti-emetic agent used clinically for the control of nausea and vomiting caused by chemotherapeutic agents. It is a racemic mixture of RR- and SS-ketones (Fig. 2) that are rapidly absorbed from the G-I tract and extensively metabolized in all species studied to date. One metabolic pathway involved in its metabolism is the stereoselective, enzymic reduction of the 9-keto moiety to yield hydroxyl metabolites. Using d_6-nabilone and d_6-carbinol metabolite as internal standards for the GC/MS determinations, the pharmacokinetics of parent and metabolite in the plasma of animals and man have been studied following oral administration of a total dose of 1 mg of ^{14}C-nabilone. Plasma concentrations of parent, total radiocarbon and carbinol metabolites in dogs given a single 100 μg/kg dose of ^{14}C-nabilone are shown in Fig. 3.

Nabilone and its carbinol metabolites accounted for 80% of the circulating radiocarbon. The apparent $t_{1/2}$ of nabilone was 2 hr while that of the carbinols was 20 hr. The ratio of SSS- to RSS-carbinol was 5/1 throughout the test period. Multiple dose studies, over 14 days, showed accumulation of these carbinols in the plasma compartment. While 90 day toxicology studies in dogs revealed no apparent toxicity at doses of 0.5, 1.0, and 2.0 mg/kg, toxicity was observed in a subsequent 1 year study. After 115 days deaths were observed at the high dose and, by day 205, deaths were observed at all dose levels. In many instances death was immediately preceded by convulsions. Since the observed CNS toxicity occurred only after chronic dosing and an accumulation of the carbinol metabolite in the plasma compartment was observed, a study was designed to determine brain concentrations of total radiocarbon, nabilone and carbinol metabolites and to compare these concentrations to those found in the plasma. In this study a single 400 μg/kg dose of ^{14}C-nabilone was administered orally to three dogs. Concentrations of radiocarbon and carbinol metabolites in the plasma and certain brain sections 24 hr after dosing were determined

Figure 2. Enzymic reduction of racemic nabilone.

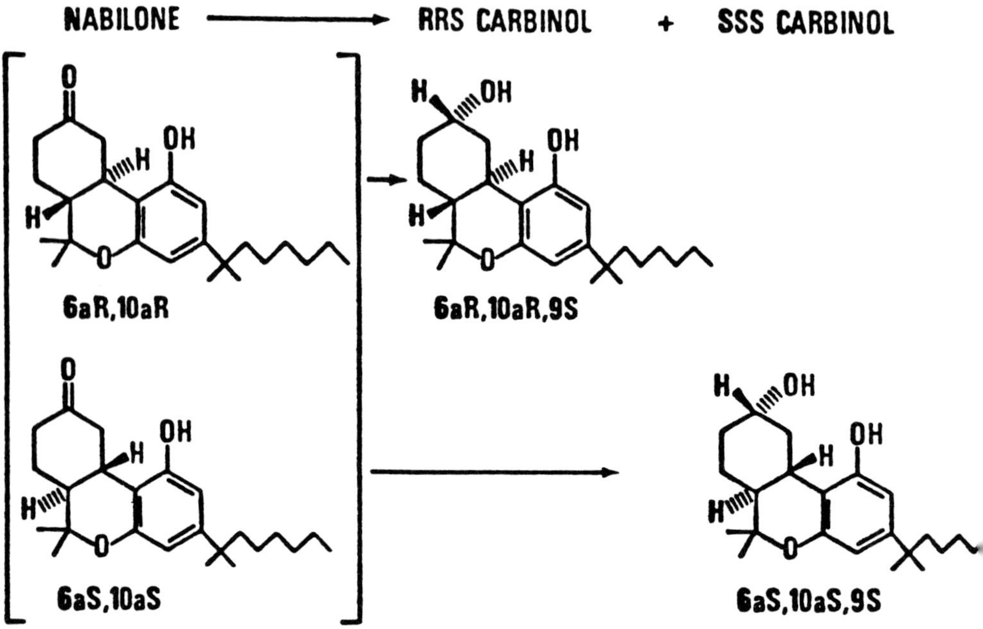

Figure 3. Dog plasma concentrations of total radiocarbon, nabilone and carbinol metabolite after oral administration.

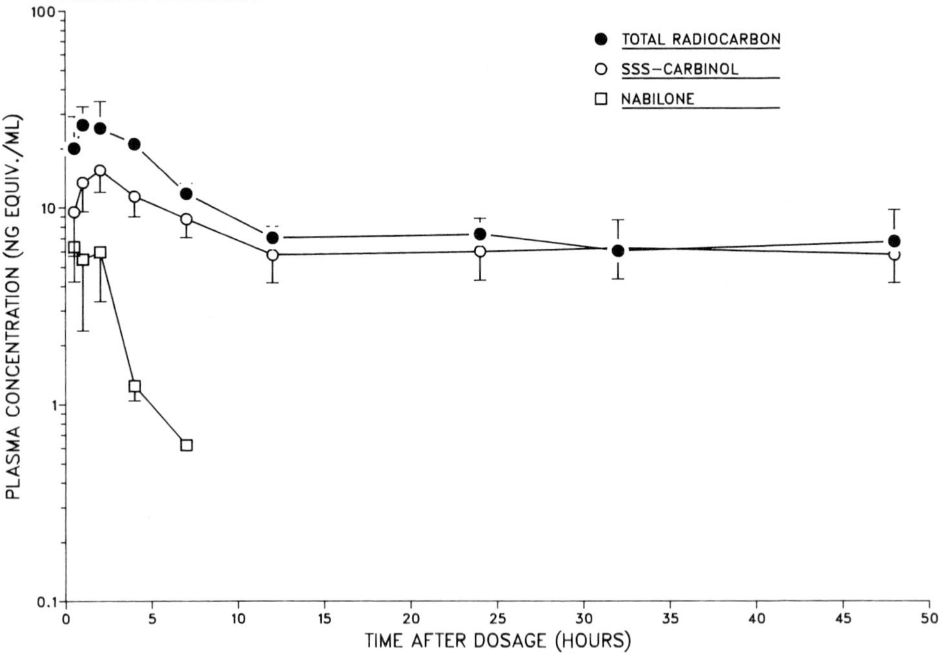

using GC/MS and deuterium labelling. No parent drug was detected in the brain. All radiocarbon found in the brain sections analyzed represented the carbinol metabolites and these concentrations were 5-fold greater than that found in the plasma. These results further implicated the sequestration of these carbinol metabolites as the causative factor for the CNS toxicity observed in the toxicity studies in the dog.

Single dose studies in man by Rubin et al. (1977), using ^{14}C-nabilone and GC/MS analysis using d_6-nabilone and d_6-carbinol metabolite as internal standards, revealed that plasma concentrations of nabilone and its carbinol metabolites were comparable and together accounted for just 20% of the circulating radiocarbon. The apparent $t_{\frac{1}{2}}$ of parent was 2 hr while that of the carbinol was 5 hr. It thus appeared that the dog was an inappropriate model for safety and toxicity studies, required prior to clinical evaluation. With the intent of finding an animal model more closely resembling man, similar studies were conducted in monkeys using the same dose of ^{14}C-nabilone. The pharmacokinetic studies showed parent to have a $t_{\frac{1}{2}}$ of 1.4 hr, while that of the carbinol metabolites was 24 hours. Combined concentrations of nabilone and carbinol metabolites, however, accounted for less than 20% of the circulating ^{14}C. This result was similar to that found in man. Concentrations of ^{14}C in the brain were significantly less than those found in the dog and, more significantly, no detectable concentrations of the carbinol metabolites could be found in the brains of these monkeys. It was apparent from these results that the monkey more closely emulated man in its metabolism of nabilone. On the basis of this judgement a 1 year toxicology study was conducted in monkeys where no significant accumulation of carbinol metabolites was observed and no obvious signs of toxicity were noted at any dose level. All animals survived the test period.

APPLICATIONS OF STABLE ISOTOPE LABELLING TO QUANTITATIVE LC/MS

Thermospray LC/MS has been successfully applied to the separation and quantitation of drug metabolites in a biological medium. The technique was applied to an *in vitro* study of the stereoselective reduction of nabilone using the 15000g rat liver fraction. LC/MS has been shown to be a very soft ionization method yielding only molecular ions with little or no fragmentaion. It appeared that LC/MS was ideally suited for the quantitation of nabilone and its carbinol metabolites in biological matrices. Excellent resolution of the diastereoisomeric carbinols was attained: signal to noise ratio was better than 100/1. It was interesting to note that the deuterated analog had a slightly shorter retention time than that of protio form. This phenomenon has been frequently seen in GC/MS work and apparently also occurs in LC/MS.

The effect of incubation time on the *in vitro* metabolism of dl-nabilone (RR/SS) and SS-enantiomer is shown in Fig. 4.

Figure 4. *In vitro* reduction of SS- and RR/SS-nabilone by rat liver supernatant fraction.

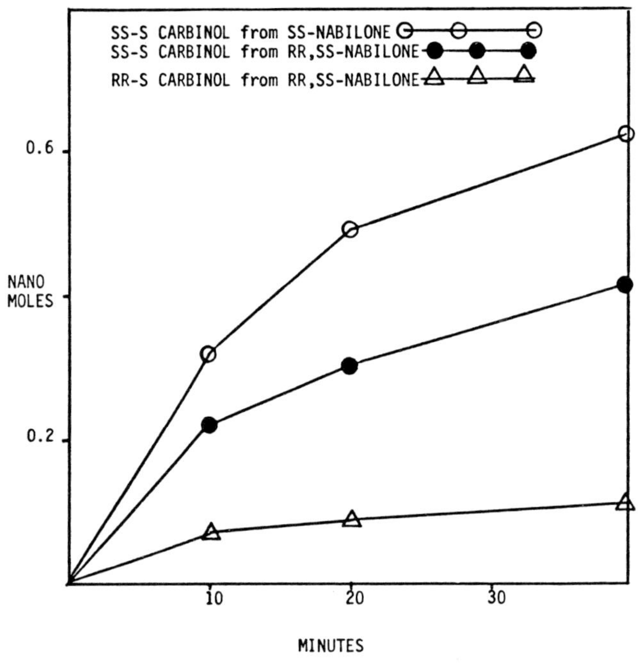

The SS-isomer appeared to be the preferred substrate. When the racemic mixture was the substrate, yield of the RRS-carbinol was the least thus indicating that the SS-isomer more nearly duplicated the natural substrate for the enzyme. The sensitivity of the assay method, 1 ng/ml, was comparable to that of the GC/MS method developed previously (Sullivan *et al.*, 1978). The method has some advantages over the GC/MS method and these are: 1) no elaborate sample purification procedure is required,

2) no derivatization prior to analysis is necessary, 3) endogenous impurities do not interfere with the assay and, 4) faster assay time.

IN VIVO REDUCTION AND REOXIDATION OF ISOMAZOLE

Isomazole (LY175326) is a potent, orally effective cardiotonic agent with vasodilator properties, currently under development at the Lilly Research Laboratories. Following its oral administration to rats and dogs, the most prominant entity in the plasma and urine was unchanged drug, although other metabolites, such as the sulfone and the sulfide, have been noted (Bernstein and Franklin, 1985; Franklin et al., 1986; Fig. 5). While reconversion of the sulfone to the parent sulfoxide has not been found to occur, the sulfide metabolite can be reoxidized to the sulfoxide (Fig. 5).

Figure 5. Metabolism of ^{18}O-isomazole.

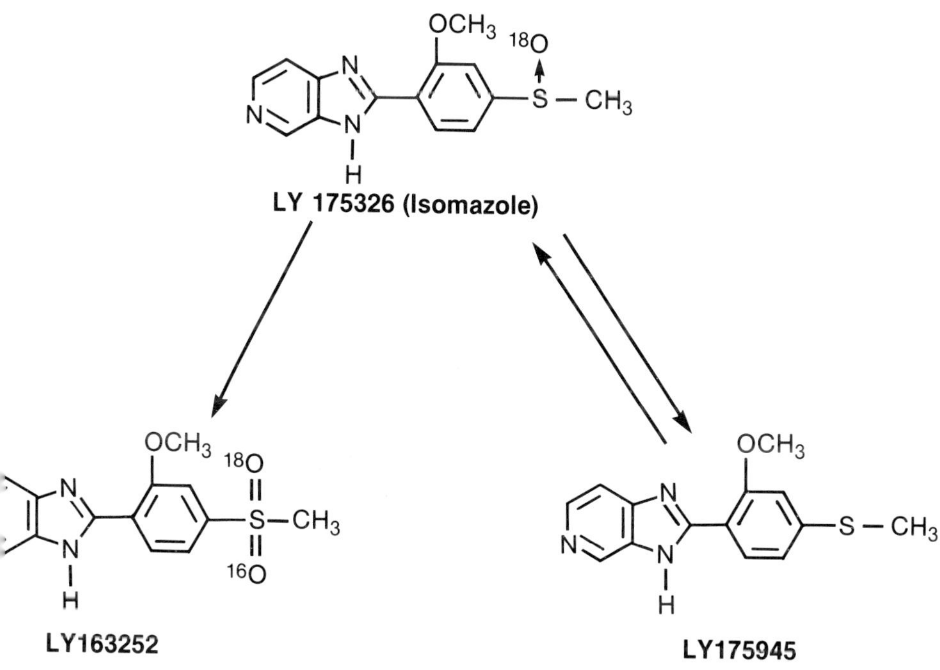

The involvement of this pathway in the metabolism has been evaluated by the insertion of an ^{18}O-label into the sulfoxide moiety. Rats were dosed orally with 20 mg/kg

^{18}O-isomazole and plasma was obtained at 0.5, 1, 2, 4, 6, 8, and 24 hours following drug administration. Metabolites were separated by HPLC utilizing a Pinkerton column and a mobile phase consisting of 0.1M ammonium acetate and THF. The HPLC was coupled via a thermospray interface to a Finnegan 4500 mass spectrometer focussed on both the ^{16}O- and ^{18}O-isomazole. Over a 6 hour period it was noted that the mean plasma ratio of ^{18}O to ^{16}O-isomazole decreased from 95%, at 0.5 hours following the dose, to 47% at 6 hours, indicating reoxidation of the sulfide metabolite to sulfoxide.

The above examples of the use of stable isotopes in drug dispostion and pharmacokinetic studies were conducted in the authors' laboratories. Needless to say there are many other excellent examples of such use in the literature (see, for example, review by Baillie, T.A., 1981). The utilization of stable isotopes in conjunction with GC/MS and LC/MS has been and will continue to be of great importance in such studies, particularly with potent drugs where total dosages are very low. This utilization can also serve as an alternate method to the clinical use of radioactive isotopes and, thereby, alleviate or eliminate entirely the limitations and requirements associated with the latter technique. The utilization of LC/MS and stable isotopes is in its infancy; however, results obtained thus far in the separation and identification of very polar and high molecular weight entities are promising.

REFERENCES

Baillie, T. A., 1981, Pharmacological Reviews, 33,81.

Bernstein, J. R. and Franklin, R. B., 1985, Journal of Chromotography, 342,228.

Franklin, R. B., Bernstein, J. R., and Bühring, K. U., 1986, 10th European Drug Metabolism Workshop, Abstract P.3/29, University of Surrey, U.K.

Guroff, G., Daly, J. W., Jerina, D. W., Renson, J., Witkop, B. and Udenfriend, S., 1967, Science, 157,152.

McMahon, R. E. and Sullivan, H. R., 1966, Life Science, 5,921.

Rubin, A., Lemberger, L., Crabtree, R. E., Sullivan, H. R., Rowe, H., Warrick, P. and Obermeyer, B. D., Clinical Pharmacology and Therapeutics, 22,532.

Sullivan, H. R., Kau, D.H.K. and Wood, P. G., 1978, Biomedical Mass Spectrometry, 5,296.

THE USE OF HPLC-LINKED MASS SPECTROMETRY IN XENOBIOCHEMISTRY

C.J.Brealey, P.B.Henry and A.Strother*

Wellcome Research Laboratories, Ravens Lane, Berkhamsted Herts., UK, and *King's College, Chelsea Department of Pharmacy, London, UK. (Permanent address: Department of Pharmacology, Loma Linda University, CA. 92354, U.S.A.)

INTRODUCTION

The study of xenobiochemistry involves the separation and identification of small amounts of xenobiotics and their metabolites present in complex biological matrices. The polarity range from the parent compound to excreted metabolites may be very wide. The technique of HPLC offers the necessary chromatographic separation power and contemporary mass spectrometry (MS) offers the required sensitivity. While fast atom bombardment (FAB) of metabolites collected off-line from HPLC is powerful, the direct linking of the HPLC flow to the MS combines these methods to the greatest effect. Moving-belt and direct liquid insertion (DLI) interfaces are successful but current interest is centred on the thermospray (TSP) technique (Vestal 1985) and the related plasmaspray interface. Not only does this technique allow pumping of typical reverse-phase eluants (1-2ml/min methanol/water mixtures) directly into the MS source but it provides a sensitive soft ionisation method particularly suitable for polar materials. Disadvantages of TSP LC/MS are its failure to detect certain compounds and the lack of information from fragmentation in many spectra. The examples from xenobiochemical studies presented here attempt to demonstrate these features with particular reference to unstable metabolites (epoxides and N-oxides) and highly polar metabolites (glucuronic acid, sulphate and amino acid conjugates).

METHODS

Thermospray spectra of polar drugs, metabolites and biochemicals were obtained using a Finnigan 4500 MS with a Finnigan TSP interface. For most studies standard conditions were used as follows: 1.2 ml/min 50/50 methanol/0.1M aq. ammonium acetate, TSP vaporiser 120°C, jet 200°C, repeller voltage tuned to maximum amplitude on the solvent spectrum. Samples (100ng) were injected via the sample loop to by-pass the LC column.

Secondly, gradient LC was performed on a 20μl sample of a 50/50 acetonitrile/water extract of a rat liver microsomal incubation used under oxidising conditions to generate metabolites of a novel insecticidal lipid amide (Black et al. 1985). A 5μm RP-8 column was used with post-column mixing to give the same TSP conditions as above.

Thirdly, the effect of varying the vaporiser temperature on the sensitivity and fragmentation of the 1- and 3-N oxides of pyrimethamine was examined. With all other parameters maintained as listed above the TSP vaporiser temperature was increased from 115° to 155° and the intensities of the ions for the N-oxide, the N-oxide dimer and the N-oxide-16 were measured.

RESULTS AND DISCUSSION

TSP of polar and apolar xenobiotics

Figure 1 shows a typical TSP spectrum of a polar xenobiotic, in this case a major metabolite of benzoic acid namely hippuric acid (Keller 1842). Many features of TSP ionisation are shown with formation of both the proton

Figure 1. TSP of hippuric acid.

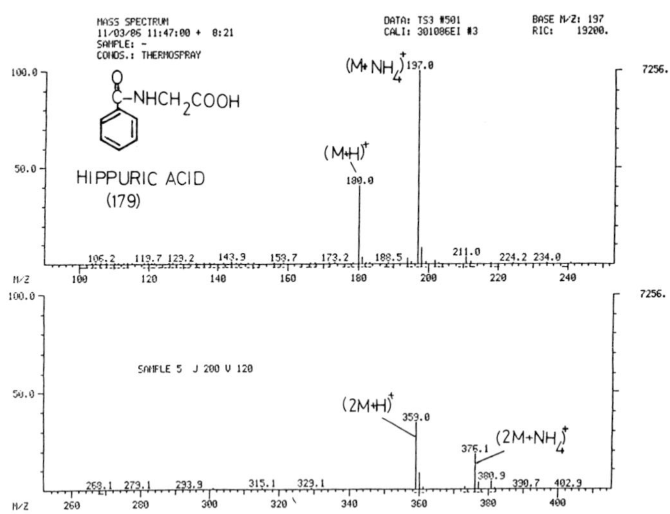

and ammonium ion adducts. In this case the dimers $2M.H^+$ and $2M.NH_4^+$ are also relatively intense. It is well known that in general, compounds of this type are very good candidates for TSP ionisation. In contrast highly apolar compounds often fail to give spectra. Recent advances in TSP interfaces to allow secondary ionisation may overcome this problem and also give information from fragmentation. Figure 2 illustrates this for the apolar insecticide permethrin. While a TSP spectrum of this compound could be obtained it was only in the plasma discharge mode in the TSP interface that fragmentation was observed, and only then in the absence of any buffer ions.

TSP of conjugates

Glucuronic acid conjugates are good subjects for TSP. The positive ion spectrum of the O-glucuronide of o-aminophenol (Figure 3) was obtained under the standard conditions (see Methods). In addition to the $M.H^+$ molecular ion there is useful fragmentation to the aglycone. Furthermore the ion at m/z 194, although weak in this spectrum, corresponds to the ammonium ion adduct of free glucuronic acid. This has been observed for other O-glucuronides in TSP (Liberato et al. 1983). In +ve ion the formation of the proton or ammonium adduct depends on the proton affinity of the glucuronides or fragments. Certain compounds (often lacking basic

Figure 2. Plasma discharge ionisation of permethrin in a buffer-free medium in a TSP interface.

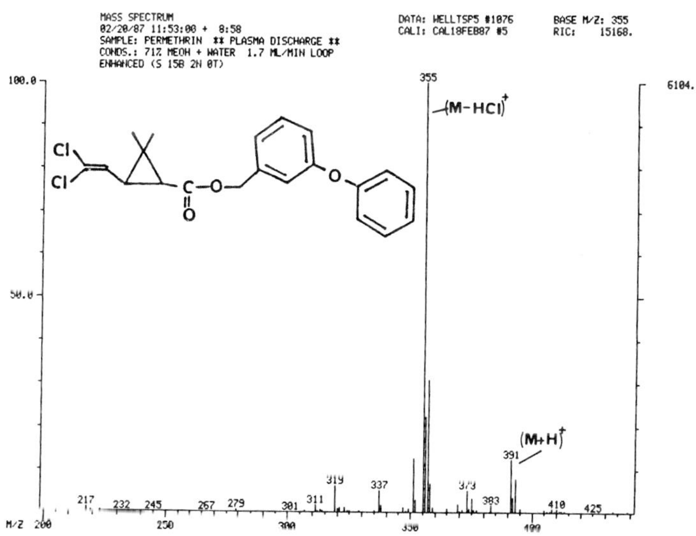

Figure 3. TSP of an O-glucuronide in positive ion mode.

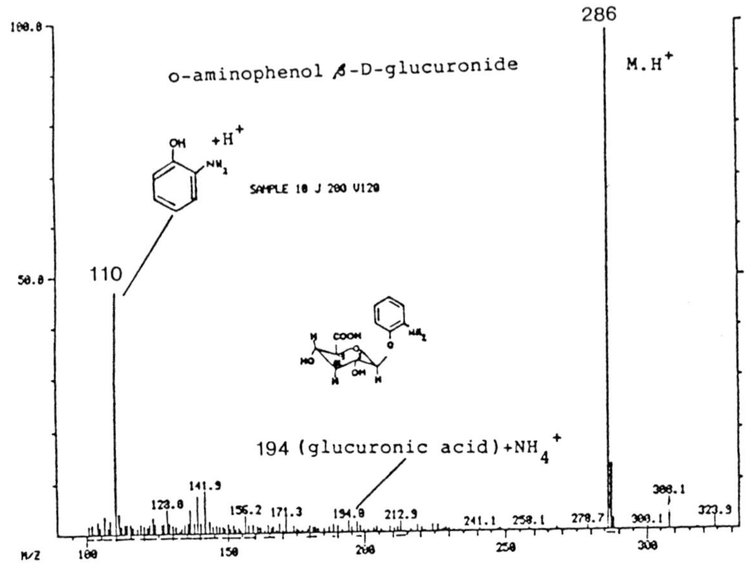

nitrogens) give more intense spectra in negative ion mode, particulaly in buffer-free solution. This was the case for phenolphthalein glucuronide in our studies when the free anion was the only ion in the spectrum. However in the case of the negative ion TSP of furosemide-1-O-acyl glucuronide the anion of the free glucuronic acid was observed (m/z 175) in addition to the parent anion and the aglycone (Rachmel et al., 1985). Negative ion spectra are very favourable for glucuronide conjugates of many steroids (Watson et al., 1986). The response of N-glucuronide conjugates may not be as good: dapsone N-glucuronide failed to give a spectrum in our studies under a wide range of conditions.

Sulphates can be observed as the free anions in negative ion TSP, usually in buffer-free systems. However these compounds appear to show marked temperature effects on sensitivity and adduct formation. For p-nitrocatechol sulphate a TSP vaporiser temperature of 110° was much more effective than 120° in our experiments. Sulphate conjugates of steroids are similarly temperature-dependent: Watson et al.(1985) observed the M^{2-} ion for 20-oxo-pregn-5-ene-3β,17α-diol disulphate at 130° but a complex set of adducts at 150°.

While we have been able to obtain intense spectra on the modified tri-peptides glutathione and S-methyl glutathione,

Table 1. Differences in adduct formation and fragmentation of aromatic and aliphatic N-oxides in thermospray.

	RELATIVE INTENSITY		
DIMER AS BASE PEAK	M.H-16	M.H	2M.H
Quinoline N-oxide	0	20	100
Nicotinamide N-oxide	0	5	100
2,4-diamino-6-diethylaminopyrimidine 3-N-oxide	11	43	100
2,4-diamino-6-chloropyrimidine 3-N oxide	9	48	100
M.H AS BASE PEAK			
Trimethoprim 1-N-oxide	9	100	12
Trimethoprim 3-N-oxide	28	100	12
Pyrimethamine 1-N-oxide	7	100	7
Pyrimethamine 3-N-oxide	16	100	11
2,4-diamino-6-piperadinopyrimidine 3-N-oxide	17	100	81
2,4-diamino-6-morpholinopyrimidine 3-N-oxide	24	100	40
Imipramine N-oxide	56	100	8
M.H-16 AS BASE PEAK			
Diethylcarbamyl-4-methyl piperazine	100	78	77
Imipramine N-oxide.HCl	100	47	8
Chlorpromazine N-oxide	100	36	0
Chlorpromazine N-oxide.malate salt	100	9	0

which showed relatively weak $M.H^+$ molecular ions and sodium adducts, but intense fragment ions from N-C bond cleavage. Also N-acetyl cysteine could be readily observed as the ammonium adduct under the standard conditions. However of several amino acid conjugates of m-phenoxybenzoic acid only the glycylvaline conjugate could be detected. A similar phenomenon has been noted in the thermospray of aromatic amino acids, where p-hydroxyphenylalanine was not detected when five other amino acids were (Games & Ramsey 1985). More studies are required to explain these deficiencies in thermospray ionisation.

TSP of N-oxides

When a range of aromatic and aliphatic N-oxides were analysed under the standard conditions at 120°C wide differences in their adduct formation and fragmentation were seen. Some N-oxides (e.g. nicotinamide N-oxide) ionised almost exclusively as the protonated dimers, other N-oxides gave the $M.H^+$ ion as the base peak with both dimer formation and loss of oxygen while a third group lost oxygen readily so that the $M.H\text{-}16^+$ ion was predominant in the spectrum (Table 1). It is suggested that simple aromatic N-oxides may dimerise more readily than aromatic

N-oxides which have more bulky ring substituents. The greater tendency of the aliphatic N-oxides to fragment is not unexpected but indicates that care must be taken not to overlook these metabolites in thermospray studies.

More detailed studies on the effect of vaporiser temperature on the stability of the 1- and 3-N-oxides of pyrimethamine (Figure 4) showed that both N-oxides fragmented more readily above 130°. However this was much more marked for the 3-N-oxide. This may be due at least in part to differences in the basicities of the two ring nitrogens. Thus by conducting TSP spectroscopy at a range of temperatures, and with the above structural considerations in mind, it should be possible to distinguish N-oxides from other mono-oxygenated metabolites.

<u>LC/TSP MS of metabolites in complex mixtures</u>

For an LC/MS technique to be useful in xenobiochemistry it must be able to detect compounds of interest in a complex biological matrix. Figure 5 shows the pattern of metabolites produced from a novel lipid amide by microsomal oxidation. No radiolabel was used in this experiment but

Figure 4. Effect of vaporiser temperature on adduct formation and fragmentation of 1- and 3-N-oxides of Pyrimethamine. 2M.H$^+$ ■ M.H$^+$ ● M.H-16$^+$ ○

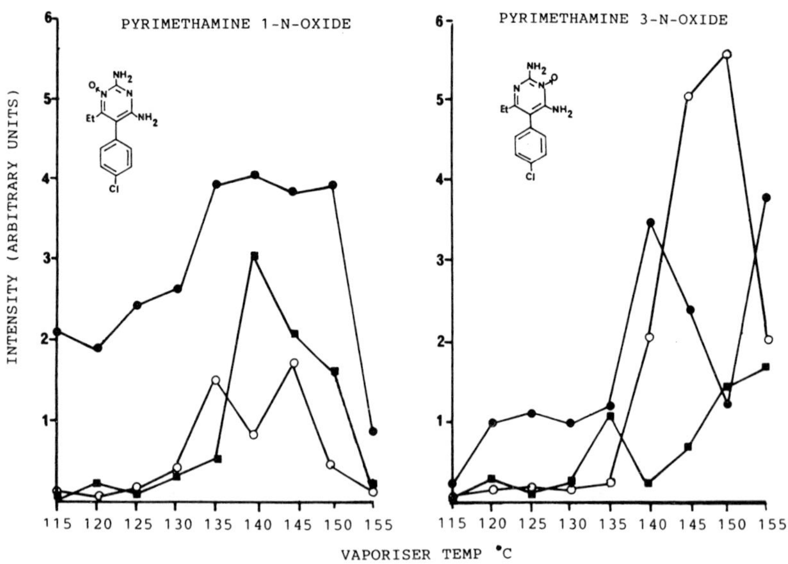

Figure 5. Detection of novel metabolites by LC/TSP MS. Products from microsomal mono-oxygenation in vitro of a lipid amide were detected by displaying ion chromatograms for putative metabolites. At least four mono-oxygenated species and one diol are present. Compounds were separated on a 20cm, 0.45cm i.d. 5μm RP-8 eluted with a gradient from 0-100% acetonitrile over 20min and then the solvent was held at 100% acetonitrile. Ammonium acetate was added by post-column mixing.

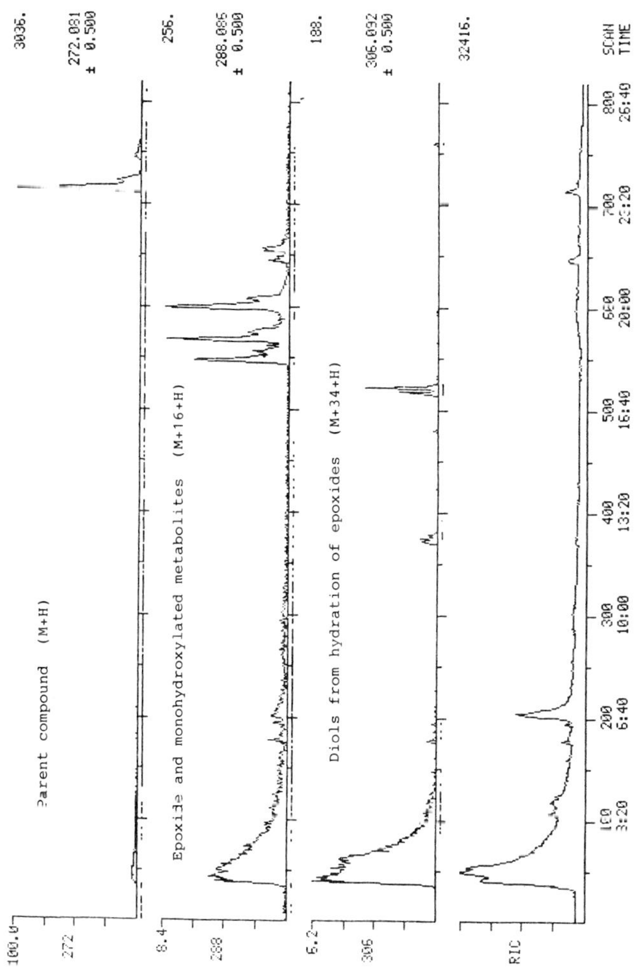

putative metabolites were detected by displaying ion chromatograms. There is clear evidence for several monooxygenated species (M+16.H) and it can also be inferred that at least two of these are epoxides since two peaks were detected with m/z M+34 corresponding to the hydration of an epoxide i.e. ($M+O+H_2O.H$).

REFERENCES

Black, M.H., Blade, R.J., Moss, M.D.V. & Nicholson, R.A. 1986, Sixth International Congress of Pesticide Chemistry, IUPAC, Ottawa, Abstract 1B-21.

Games, D.E. & Ramsey, E.D., 1985, Journal of Chromatography, 323, 67.

Keller, W., 1842, Annalen der Chemie, 43, 108.

Liberato, D.J., Feneslau, C.C., Vestal, M.L. & Yergey, A.L., 1985, Analytical Chemistry, 55, 1741.

Rachmel, A., Hazelton, G.A., Yergey, A.L. & Liberato, D.J., 1985, Drug Metabolism and Disposition, 13, 705.

Vestal, M.L., 1985, European Spectroscopy News, 63, 22.

Watson, D., Taylor, G.W. & Murray, S., 1985, Biomedical and Environmental Mass Spectrometry, 12, 610.

Watson, D., Taylor, G.W. & Murray, S., 1986, Biomedical and Environmental Mass Spectrometry, 13, 65.

Acknowledgements. Prof. J.W.Gorrod is thanked for advice and supply of several samples. Finnigan (UK) are thanked for plasma discharge TSP.

RECENT DEVELOPMENTS IN THE APPLICATION OF HPLC TO XENOBIOCHEMISTRY

Edward S. Yeung

Department of Chemistry
Iowa State University
Ames, IA 50011

Inherent in any application of liquid chromatography (LC) is the problem of detection. Except in the case of preparative separations, the LC detector is the key to obtaining qualitative and quantitative information about the analytes separated. Even though significant advances in chromatographic instrumentation and applications have been made in recent years, most of the systems in use today are still based (in decreasing order of popularity) upon the absorption detector, the refractive index (RI) detector, or the fluorescence detector.

For the development of pharmaceuticals, very often there are special problems of detection in LC. High sensitivity is needed to screen for impurities or to follow metabolic products in serum or in urine. Because good chromophores must be present to use an absorption or fluorescence detector, derivatization may be necessary if chromophores are lacking. In addition to the tedious sample preparation that is involved in derivatization, the sample of interest may be altered during the process. It is thus of interest to develop special detectors that are more sensitive than standard detectors for LC.

Because of the complexity of the samples in drug analysis is general, interferences must be minimized to obtain reliable information, which calls for highly selective LC detectors. Even if the chromatographic separation does not clearly isolate the component of interest, a highly selective detector can provide essentially the same information about the component as when interferences are absent. It is beyond the scope of this presentation to review the many uses of LC detectors in the development of pharmaceuticals. Instead, emphasis will be placed on several distinct detection schemes that address some of the special needs described above.

1. Fluorescence

It is obvious that for a higher excitation intensity (laser source), a larger fluorescence intensity will be observed in the same sample. However, this does not immediately lead to better detectabilities unless the noise is intensity independent. The most common sources of noise in fluorometric LC detectors are stray light, fluorescence from the cell walls or cell windows, and fluorescence or Raman scattering from the eluent. Most of these sources are dependent on the excitation intensity, but can be reduced to some extent by spatial filtering, since laser light is highly collimated. Particularly relevant to microcolumn LC is that as the volume of the detector is reduced, the ratio of analyte molecules to eluent molecules remains constant. Thus, if solvent fluorescence or solvent Raman scattering is the limiting factor, the concentration detectability of the analyte can be maintained in fluorescence, and its mass detectability can be substantially better in microcolumn LC as compared to conventional LC.

To eliminate the effects of stray light altogether, one can use a thin optical fiber inserted through the open end of the capillary in order to collect light emitted from the excitation region defined by a laser beam properly focused at the center of the capillary through the cell wall. This is because the optical fiber has a well-defined acceptance angle for light (Sepaniak & Yeung, 1980), and proper placement of the fiber relative to both the optical region and the cell walls can selectively transmit fluorescence from the liquid. A version of this system designed for microbore LC is shown in Figure 1. There, the internal diameter of the quartz capillary is 300μ, and the outer diameter of the optical fiber is 150μ. The volume of the detector is only 10 nL.

The use of laser fluorometric detection in the study of biological fluids has been reported for the antitumor agents adriamycin (A_1) and daunorubicin (D_1). A 20-μL sample of human urine is injected directly and separated by reversed phase HPLC coupled to an optical-fiber-based fluorometric detector. Figure 2 shows the chromatograms of a urine blank and a urine sample spiked with 63 pg (total amount) each of A_1 and D_1. Detection in the 10-pg range with no noticeable interference is achieved. The unique aspect is that visible laser at 488 nm is used to

Figure 1. Fiber optic fluorescence detector for LC.

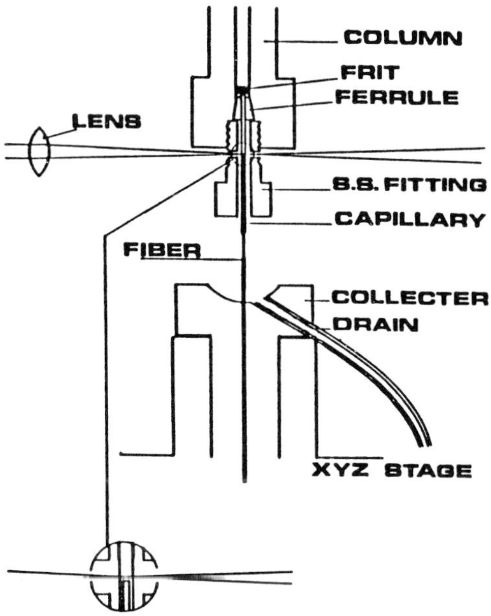

Figure 2. Determination of antitumor drugs A_1 and D_1 by direct injection of human urine. The blank (a) shows little interference during the elution of 63 pg each of the two drugs (b).

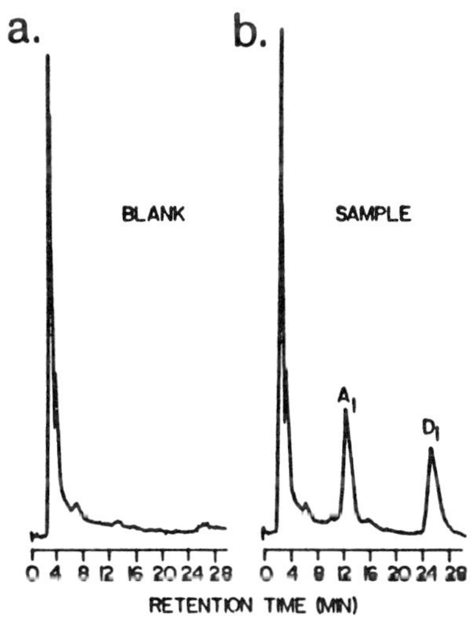

excite visible fluorescence at 590 nm. The complex chromatograms normally associated with the HPLC of untreated urine using either UV absorption or UV fluorescence are avoided. The use of a laser has improved the signal-to-noise level sufficiently to deal with these low concentration levels, typical of patients receiving such drug treatment. It is also found that interference-free determinations at comparable concentration levels are possible in unextracted human blood serum. There, however, chemical changes to the drugs do occur in time so that more careful controls are necessary.

2. Two-Photon Excited Fluorescence

The simultaneous absorption of two photons by atoms or molecules to reach an excited state at the sum of energies of the two photons is a weak process. Using high power lasers the absorption process is enhanced, and using the high sensitivity associated with fluorescence monitoring, detection of species at concentration levels typical of HPLC becomes possible.

The instrumentation for two-photon excited fluorescence detection cannot be more simple. Some means of introducing the focused laser beam into the chromatographic flow stream is needed. Collection of fluorescence using cut-off filters and phototubes is no different from other fluorometric detectors. In fact, there is no reason why the same laser beam cannot be used to excite both one- and two-photon states, simultaneously gathering the two types of information through separate filter/monochromator combinations.

The unique features of a two-photon excited fluorometric detector have been demonstrated in the separation of three oxadiazoles (Sepaniak & Yeung, 1977). These compounds are related to certain anti-inflammatory agents. Simplification of the chromatogram in the analysis of a mixture of compounds that normally are not resolved using UV absorption or fluorescence is illustrated in Figure 3. An interesting application is in the study of biological fluids by HPLC. Normal human urine and blood plasma, although they are complex mixtures, do not show any signal in two-photon excited fluorescence, even at high sensitivity settings. Drugs such as A_1 and D_1, however, show good two-photon response and can be detected at the 10-ng level with a 2W argon ion laser by direct injection of untreated samples.

Figure 3. Simplification of chromatograms by two-photon excited fluorometry. All seven compounds in a mixture show up and interfere with one another in a standard UV absorption detector (a), while only the oxadiazoles appear in the two-photon detector (b).

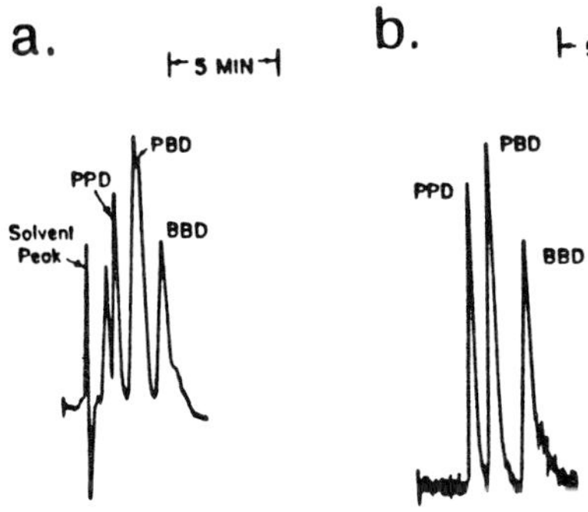

Figure 4. Separation of cholesterol and cholesterol esters in human serum. Peaks: A, cholesterol and cholestanol; B, cholesteryl linolenate and arachindonate; C, cholesteryl palmitoleate and linoleate; D, cholesteryl palmitate and oleate; E, cholesteryl stearate. Mobile phase, tetrahydrofuran-water (76:24, v/v); flow-rate, 0.5 ml/min.

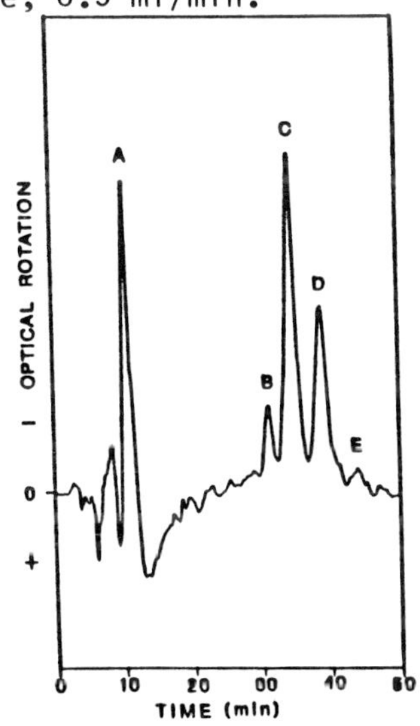

Since the two-photon excitation rate depends on laser power, a pulsed laser with high repetition rate should produce even better detection limits. Recently (Pfeffer & Yeung, 1986), we have been able to use a copper vapor laser for excitation. The output at 510 nm is 7W average power, or 1.4 mJ pulses at 30 ns pulse widths and repeated at 5 kHz. For the exact same compounds shown in Figure 3, using microbore columns (5-μm C_{18}, 1 mm i.d., 25 cm long, 90/10 acetonitrile/H_2O eluent, 30 μL/min, 1 μL injection loop), we are able to detect 250 fg of injected material. This means that sensitivity is approaching that of normal fluorescence detection. The complementry information makes two-photon excitation a valuable tool for identification of trace levels of xenobiotics.

3. Optical Activity

Optical activity is an interesting property of chiral molecules because the rotation of the polarization direction of light is usually an indication of biological activity. In complex samples of clinical, geological, or biological importance, this type of selectivity is useful. Commercial polarimeters, however, do not have the sensitivity required for and cannot handle the small volumes required in liquid chromatography. A laser-based polarimeter has been used for detection in the study of sugars in urine, cholesterol in serum, and chiral components in coal extracts after liquid chromatographic separation. A small, collimated laser beam that provides good rejection of stray light and the reduction of birefringence in the optical components is essential to the success of the laser-based polarimeter (Yeung, et al., 1980). For analytical scale LC applications, a 5-cm path-length cell with a volume of 100 μL seems to be the best compromise between sensitivity and volume in designing such a system. The most recent version has been interfaced to a microbore LC system that has a detector volume of 1 μL and an optical path length of 1 cm. The actual optical volume is even smaller; the machining process limits the volume to 1 μL. The applicability of the miniaturized version of the detector was tested in a reversed-phase elution of fructose using water as the eluent. The peak did not show any broadening beyond the specified efficiency of the column used (N = 25,000 plates) at a k' of 2.1. The most recent version of the polarimeter (Bobbitt & Yeung, 1986) allows the detection of 1 ng of material, i.e. 1 microdegree of rotation. The entire instrument can be assembled at a cost comparable to some LC detectors. In fact, several prototypes now exist in various research laboratories in the chemical and pharmaceutical industry.

The unique nature of the information that can be obtained can be illustrated in Figure 4. Cholesterol is a major component of all mammalian plasma membranes. Though it is vital to cell growth and survival, there is a statistically significant correlation between elevated serum cholesterol levels and cardiovascular diseases in general and atherosclerosis in particular. Cholesterol is found in two forms in the serum: either as free cholesterol, or esterified with long-chain fatty acids such as palmitic acid. Typically about 75% of the serum cholesterol is esterified. The ratio has been shown to be related to hormones, diets, toxic conditions such as ethanol poisoning, and disorders like familial lecithin:cholesterol acyltransferase deficiency.

We have devised a simple procedure (Kuo & Yeung, 1982), in which about 50 μL of blood is converted into serum. Tetrahydrofuran (150 μL) was then added and the supernatant liquid is injected into an LC with optical activity detection. Figure 4 shows that the bound cholesterol species are well separated from the free cholesterol fraction. This procedure will facilitate future clinical tests and development of potential correlations with heart disease.

Another important use of optical activity (OA) is the determination of enantiomeric ratios of chiral substance. This have applications in amino acid dating, quality control in pharmaceuticals, and for monitoring degradation and denaturization in proteins. We note that a UV or RI detector responds to the concentration of the species while the OA detector responds to both the concentration and the enantiomeric ratio of the species. It is easy to see that the response OA/UV will give an indication of the enantiomeric purity of the material (Reitsma & Yeung, 1986). For example, a totally racemic mixture will show a response of zero for OA/UV. Table I shows the result of plotting the OA/UV or OA/RI response for 4 different amino acids vs the fraction of the ℓ form present. Excellent correlation with enantiomeric purity is obtained. The slopes are related to the individual specific rotations. The racemic response should be zero in each case, and the percent deviation from zero is an indication of bias in the measurements. Table I shows the bias is small, i.e. within experimental errors. For situation where chiral separation is not possible or inconvenient, this technique offers the same information without added complexity.

Summary

Laser detectors for xenobiotics have allowed improvements in sensitivity and selectivity. Although there are no commercial versions of these yet, there is no reason why any of these cannot be packaged into routine instruments. For the research laboratories, the techniques described here offer unique information and capabilities for the study of xenobiotics.

Table 1. Determination of enantiomeric ratios using dual detectors.

Species	Mode	No. pts.	Correlation coefficient	Slope(s)	Racemic* response	RR/S (%)
Thr	OA/RI	12	0.998	15.0	-0.40	-2.7
Pro	OA/RI	12	0.991	6.54	0.17	2.6
Tyr	OA/UV	9	0.995	135	1.0	0.7
Phe	OA/UV	9	0.998	241	3.5	1.5

*Racemic response (RR) is defined as the value for a sample with a fractional concentration of 0.5ℓ.

ACKNOWLEDGMENTS

Research support of the work leading to this manuscript is derived from the Director of Energy Research, Office of Basic Energy Sciences. The Ames Laboratory is operated for the U.S. Department of Energy by Iowa State University under Contract. No. W-7405-Eng-82.

REFERENCES

Kuo, J. C. & Yeung, E. S., 1982, Journal of Chromatography, 229, 293.

Pfeffer, W. D. & Yeung, E. S., 1986, Analytical Chemistry, 58, 2103.

Reitsma, B. H. & Yeung, E. S., 1986, Journal of Chromatography, 362, 353.

Sepaniak, M. J. & Yeung, E. S., 1977, Analytical Chemistry, 49, 1554.

Sepaniak, M. J. & Yeung, E. S., 1980, Journal of Chromatography, 190, 377.

Yeung, E. S., Steenhoek, L. E., Woodruff, S. D. & Kuo, J. C., 1980, Analytical Chemistry, 52, 1399.

5. Amide-bond: formation and cleavage

ALTERNATIVE ROUTES TO THE FORMATION OF AMIDE BONDS IN BIOLOGICAL SYSTEMS

J. W. Gorrod

Chelsea Department of Pharmacy,
King's College London (KQC),
Chelsea Campus, Manresa Road,
London SW3 6LX, U.K

Apart from the formation of amide bonds by the classical method of acyl transfer from a donor, usually acylcoenzyme A, to a suitable acceptor nitrogen containing group, it is now clear that amides can arise during the metabolism of a variety of nitrogenous compounds.

It was early recognised that the tobacco alkaloid nicotine was converted to the corresponding cyclic amide cotinine. This amide is a major metabolite in all species studied, both _in vitro_ and _in vivo_ (Gorrod & Jenner, 1975, and references therein). Initial studies by Hucker, Gillette and Brodie (1960) showed that this compound was formed by hepatic preparations and it was suggested that it arose via a two step reaction involving first hydroxylation at the 5'-carbon to produce the corresponding carbinolamine which was then oxidised to give the amide by a dehydrogenase present in the cytosolic fraction. Indeed the inhibition of cotinine formation by cyanide supported this idea. 5'-Hydroxynicotine has never been isolated in the pure state and, whilst it has been detected in ethereal solutions of cotinine that have been treated with $LiAlH_4$, its total metabolic fate has never been determined. During their studies on the metabolism of nicotine, Booth and Boyland (1971) detected the formation of a new compound in the presence of cyanide. The structure of this compound was later established as 5'-cyano nicotine (Murphy, 1973a, Saunders et al., 1975) and from elegant studies using isotopic oxygen it was proposed that nicotine $\Delta 1'(5')$ iminium ion was an obligatory intermediate in the biosynthesis of cotinine. The synthesis of nicotine Δ 1'(5') iminium ion and subsequent metabolic studies by Brandange & Lindblom (1979a) and, Hibberd and Gorrod (1978,1980) confirmed the role of this compound in the formation of cotinine. It is of interest that the oxygen of the carbonyl group of cotinine is not derived from molecular oxygen (Murphy, 1973a) despite the reaction being initiated via the cytochrome P-450 system. The conversion of the iminium ion to cotinine is catalysed by aldehyde oxidase (Brandange and Lindblom, 1979b). Murphy (1973b) used the reactivity of nicotine Δ 1'(5') iminium ion with cyanide as the basis of a study designed to see whether this type of intermediate could be formed from other compounds which were known to yield a cyclic amide as a metabolite. The finding of a cyano adduct being strong evidence for the involvement of an iminium ion presumably derived from cytochrome P-450 mediated α-hydroxylation. Using this cyanide trapping technique, Murphy was able to show the formation of cyanide adducts during the microsomal metabolism of tremorine, N-methyl-4-phenyl piperidine, pethidine and thebaine, carried out in the presence of cyanide. By the use of ^{14}C-cyanide, Murphy developed a simple assay for the α-hydroxylase activity and showed that it occurred in rabbit, guinea pig and rat liver microsomes and in rabbit lung, brain and kidney microsomes.

Considerable species and organ variation in activity was observed. Such variation depended on the substrate being examined. Cyanide adducts were also formed from 4-phenylpiperidine and the N-ethyl, N-butyl, N-phenylethyl, N-phenylpropyl and N-allyl derivatives. No clear structure activity relationships have yet emerged. The amount of cyanide adduct formed was enhanced when microsomes prepared from a rabbit pretreated with phenobarbitone were used.

Analogous amides have been recognised as metabolites from other compounds containing a pyrrolidine ring system. Tremorine is a convulsant that contains two pyrrolidine rings and because of its interesting pharmacological properties, has been the subject of numerous studies. Cho et al., (1961) recognised that tremorine was converted to a pyrrolidone by metabolic oxidation and that this compound was the active agent. Further studies by Hammar et al.,(1969) showed that this compound was also metabolised and that the other pyrrolidine moiety was also converted to a pyrrolidone. It is of interest that this compound could be formed by the cyclisation of N-(4-pyrrolidino-γ-butynyl)-γ-aminobutyric acid previously recognised as a metabolite (Hammer et al., 1968).

Similar pyrrolidone metabolites have been detected from prolintane (Yoshihara & Yoshimura, 1974), sulpirid (Dross, 1978) and N-(5-pyrrolidinopent-3-ynyl)-succinimide(BL14), (Hallstrom, Lindeke and Anderson, 1981). In the latter case, cyanide was shown to inhibit pyrrolidone formation although no cyano adduct could be detected; suggesting either an alternative mechanism of amide formation or reflecting a wide range of reactivities of iminium ion intermediates.

Drugs containing other alicyclic amines are also converted to cyclic amides. These include mepivocaine, which contains a piperidino ring (Meffin et al., 1973) and meptazinol, which contains a seven membered ring (Franklin et al., 1976). Amide formation has also been recognised in aliphatic ring systems containing a second heteroatom. Thus, perazine and lidoflazine which contain piperazine groups are converted into the corresponding α-keto compounds (Breyer & Gaertner, 1973; Meuldermans et al., 1977). In the case of perazine, a unique cyclic diamide is also formed (Kraus et al., 1969). Formacaine and indeloxazine which contain morpholino groups are both converted to the corresponding cyclic amides in a variety of species and systems (Oelschlager, 1985; Kanimura et al., 1987). Studies on the metabolism of clonidine carried out in dog, man and rat (Darda et al., 1978) have shown that this imidazole containing compound is converted to a cyclic amide, and a ring hydroxylated amide.

As far as can be ascertained, no in vitro studies have been carried out with a view to elucidating the enzymology of the processes involved in cyclic amide formation from the latter compounds. Cyclic amides can be formed during the metabolism of a number of aza hetero aromatic compounds. These are often tautomers of the corresponding hydroxy compounds; their formation had been discussed by Beedham (1985) and will not be considered here.

A novel mechanism of cyclic amide formation results during the metabolism of hydralazine. This drug is converted to phthalazinone both in vivo and in vitro. This removal of the hydrazino group was thought to be carried out by hydrolytic enzymes (McClean et al., 1977) but is probably oxidative and mediated by a microsomal cytochrome system (Streeter & Timbrell, 1985). This oxidative pathway is involved in the protein binding observed with this compound and its associated toxicity (Streeter & Timbrell, 1983). Recently, the formation of a N-methylformamido compound has been observed during the metabolism of caffeine (Guaitani et al., 1981). An analogous compound, 6-amino-5-(N-methylformylamino)-1-methyluracil is formed as a major urinary metabolite of theobromine (Shively & Vessel, 1987). These metabolites are formed via oxidative cleavage of the heterocyclic ring by a β-naphthoflavone and 3-methylcholanthrene inducible cytochrome P-450 system (Bonate et al., 1987) and represents a novel route to the formation of an amide bond.

Recently, the metabolism of a number of N-benzylanilines have been investigated in vitro (Gorrod & Gooderham, 1982; 1985; 1987). These studies, which were designed to investigate the microsomal C-& N-oxidation of these substrates required the preparation of relatively unstable hydroxylamines and nitrones and the development of sensitive specific analytical techniques (Gorrod & Gooderham 1986, Gooderham & Gorrod 1984). During this study, new metabolites were recognised in which the methylene groups of the aralkyl moiety in N-benzylaniline, N-benzyl-4-chloro aniline and N-benzyl-4-toluidine were converted into a carbonyl function (Gorrod & Gooderham, 1985). The enzymology of formation of these amide bonds has not been fully established. In line with our understanding of the processes involved in N-dealkylation (McMahon, 1966; Gorrod & Temple, 1976), it would be easy to assume that N-benzylanilines were first converted to the corresponding carbinolamine which underwent dehydrogenation to yield the amide. However, experiments in which various potential inhibitors or activators were incorporated into the incubation media or when the animals were treated with inducing agents, failed to fully substantiate this pathway (Gooderham & Gorrod, 1986; Gorrod & Gooderham, 1987). The formation of amides from the amines was unaffected by SKF525A, and enhanced in the presence of DPEA. This would indicate that the flavin containing mono oxygenase rather than cytochrome P-450 was involved. However, the process was inhibited by the presence of octylamine or methimazole and when the incubations were carried out in an atmosphere containing carbon monoxide. The formation of the amides was enhanced when microsomes were used that had been prepared from hamsters that had been pretreated with 3-methylcholanthrene (but not phenobarbitone).

My current view is that the primary step in the formation of amides involves microsomal N-oxidation to give the N-hydroxy-N-benzylaniline. This is then further oxidised to a nitrone which rearranges via an oxaziridine intermediate to yield the amide. Abbot et al., 1985, have identified an N-formyl dervative as a metobolite of methadone and implicated both nitrone and oxaziridine intermediates in its formation. Their proposals are compatible with the route presented above. However, an alternative mechanism involving the metabolic formation of an imtermediate iminium ion in the metabolism of secondary anilines and cyclic amines is currently being investigated in my laboratories. Such an intermediate would fit into the proposals for an iminion ion intermediate in N-dealkylation (Nguyen et al., 1976) and in the metabolism of cyclic amines (Murphy 1973).

The production of reactive intermediates during the formation of amides by metabolic processes may indicate potential mechanisms for initiating toxic processes. In view of the widespread occurence of nitrogen containing groups that can form amides in drugs and other xenobiotics, it is important that the nature of any intermediates be established and their reactivity with cellular macromolecules be determined.

Acknowledgement I would like to record my thanks to Dr. P.J. Murphy, Lilly Research Laboratories, Indianapolis, U.S.A., for making available details of his unpublished observations relating to cyanide adduct formation.

REFERENCES

Abbot, F.S., Slatter, J.G., Burton, R. & Kang, G.I., 1985, Xenobiotica, 15,129.

Beedham, C. 1985, Drug Metabolism Reviews, 16, 119.

Booth, J. & Boyland, E., 1971, Biochemical Pharmacology, 20, 407.

Brandange, S. & Lindblom, L., 1979a, Acta Chem Scand B33, 187.

Brandange, S. & Lindblom, L., 1979b, Biochemical & Biophysical Research Communications, 91, 911.

Breyer, U.K., & Gaertner, H.J., 1973, Excerpta Medica International Congress Series, 288, 59.

Cho, A.K., Haslett W.L. & Jenden D.J., 1961 Biochemical Biophysical Research Communications, 5, 276.

Darda,S., Forster, H.J. & Stahle,H., 1978, Arzneimittel Forschung, 28, 255.

Dross, K., 1978, Arzneimittel Forschung, 28, 824.

Franklin, R.A., Aldridge, A. & White, C. de B., 1976, British Journal of Clinical Pharmacology, 3, 497.

Gaertner, H.J. & Breyer U., 1972, Arzneimittel Forschung, 22, 1084

Gooderham, N.J. & Gorrod, J.W., 1984, Journal of Chromatography, 309,339.

Gooderham, N.J. & Gorrod, J.W., 1986, In Development of Drugs & Modern Medicines, edited by J.W.Gorrod, G.G.Gibson & M. Mitchard. Ellis Horwood Ltd., Chichester, p318.

Gorrod, J.W. & Gooderham, N.J., 1982, In Microsomes, Drug Oxidations and Drug Toxicity, edited by Sato, R. & Kato, R., Wiley Interscience, New York, USA, p565.

Gorrod, J.W. & Gooderham, N.J., 1985, Xenobiotica, 15, 1021.

Gorrod, J.W. & Gooderham, N.J., 1987, Xenobiotica, 17, 165.

Gorrod, J.W. & Gooderham, N.J., 1986, Archives der Pharmazie (Weinheim), 319, 261.

Gorrod, J.W. & Temple, D.J., 1976, Xenobiotica,6, 265.

Gorrod, J.W. & Jenner, P. 1975, Essays in Toxicology, 6, 35.

Gorrod, J.W., & Temple, D.J., 1976, Xenobiotica, 6, 265.

Guaitani, A Abbruzzi R., Bastone, A., Bianchi, M., Bonati, M., Catalani, P., Latani., R., Pantarotto, C., & Szcawinska, K., Toxicology Letters, 38, 55.

Hallstrom, G., Lindeke, B. & Anderson, E., 1981, Xenobiotica 11, 459.

Hammar, C.G., Hammer, W. & Holmstedt, B., 1969 Biochemical Pharmacology, 18, 1549.

Hammer, W., Holmstedt, B., Karlen, B., Sjoquist, F. & Vessman, J., 1968, Biochemical Pharmacology, 17, 1931.

Hibberd, A.R. & Gorrod, J.W., 1978, Proceedings of 7th International Pharmacology Congress Paris p.651 (Absract No. 2082).

Hibberd, A.R. & Gorrod, J.W., 1980, Advances in Experimental Medicine & Biology, 136B, 1121.

Hucker, H.B., Gillette, J.R. & Brodie, B.B., 1960, Journal of Pharmacology & Experimental Therapeuties, 129, 94.

Kanimura, H., Enjoji, Y., Sasaki, H., Kawai, R., Kaniwa, H., Niigata, K. & Kageyama, S., 1987, Xenobiotica, 17, 645.

Latini, R., Bonati, M., Marzi, E. & Garattini, S., 1981, Toxicology Letters, 7, 1931.

McClean, A.J., Haegele K.D., duSouich, P., & McNay, J.L., 1977, European Journal of Drug Metabolism & Pharmacokinetics, 2,17.

McMahon, R.L., 1966, Journal of Pharmaceutical Sciences, 55, 457.

Meuldermans, W., Lauwers, W., Knaepa, A. & Heykants, J., 1977, Arzneimittel Forschung, 27, 828.

Murphy, P.J., 1973a, Journal of Biological Chemistry, 248, 2796.

Murphy, P.J., 1973b, Proceedings of International Congress of Biochemistry Stockholm, (Abstract No.).

Nguyen, T.L., Gruenke, L.D., Castagnoli, N., 1976, Journal of Medicinal Chemistry, 19, 1168.

Saunders, E.B., DeBardeben J.F. & Osdene, T.S., 1975, Journal of Organic Chemistry, 40, 2848.

Shively, C.A. & Vessell, E.S., 1987, Drug Metabolism & Disposition, 15, 217.

Streeter, A.J. & Timbrell, J.A., 1983, Drug Metabolism & Disposition 11, 179.

Streeter, A.J. & Timbrell, J.A., 1985, Drug Metabolism & Disposition, 13, 255.

Walkenstein, S., MacMullen, J.A., Knebel, C & Seifter, J., 1958, Journal of the American Pharmacy Association, Science Edition, 47, 20.

Yoshihara S. & Yoshimura H., 1974, Xenobiotica, 4, 529.

Acetylation

K.J. NETTER

Department of Pharmacology and Toxicology,
University of Marburg, Lahnberge,
3550 Marburg (Lahn), FRG

In this paper several aspects of acetylation are dealt with. These are firstly historical aspects, since the phenomenon of acetylation cannot be understood without knowledge of the activation of acetic acid which was discovered in the late 1940s and culminated in the discovery of the central role of acetyl-coenzyme A (acetyl-S-CoA). This is followed by a consideration of the acetylation of xenobiotics, which constitutes an important conjugative pathway of drug inactivation. There are also examples of acetylation leading to activation of certain foreign compounds. As is generally known, acetylation plays a major role in basic biochemical processes such as energy supply (Krebs cycle) or fatty acid synthesis. Moreover, cellular proteins are acetylated, notably the histones. It is estimated that a large proportion (around eighty per cent) of the cytosolic proteins are acetylated at the N-terminal group. Acetylation also affects the activity of hormones and mediators.

Distinct from the biological mechanisms, a foreign compound or drug, namely acetylsalicylic acid (aspirin), is capable of inducing a rapid acetyl transfer leading to acetylated products.

In table 1 the historical development of our knowledge on biological acetylations is summarized. As early as 1938, i.e. approximately one year after the discovery of the antibacterial properties of sulfonamides, Klein & Harris incubated tissue slices with sulfanilamide and found that this is converted to the corresponding acetylated compound. It should be noted that the acetylation takes place on the para amino group of the aromatic ring and not on the sulfonylamine moiety of the molecule.

Table 1. Summary of historical development of biological acetylation research.

Investigational history of acetyl group transfer	
1938	Tissue slices of guinea pig liver: sulfanilamide transformed to acetyl sulfanilamide: Klein & Harris
1940	Labeled acetate + sulfanilamide in vivo transformed to labeled acetylsulfanilamide in rabbits and rats: Bernhard
1943	Choline acetylation requires ATP, acetate activation: Nachmansohn & Machado
1945	Sulfonamide acetylation requires ATP: Lipmann
1946	Extract from liver and brain Kochsaft reactivate dialysed choline acetylase: Nachmansohn & Berman
1947	Coenzyme for acetylation (CoA), a pantothenic acid derivative: Lipmann, Kaplan, Novelli, Tuttle, Guirard
1951	Acetate is activated by ester formation with -SH of CoA: Lynen & Reichert
1956	Mechanisms of acetate activation: Berg
1957	Genetic basis for the variation in isoniazid acetylation (slow, rapid inactivators): Bönicke et al., Price-Evans et al., twin studies, pharmacogenetics
1958	N-terminal acetylation of proteins (TMV coat protein): Narita Acetylation of serotonin to melatonin: Lerner
1963	The presence of acetyl groups in histones: Philipps
1971	Aspirin inhibits prostaglandin synthetase: Vane
1972	Metabolic activation by acetylation: 2-acetylaminofluorene Bartsch, Dworkin, Miller, Miller
1975	Aspirin acetylates the active site of prostaglandin synthetase: Roth et al., Stanford and Majerus
1976	Bioactivation of isoniazid: Nelson et al.
1986	Acetylation of leukotriene E_4: Örning et al.

The following years marked the fascinating stepwise discovery of the energy requirement and mechanism of acetyl transfer through the investigations of several laboratories. This development was characterized by the simultaneous description of the acetylation mechanism of sulphanilamide and choline and the final revelation that the same mechanism of bioactivation is involved in both reactions: acetyl-S-CoA. The activity of CoA in providing group transfer energy is not located in an acetyl-phosphate bond, as was expected by all investigators at that time because of the well known properties of the energy-rich phosphate bond. Rather it was found in 1951 by Lynen & Reichert that the sulfhydryl moiety of CoA forms an energy-rich bond with acetate. With these developments the N-acetyltransferase acquired a pivotal role in conjugative xenobiotic metabolism and the active acetate became a biological substance of far greater general importance. This was soon extended to the study of acetylation in humans and an enzyme polymorphism was discovered which manifests itself in the existence of rapid and slow inactivators of isoniazid. This has first been summarized in the monograph of Kalow (1962) and later in the review by Weber & Hein (1985). During the last twenty years acetylation has become a general biochemical phenomenon with the discovery that many proteins are acetylated at their amino terminals. An important change in our thinking occurred, when it turned out that a very common drug, namely aspirin is also able to transfer acetyl groups to proteins and thereby to evoke particular pharmacological phenomena. Prior to this it had become known that the pineal hormone regulating the chromatophores, melatonin, is produced through the acetylation of serotonin. Recently acetylation has been described also as an inactivation pathway for leukotriene E4. Finally it may be mentioneed that the gene for chloramphenicol acetyl transferase has been successfully used to help in the elucidation of the cytochrome P-450 gene expression modification by dioxin (Jones et al., 1985). The melatonin-forming N-acetyltransferase in the pineal gland shows extensive variation in activity and increases (especially in the chicken) very drastically during darkness; it seems as if the enzyme is part of a biological clock regulating endocrinological change. This was reviewed by Binkley (1979).

Acetylation of xenobiotics

A number of xenobiotic compounds can be acetylated, according to the mechanism of acetate activation and transfer. The source of acetate can be, to a very small extent, administered (e.g. labelled) acetate but is mostly cellular acetyl-S-CoA.

Figure 1. Acetate activation and transfer to an acceptor.

Figure 1

Acetate activation and transfer to an acceptor

$$\text{Acetate} + \text{ATP} \rightleftharpoons \text{acetyl adenylate} + \text{PP}$$

$$\text{Acetyl adenylate} + \text{CoASH} \rightleftharpoons \text{acetyl CoA} + \text{AMP}$$

$$\text{Enzyme} + \text{AcCoA} \rightleftharpoons \text{Ac-enzyme} + \text{CoA}$$

$$\text{Ac-enzyme} + \text{substrate} \rightleftharpoons \text{Ac-substrate} + \text{enzyme}$$

$$\text{AcCoA} + \text{substrate} \longrightarrow \text{Ac-substrate} + \text{CoA}$$

enzyme = N-acetyltransferase

In the case of acetate activation it is important that the equilibrium is destabilized in the direction of acetyl-S-CoA; this is accomplished by the rapid hydrolytic elimination of pyrophosphate through the activity of pyrophosphatase. This will suppress the reverse reaction of acetyl adenylate to ATP and acetate. The N-acetyltransferase reaction is under genetic control leading to two phenotypes, either slow or rapid inactivators. Studies in different mouse strains have pointed to the fact that possibly differences in K_m are responsible. But conversely attempts to separate different enzyme proteins have not lead to conclusive results; the enzyme(s) so far have resisted attempts at separation with conventional protein chemical procedures (Weber & Hein, 1985). Nevertheless, substrates for acetylation may be divided into two groups, namely monomorphic (unimodal - such as sulphanilamide) and polymorphic (bimodal - such as isoniazid and sulphamethazine), as has recently been pointed out by Caldwell, 1986, in his chapter on conjugation mechanisms.

Xenobiotic substrates for acetylation are aromatic amines (e.g. *para* amino benzoic acid), sulphonamides (e.g. aliphatic amines. It is notable that there are conspicuous defects in acetylation. For example, the guinea pig cannot acetylate the alpha amino group of S-substituted cysteine and hence cannot excrete mercapturic acids, although it can readily synthesize glutathione conjugates. On the other hand, dog, fox and hyena can form mercapturic acids but cannot acetylate most other substrates. Various species of frogs and some reptiles such as the green lizard and the turtle cannot acetylate *para* amino benzoic acid and some sulphonamides (Smith 1964, Caldwell 1986). While all other animals acetylate sulphanilamide at the aromatic amino group in *para* position the dog seems to acetylate the moleculre at the other end, namely the sulphamido-N. Farah et al. (1977) have found the increasing age does not affect the ability to acetylate isoniazid in elderly humans over 65 years; this was found to be in contrast to the oxidation of acetanilide, the metabolic conversion rate of which is dependent on age. Acetylation does not only lead to inactivation of the particular xenobiotic but also may give rise to reactive intermediates: acetylisoniazid is hydrolysed to acetyl hydrazine which in turn through a hydroxylation step is converted to reactive species which bind covalently to cellular macromolecules (Nelson et al. 1976).

Acetylation of proteins

As early as 1977 Bloemendal had compiled a list of proteins of eukaryotic and viral origin that are acetylated at the amino terminal. The list contains more than forty defined proteins which are acetylated at N-terminal alanine, serine, glycine, threonine and methionine residues. Similarly Brown & Roberts in 1976 deduced from their determinations of N-terminal amino acids that no less than eightly per cent of the soluble cellular protein may be acetylated and they suggest that N-acetylation is a common type of post-initiation modification and may account for a significant percentage of the blocked N-terminal residues in eukaryotic protein. Thus, it seems that acetylated proteins are the role rather than the exception. Wold (1984) explains the fact that this phenomenon had not been observed earlier with the experiments of rabbit muscle aldolase when it was isolated in the presence of a protease inhibitor (phenylmethanesulphonylfluoride, PMSF): in this case the isolated produce has a blocked N-terminus. Treatment of this blocked form of the enzyme with CNBr yields a peptide with N-terminal Pro-His-... which is identical to the peptide isolated without PMSF. Since CNBr specifically cleaves methionyl peptide bonds and since the known mRNA codes for Met-Pro-His-... the blocked terminus must be X-Met where X represents in all probability acetyl. Thus it seems that a synthesized protein is N-acetylated soon after its emergence from the ribosome. Rubenstein et al., 1981, have determined the rate of acetylation of actin in a cell-free protein-synthesizing system. Non-acetylated actin was initially produced by depriving the system of acetyl-S-CoA and additionally deceiving the transferase by S-acetonyl-CoA; reconstitution of the acetylating system lead to a rapid acetylation of actin with a time constant of 15 minutes for half-acetylation.

In their review on the acetylation of histones in nucleosomes Doeneke and Gallwitz (1982) record that calf and trout histones are acetylated not only at the N-terminal serine but also very extensively in the lysine molecules along the peptide chain. On hydrolysis, epsilon-N-acetyllysine was identified as the modified amino acid. Furthermore they correlate acetylation of histones with an increased transcriptional activity of the respective tissues. This is exemplified by the observation that the genome of the lower eukaryote yeast appears to be entirely de-repressed and also hyperacetylated. Thus it seems that histone acetylation changes the internal structure of the nucleosomes and thus may be regulating the availability fo DNA and mRNA formation. At this point the modification of the system by inhibition of the de-acetylation through short-chain fatty acids seems of great importance (Kruh, 1982). In his review as well as in Cousens et al. (1979) evidence is found that particularly butyric acid inhibits the deacetylation process of calf thymus histone non-competitively and reversibly. In cell culture hyperacetylated histones return to the normally acetylated form 15 minutes after the removal of butyrate, and pulse labelling experiments show that about 70 per cent of acetyl histones are hydrolysed with $t_{1/2}$ of three minutes. Propionic acid exerts the same effect, only weaker. It remains open whether the hyperplasias observed in the rat forestomach after excessive feeding of propionate can be explained by the phenomenon of hyperacetylation of histones and ensuing derepression.

Recently Augen & Wold (1986) considered the available evidence on protein acetylation and developed a computer programme answering the question of which amino acids (counting from the N-terminal end of peptides) are responsible for the triggering of acetylation. By comparing the first 40 residues evolving from the ribosome they come to the conclusion that the distinguishing features for acetylation appear in the sequence ranges 1 - 10, 16 - 24 and 30 - 40; obviously the precise nature of the distinguishing characteristics are unknown.

Acetyl transfer from aspirin

Figure 2 shows the two mechanisms by which acetyl salicylic acid can transfer the acetyl group to a nitrogen atom, either by base catalyzed transfer or by the intermediate formation of an intramolecular anhydride. This non-enzymatic acetylation occurs with proteins, some of which have an important enzymatic function: oxygenation of arachidonic acid to form prostaglandins (Vane, 1971). It must be noted however that the acetate is attached to the aspirin molecule by an ester bond. This is not so in various other non-steroidal anti-inflammatory compounds where a carbon-bond is found. Hack et al. (1984) investigated the time course and degree of acetylation of a 72 kDa polypeptide from platelet intercellular membranes; they found, similar to the "biological" acetylation of actin, a rather rapid acetylation by 100 µM aspirin leading to half-acetylation after about three minutes. This means that both very different mechanisms of acetylation proceed with comparable rapidity. Analysing the acetylated amino acids in prostaglandin synthethase, Roth et al. (1983) have determined an acetylated serine moiety in position 8 of the N-terminal sequence and have further observed that this polypeptide sequence constitutes part of the active site of the enzyme. Thus, it seems as if aspirin is able to "specifically" acetylate a critical region of this oxygenating enzyme. Similarly, a hydrogen transferring enzyme, namely yeast glucose-6-phosphate dehydrogenase, is also affected by aspirin. Jeffery et al. (1985) found that in this enzyme a reactive lysine (not serine) is acetylated by aspirin. In fact, acetylation can be used as a tool to characterize the structure of the active centres of various dehydrogenases. 50 per cent inactivation in the presence of 3 mM aspirin is achieved after about 80 minutes. As a final note it may be added that calf eye lens proteins are covalently acetylated as measured by adding acetyl labelled aspirin and separating the main proteins by column chromatography (Rao et al., 1985). Aspirin leads to a decrease in epsilon-amino groups by about 20 per cent.

Figure 2.

Acetyl Transfer from Acetylsalicylic Acid

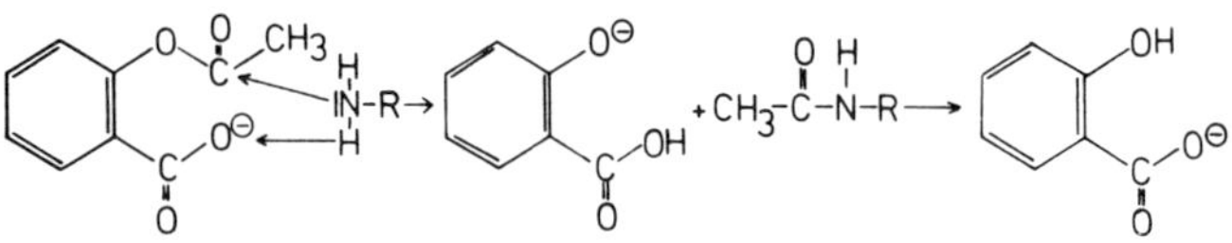

Base catalysed acetyl transfer

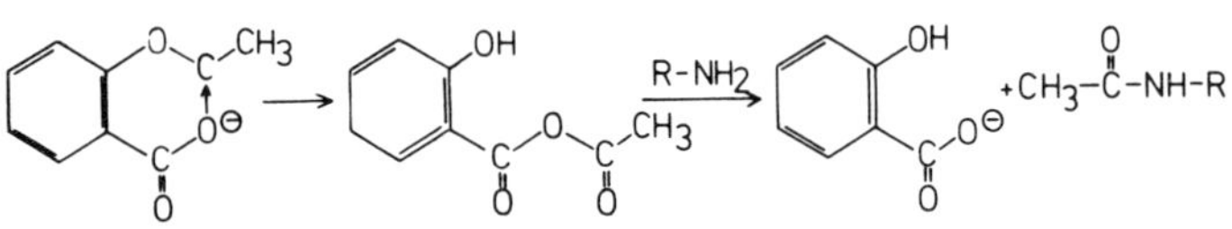

Acetylation of amino groups with intermediary formation of an anhydride: intramolecular nucleophilic catalysis

CONCLUSION

The formation of the C-N bond by acetylation is an important biological tool to modify xenobiotics as well as functional proteins. Acetylation can be achieved not only via biochemical mechanisms using activated acetate in the form of acetyl-S-CoA. Rather, a commonly used drug, namely aspirin, has turned out to be a potent acetylator of various enzymes.

REFERENCES

Augen, J. & Wold, F., 1986, *Trends in Biochemical Sciences*, 11, 494-497.

Bartsch, H., Dworkin, M., Miller, J.A., & Miller, E.C., 1972, *Biochimica et Biophysica Acta*, 186, 272-298.

Berg, P., 1956, *Journal of Biological Chemistry*, 222, 991-1013.

Bernhard, K., 1940, *Hoppe-Seylers Zeitschrift fur Physiologische Chemie*, 267, 91-98.

Binkley, S., 1979, *Scientific American*, 240, 66-72.

Bloemendal, H., 1977, *Science* 197, 127-138.

Bonicke, R. & Lisboa, B.P., 1957, *Naturwissenschaften*, 44, 314.

Brown, J.L. & Roberts, W.K., 1976, *Journal of Biological Chemistry*, 251, 1009-1014.

Caldwell, J., 1986. In *Xenobiotic Conjugation Chemistry*, edited by G.D. Paulson, J. Caldwell, D.H. Hutson & J.J. Menn, American Chemical Society Symposium Series, 299, p.2-28, Washington, DC.

Cousens, L.S., Gallwitz, D. & Alberts, B.M., 1979, *Journal of Biological Chemistry*, 254, 1716-1723.

Doenecke, D. & Gallwitz, D., 1982, *Molecular and Cellular Biochemistry* 44, 113-128.

Farah, F., Taylor, W., Rawlins, M.D. & James, O., 1977, *British Medical Journal*, 2, 155-156.

Hack, N., Carey, F. & Crawford, N., 1984, *Biochemical Journal*, 223, 105-111.

Jeffery, J., Hobbs, L. & Jornvall, H., 1985, *Biochemistry*, 24, 666-671.

Jones, PB.C., Galeazzi, D.R., Fisher, J.M. & Whitlock Jr, J.P., 1985, *Science*, 227, 1499-1502.

Kalow, W., 1962, *Pharmacogenetics: Heredity and the response to drugs*. Saunders, Philadelphia, London.

Klein, J.R. & Harris, J.S., 1938, *Journal of Biological Chemistry*, 124, 613.

Kruh, J., 1982, *Molecular and Cellular Biochemistry*, 42, 65-82.

Lerner, A.B., Case, J.D. & Takahashi, Y., 1960, *Journal of Biological Chemistry*, 235, 1992-1997.

Lipmann, F., 1945, *Journal of Biological Chemistry*, 160, 173-190.

Lipmann, F., Kaplan, N.O., Novelli, G.D., Tuttle, L.C. & Guirard, B.M., 1947, *Journal of Biological Chemistry*, 167, 869-870.

Lynen, F. & Reichert, E., 1951, *Angewandte Chemie*, 63, 47-48.

Nachmansohn, D. & Machado, A.L., 1943, *Journal of Neurophysiology*, 6, 397-403.

Nachmansohn, D. & Berman, M., 1946, *Journal of Biological Chemistry*, 165, 551-563.

Narita, K., 1958, *Biochimica et Biophysica Acta*, 30, 352-359.

Nelson, S.D., Mitchell, J.R., Timbrell, J.A., Snodgrass, W.R. & Corcoran III, G.B., 1976, *Science*, 193, 901-903.

Orning, L., Norin, E., Gustafsson, B. & Hammerstrom, S., 1986, *Journal of Biological Chemistry*, 261, 766-771.

Philipps, D.M.P.,1963, *Biochemistry Journal*, 87, 258-263.

Price-Evans, D.A., Manley, K.A. & McKusick, V.A., 1960, *British Medical Journal*, 2, 485-491.

Rao, G.N., Lardis, M.P. & Cotlier, E., 1985, *Biochemical and Biophysical Research Communications*, 128, 1125-1132.

Roth, G.J., Stanford, N & Majerus, P.W., 1975, *The Proceedings of the National Academy of Science USA*, 72, 3073-3076.

Roth, G.J., Machuga, E.T. & Ozols, J., 1983, *Biochemistry*, 22, 4672-4675.

Rubenstein, P., Smith, P., Deuchler, J. & Redman, K., 1981, *Journal of Biological Chemistry*, 256, 8149-8155.

Smith, J.N., 1964. In *Comparative Biochemistry*, edited by M. Florkin & H.S. Mason, Vol.VI, 403-457.

Vane, J., 1971, *Nature* (New Biology), 231, 232-235.

Weber, W.W. & Hein, D.W., 1985, *Pharmacological Reviews*, 37, 25-79.

Wold, F., 1984, *Trends in Biochemical Sciences*, 11, 494-497.

IDENTIFICATION, LOCALIZATION AND SPECIFICITY OF DETOXIFYING HYDROLASES IN RAT TISSUES.

Eberhard Heymann and Rolf Mentlein

Medical Chemistry, University of Osnabrück, D-4500 Osnabrück, GFR.

Presently, the nomenclature of carboxylesterases is highly confusing. The confusion results from the widespread use of xenobiotic substrates of all possible types. If someone starts characterizing an enzyme using a certain type of xenobiotic ester , it is almost impossible for him to recognize that others have characterized the same esterase before, using other esters, thioesters, amides or even an acyl transfer reaction. This situation has made enzymologists believe that an immense number of individual specific esterases exist . The view was supported by the detection of countless electrophoretic esterase bands in all tissues. In contrast, 20 years earlier it was believed that almost all xenobiotic esterase activity was combined in a single enzyme: the so-called non-specific carboxylesterase which was most active in the liver. The truth seems to be somewhere between these extremes. About 10 to 15 differing true carboxylesterases appear to exist in every mammal. All of these have differing specificities, but all are active with simple xenobiotic esters. The natural task of these esterases is probably to cleave physiological carboxyl esters, like lipids or sialic acid esters. The highest esterolytic activity with xenobiotics is found in membrane bound fractions from all tissues, especially in the liver. The objective of this paper is to identify four of the membrane bound carboxylesterases of rat tissues which seem to be responsible for most of the xenobiotic esterase activity in rats. Numerous data not reviewed here, indicate that the same types of esterases seem to exist in other mammals as well. Identification means correlation of the numerous existing data on the specificity, the cellular localization and the organ distribution of these enzymes. These data have been reported either for a universal non-specific esterase or, more frequently, for a more or less specific enzyme named according to the substrate preferred by the author. Identification means also to correlate the existing genetical nomenclature for rat carboxylesterases with the biochemical and pharmacological reports.

IDENTITY OF THE FOUR CARBOXYLESTERASES

Tentatively, we have named the enzymes according to one of their actions on natural intracellular substrates, namely lipoids. However, we do not know whether these actions represent the most important physiological function of these enzymes. In addition, we always give the ES-number according to the genetic nomenclature as recommended by van Zutphen (1983). The correlation between genetic and biochemical nomenclature has been established by comparing purified enzyme preparations from differing laboratories with genetically defined electrophoretic esterase bands in organs from a number of reference strains of rats (Mentlein et al. 1987). The varying biochemical and pharmacological names of rat esterases have been assigned to the four individual esterases either by direct chemical comparison of preparations from differing laboratories (Mentlein et al. 1980, Mentlein et al. 1984a, Mentlein et al. 1985a, Mentlein et al. 1987) or by evaluation of the reported data. Table 1 does not refer to all of the reported names for the individual carboxylesterases, however, in many cases the data of this table should allow a decision, whether an unknown esterase can be identified with one of those described here.

Table 1. Features of the carboxylesterases from rat ER involved in the hydrolysis of xenobiotics

A.Lysophospholipase

Genetic nomenclature: ES-3 (Mentlein et al. 1987).

Other names: Esterase pI 5.6 (Mentlein et al. 1984b). Esterase EA (Arndt et al. 1978). Butyrylesterase L-1 (Kaneko et al. 1979). ß-Glucuronidase-complexing protein = Egasyn (Medda et al. 1987).

Organ distribution: Liver, small intestine, (kidney, lung, tongue, epididymis); low activity in the liver of newborn rats; (Mentlein et al. 1987).

Chemical properties: Monomeric serine enzyme, M_r 61000, multiple forms (Mentlein et al. 1984a).

Natural substrates: Lysophospholipids, monoglycerides, long-chain acylcarnitines (Mentlein et al. 1984b, 1985b).

Prominent xenobiotic substrates: Acetanilide, phenacetin, retinyl acetate, steroid acetates(?) (Mentlein and Heymann 1984, Mentlein and Heymann 1987, Hattori et al. 1981).

B. Long-chain acyl-CoA hydrolase

Genetic nomenclature: ES-4 (Mentlein et al. 1987).

Other names: Esterases pI 6.2/6.4 (Mentlein and Heymann 1981). Ethanol acyltransferase (Polokoff and Bell 1978, Mentlein 1984). Cholesterolester hydrolase (Deykin and Goodman 1962, Nilsson 1976). Monoacylglycerol lipase (Ikeda et al. 1977, Oerlemans et al. 1977). Palmitoyl-CoA hydrolase (Mentlein et al. 1985a, Berge 1980, Jamdar 1979).

Organ distribution: Liver, kidney, (brown fat); activity high in kidney of newborn rats (Mentlein et al. 1987).

Chemical properties: Monomeric serine enzyme, M_r 61000, at least two forms (Mentlein et al. 1984a).

Natural substrates: Long-chain acyl-CoA, monoglycerides, retinyl palmitate, cholesterol esters.

Prominent xenobiotic substrates: Aspirin, propanidid, malathion, pyrethroid esters, dibutyl phthalate (Mentlein 1984, Mentlein and Heymann 1984, Mentlein et al. 1987).

C. Medium-chain monoacylglycerol lipase

Genetic nomenclature: ES-8/ES-10 (Mentlein et al. 1987).

Other names: Esterase pI 6.0 (Mentlein et al. 1984b). Esterase E1 (Arndt et al. 1973). Monoglyceridase (Oerlemans et al. 1977, Mentlein et al. 1984a).

Organ distribution: Liver, small intestine, lung, tongue, testis, brown fat, (heart, epididymis); absent in the liver of newborn rats (Mentlein et al. 1987).

Chemical properties: Serine enzyme, three identical subunits of M_r 58000 (Mentlein et al. 1984a).

Natural substrates: Monoglycerides of medium-chain fatty acids (Mentlein et al. 1984b).

Prominent xenobiotic substrates: Clofibrate, procaine, octanoyl amide, isoarecaidine esters (Mentlein and Heymann 1984); dimethylbilirubin, malathion, pyrethroid esters, isocarboxazid, meperidine, palmitoyl ethanediol (reviews: Heymann 1982, Mentlein et al. 1987).

D. Diacylglycerol lipase

Genetic nomenclature: ES-15 (Mentlein et al. 1987).

Other names: Esterase pI 5.0 (Robbi and Beaufay 1983). Esterase pI 5.2 (Mentlein and Heymann 1981). Carnitine ester hydrolase (Mentlein et al. 1985b).

Organ distribution: Liver; no activity in the liver of newborn rats, (Mentlein et al. 1987).

Chemistry: Monomeric serine enzyme of M_r 61000, multiple forms (Mentlein et al. 1984a, Robbi and Beaufay 1986).

Natural substrates: Medium- and long-chain acylcarnitines, diacylglycerols (Mentlein et al. 1985b).

Xenobiotic substrates: Phorbol esters (Mentlein 1986).

The lysophospholipase that is first in the order of the genetic nomenclature (ES-3, compare part A of Table 1) corresponds to the well-known acetanilide-cleaving carboxylesterase of rat liver. Surprisingly, the enzyme proved to be identical with the ß-glucuronidase-complexing protein found in rat (Medda et al., 1987). It is responsible for attaching ß-glucuronidase to the ER-membrane. The homologous protein which determines the subcellular distribution of ß-glucuronidase in mouse liver has been termed egasyn. Rat strains lacking esterase ES-3 have no ß-glucuronidase in the ER. The purified enzyme from rat liver and mouse egasyn (which also has esterase activity) are immunologically cross-reactive. The lysophospholipase ES-3 exists in multiple forms, usually five bands can be demonstrated by isoelectric focussing.
The next esterase to be identified here is the microsomal long-chain acyl-CoA hydrolase ES-4, (Tab. 1B). It also has been characterized extensively as an ethanol acyltransferase. Although the chemical properties of this esterase are very similar to those of the lysophospholipase ES-3 both have marked differences in their amino acid sequence (Mentlein et al., 1984a). The whole group of membrane-bound carboxylesterases may have evolved from one another by gene duplication.
The third membrane-bound carboxylesterase is the one that accounts for most of the esterase protein in rat liver microsomes. We tentatively name it a medium-chain monoacylglycerol lipase, (Tab. 1C). Surprisingly, it turned out to be identical with two genetically defined esterases, namely with ES-10 in the predominant trimeric form and with ES-8 as a monomer. This interrelationship could clearly be demonstrated by crossbreeding of rat strains with differing alleles of ES-10 and ES-8 (Mentlein et al., 1987): The crossbred animals showed exactly the numbers of hybrid esterases to be expected for trimers or monomers. The fact that two numbers exist for a single gene product makes the present genetic nomenclature a bit problematic. Perhaps, the serum esterase ES-2 may also be identical with ES-8/ ES-10; at least it strongly cross-reacts with antibodies against ES-10 (E. Heymann et al., unpublished).
The last one of the four membrane bound esterases cleaves two important groups of natural lipids. So far, we cannot decide whether the hydrolysis of diacylglycerols or of medium-chain acylcarnitines may be more significant in vivo. The diacylglycerol lipase (ES-15) resembles ES-3 and ES-4 in its chemical properties, but it clearly is a different protein (Mentlein et al., 1985b). Recently, it has been shown that this diacylglycerol lipase cleaves phorbol esters that

interfere with the regulatory function of diacylglycerols in vivo (Mentlein, 1986).

SPECIFICITY

All of the four esterases are able to hydrolyze esters, thioesters and acid amides. One might believe that - aside from the stereochemistry of the substrates - the hydrolysis rates might depend mainly on the chemical stability of the ester or amide bond. However, if one compares the hydrolysis rates of acetanilide, phenyl acetate and thiophenyl S-acetate it appears that the linking atom has a very selective influence on the individual esterases. In this case the esterases ES-15 and ES-10 prefer the thioester over the oxygen ester, but it is opposite with the other enzymes. We favour the hypothesis that the ratio of the hydrolysis rates of such pairs of corresponding substrates is constant for a given enzyme. Comparing other pairs of esters and amides with identical hydrocarbon structures, this principle seems to prove true.

It has been demonstrated for chymotrypsin and for other hydrolytic enzymes that the formation of the enzyme-substrate complex mainly depends on the lipophilicity of the substrates. A similar correlation exists for the monoacylglycerol lipase ES-10. The pKm-values of ES-10 correlate linearly with the substrate lipophilicity lg P. Thioesters and amides fit neatly in the curve. However, the linearity seems to end if the lipophilicity of the alcohol moiety of the substrates exceeds the value of a propyl residue. This view is confirmed if we compare the catalytical constant (k_{cat}/K_m) with the lipophilicity of the alcohol moiety in a series of butyric and acetic acid esters. Qualitative observations suggest that ES-10 prefers esters of hydrophilic alcohols with lipophilic acids, provided that the substrate is water-soluble. There exists no simple correlation between the K_m-values of the lysophospholipase ES-3 and the lipophilicity of its xenobiotic substrates. Probably, the steric form of the substrates influences the activity of these esterases more than such a simple physicochemical parameter. We assayed a series of isomeric butyl propionates with three of the four purified enzymes. In all cases, the enzymes preferred the esters of the primary alcohols over sec-butyl propionate. As it could be expected, t-butyl propionate was not hydrolyzed in any case.

Any electric charge in the substrate, both positive and negative, seems to inhibit the activity of these esterases almost completely. It does not matter whether the charge is located in the alcohol moiety as in procaine, or in the acyl moiety as in hostacain or in isoarecaidine esters.

Zwitterionic substrates, however, like carnitine esters or lysophospholipids obviously are an exception to this rule (Mentlein and Heymann 1984, Mentlein et al.,1985b).

Table 2. Selective inhibition by organophosphates of esterases from rat ER, (Brandt et al. 1980, Mentlein 1984).

Organophosphate	Remaining arylesterase activity (%) after preincubation with 0.1 mM inhibitor for 30 min at 30°C, pH 8.			
	ES-15 (pI 5.2)	ES-3 (pI 5.6)	ES-10 (pI 6.0)	ES-4 (pI 6.2/6.4)
Paraoxon	0	0	0	0 / 0
Bis(4-nitrophenyl) phosphate	3	2	4	33 / 56
Bis(4-cyanophenyl) phosphate	76	6	64	97 /100
2-Nitrophenyl-phenyl phosphate	61	58	73	100 /100
4-Nitrophenyl-phenyl phosphate	42	35	52	92 / 67
4-Nitrophenyl-phenyl-phosphonate	n.d.	51	2	47 / 38

All of these membrane-bound carboxylesterases are very sensitive to inhibition by organophosphates (Table 2). The phosphorylation of the active sites is very rapid with paraoxon. Complete inhibition in vitro - although at lower rates - can also be achieved with the organophosphorus diester bis(4-nitrophenyl) phosphate. This inhibitor can also be used for in-vivo studies, because of its low toxicity. Two similar compounds, namely bis(4-cyanophenyl) phosphate and 4-nitrophenyl phenylphosphonate can be used for a selective inhibition of ES-3 and of ES-10. Bis(4-cyanophenyl) phosphate has already been used to inhibit ES-3 in vivo (Brandt et al., 1980).

LOCALIZATION

As shown in Table 1, the four esterases exhibit the highest activities in rat liver, except for ES-4 which is equally active in kidney. To be sure that these enzymes are localized in liver parenchyme and not in macrophages or other liver cells, we separated hepatocytes from non-hepatocytes and labelled the two cell populations with radioactive. bis(4-nitrophenyl) phosphate, the above-mentioned inhibitor which specifically phosphorylates this type of carboxylesterases. As expected, the radioactivity was bound almost exclusively in hepatocytes and the labelled carboxylesterases could be identified by dodecylsulphate electrophoresis (E. Brandt et al., unpublished). To investigate the subcellular distribution of the esterases we separated rat liver homogenates into all possible subcellular fractions according to the procedure of Fleischer and Kervina (1974). The characteristic hydrolase activities for three of the four esterases are enriched about 2-3-fold in both the rough and the smooth ER fraction. Glucose-6-phosphatase, the marker enzyme of the ER increases by about the same factor. The esterases may also occur in the golgi apparatus, but our results do not point to their presence in any of the other cell compartments (Mentlein 1984). The diacylglycerol lipase ES-15 was not included in this study, but Robbi and Beaufay (1983) reported a very similar subcellular distribution for this esterase too.

The internal or external localization of enzymes in the microsomal membrane can be concluded from observations whether membrane impermeable substrates and enzyme-destroying agents have access to the enzyme or whether they cannot reach it. To evaluate the sidedness of the esterases we tried to destroy their activity with several proteinases. In all cases a disruption of the microsomal vesicles by desoxycholate increased the access of the proteinases indicating that the esterases probably are not exposed at the cytosolic surface. Although we have no definite proof it appears that all of these esterases may be located at the lumenal surface of the ER (Mentlein 1984). In this context it seems to be of note that all of the corresponding ester-forming enzymes are found on the opposite cytosolic side of the ER-membrane (Table 3).

Table 3. ER carboxylesterases as parts of substrate cycles.

Lumenal side	Ref.	Cytoplasmic side	Ref.
ES-3, Lysophospholipase	a	Enzymes of phospholipid synthesis	e
ES-4, Palmitoyl-CoA hydrolase	a,b	Fatty acid-CoA ligase	e
Cholesterol esterase	a	Acyl-CoA cholesterol acyltransferase	f
Retinol palmitate hydrol-	c	Acyl-CoA retinol acyltransferase	g
ES-15, Medium-chain acylcarnitine hydrolase	a,d	Carnitine octanoyltransferase	e
Diacylglycerol lipase	a	Enzymes of fat synthesis	e

a, Mentlein (1984); b, Jamdar (1979); c, Mentlein and Heymann (1987); d, Robbi and Beaufay (1983); e, Bieber et al. (1981); f, Lichtenstein and Brecher (1980); g, Ross (1982, sidedness not determined).

There seem to exist substrate cycles across the ER-membrane. These cycles may be involved in the regulation of lipid storage in the liver, for example of retinol esters, cholesterol esters and triglycerides. Another function of these cycles might be a transport of metabolites like retinol or free carnitine across the membrane. (Mentlein et al., 1985b). While free carnitine cannot cross the membrane, the medium-chain fatty-acyl derivative readily penetrates it. These esters are formed by a specific acyltransferase on the cytosolic side and are hydrolyzed specifically by ES-15 on the other side. Carnitine that is only synthesized in the liver in rats may be transported out of this organ by such a mechanism. The medium-chain fatty acids are able to diffuse back across the membrane. Similar mechanisms may help xenobiotic esters to cross the intestinal mucosa, but the same mechanisms would hinder such esters entering the cytosol of liver cells (or cells of other esterase-containing tissues). Another aspect of the natural function of these esterases is that they exert a membrane-stabilizing effect by detoxifying natural cytolytic lipids as lysophospholipids, monoglycerides, carnitine esters and CoA esters (Mentlein et al. 1985b). These lipids are very effectively hydrolyzed if their concentration exceeds the K_m-values of the esterases of about 10^{-5} M.

Arndt, R., Heymann, E., Junge, W. and Krisch, K., 1973, European Journal of Biochemistry, 36, 120-128.

Arndt, R., Schlaak, H.E., Uschtrin, D., Südi, D., Michelssen, K. and Junge, W., 1978, Hoppe Seylers Zeitschrift für Physiologische Chemie, 359, 644-651.

Berge, R.K., 1980, European Journal of Biochemistry, 111, 67-72.

Bieber, L.L., Krahling, J.B., Clarke, P.R.H., Valkner, K.J. and Tolbert, E., 1981, Archives of Biochemistry and Biophysics, 211, 599-604.

Brandt, E., Heymann, E. and Mentlein, R., 1980, Biochemical Pharmacology, 29, 1927-1931.

Deykin, D. and Goodman, D.S., 1962, Journal of Biological Chemistry, 237, 3649-3656.

Fleischer, S. and Kervina, M., 1974, Methods in Enzymology, 31, 6-41.

Hattori, K., Kamio, M., Nakajima, E., Oshima, T., Satoh, T. and Kitagawa, H., 1981, Biochemical Pharmacology, 30, 2051-2056.

Heymann, E., 1982, in Metabolic Basis of Detoxication, ed. W.B. Jakoby (Academic Press, New York), p. 229-245.

Ikeda, Y., Okamura, K. and Setsuro, F., 1977, Biochimica Biophysica Acta, 488, 128-139.

Jamdar, S.C., 1979, Archives of Biochemistry and Biophysics, 195, 81-94.
Kaneko, A., Yoshida, Y., Enomoto, K., Kaku, T., Hirata, K. and Onoe, T., 1979, Biochimica Biophysica Acta, 582, 185-195.
Lichtenstein, A.H. and Brecher, P., 1980, Journal of Biological Chemistry, 255, 9098-9104.
Medda, S., Takeuchi, K., Devore-Carter, D., von Deimling, O., Heymann, E. and Swank, R.T., 1987, Journal of Biological Chemistry, in press.
Mentlein, R., 1984, Habilitationsschrift, University of Kiel.
Mentlein, R., 1986, Journal of Biological Chemistry, 261, 7816-7818.
Mentlein, R., Berge, R.K. and Heymann, E., 1985a, Biochemical Journal, 232, 479-483.
Mentlein, R., Heiland, S. and Heymann, E., 1980, Archives of Biochemistry and Biophysics, 200, 547-559.
Mentlein, R. and Heymann, E., 1981, Methods in Enzymology, 77, 333-344.
Mentlein, R. and Heymann, E., 1984, Biochemical Pharmacology, 33, 1243-1248.
Mentlein, R. and Heymann, E., 1987, Biochemical Journal, in press.
Mentlein, R., Reuter, G. and Heymann, E., 1985b, Archives of Biochemistry and Biophysics, 240, 801-810.
Mentlein, R., Ronai, A., Robbi, M., Heymann, E. and von Deimling, O., 1987, Biochimica Biophysica Acta, in press.
Mentlein, R., Schumann, M. and Heymann, E., 1984a, Archives of Biochemistry and Biophysics, 234, 612-621.
Mentlein, R., Suttorp, M. and Heymann, E., 1984b, Archives of Biochemistry and Biophysics, 228, 230-246.
Nilsson, A., 1976, Biochimica Biophysica Acta, 450, 379-389.
Oerlemans, M.C., Geelhoed-Nieras, M.M. and Hülsmann, W.C., 1977, Biochemical and Biophysical Research Communications, 78, 1130-1137.
Polokoff, M.A. and Bell, R.M., 1978, Journal of Biological Chemistry, 253, 7173-7178.
Robbi, M. and Beaufay, H., 1983, European Journal of Biochemistry, 137, 293-301.
Robbi, M. and Beaufay, H., 1986, European Journal of Biochemistry, 158, 187-194.
Ross, A.C., 1982, Journal of Biological Chemistry, 257, 2453-2459.
Van Zutphen, L.F.M., 1983, Transplantation Proceedings 15, 1687-1688.

TRANS ACETYLATION AND FORMYLATION

Werner Lenk

Walther Straub-Institut für Pharmakologie und Toxikologie
der LM-Universität München, D-8000 München 2, Nußbaumstr.26
F.R.Germany

INTRODUCTION

The mechanism of biochemical activation of N-arylacetamides is illustrated in Scheme 1. In the primary step of this complex mechanism, the N-arylacetamide, such as 2-AAF(1), either injected as such or formed in vivo from the parent arylamine, is N-hydroxylated(A) to the corresponding N-arylacetohydroxamic acid(2). N-Hydroxylation is obligatory for the formation of the proximate carcinogen. Further activation is required for the production of reactive electrophilic molecular species which react at physiological pH with certain nucleophiles, such as N-acetyl methionine or the guanine residues of guanosine.

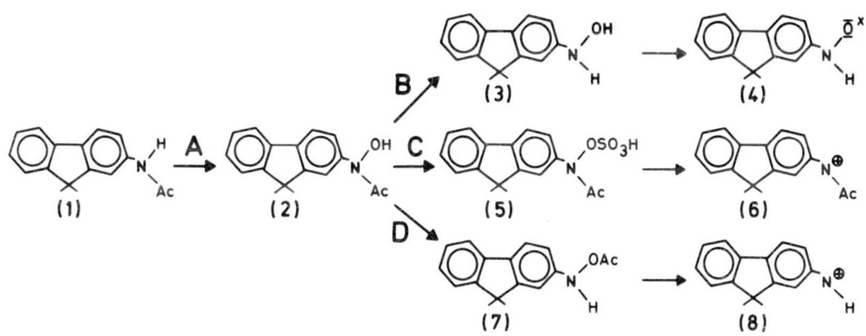

Scheme 1. Biochemical activation of N-arylacetamides

Microsomal and(or) cytosolic N-arylamidases(esterases) convert N-hydroxy-2AAF(2) by hydrolysis(B) to the reactive N-hydroxy-2AF(3), which undergoes autoxidation to give, i.a., the corresponding primary nitroxide(4) or nitrosoarene. Since neither of them readily reacted with guanosine or t-RNA at pH 7.0 or 7.4, other routes of activation were searched for.

O-acyl derivatives of N-hydroxy-2AAF, such as the sulphate(5), formed by PAPS and the cytosolic enzyme sulphotransferase(C), are labile compounds, which are spontaneously converted to N-acyl-arylamidonium ions(6), that react with nucleophiles. Alternatively N-arylacetohydroxamic acids can be converted by the cytosolic enzyme N,O-acyltransferase(D) to the putative N-acetoxy-arylamine(7), which spontaneously undergoes cleavage to the N-arylnitrenium ion(8). This very reactive electrophile is believed to combine with critical cell nucleophiles, such as the guanine residues of t-RNA. Adduct formation is considered a prerequisite for the mutagenic and carcinogenic properties of certain N-arylacetohydroxamic acids.

Acetyltransferase was discovered by Booth(1966) in rat tissues, that transfers acetyl from N-arylacetohydroxamic acids, such as N-hydroxy-4AABP, to 4-aminoazobenzene.

N,O-ACETYLTRANSFERASE ASSAY

Booth(1966) measured acetyltransferase activity by the rate of acetyl transfer from N-hydroxy-4AABP to 4-aminoazobenzene to produce 4-acetylaminoazobenzene and N-hydroxy-4ABP. At the end of a 15min incubation, the absorbance of the incubates was read at 497 nm; a decrease in the molar extinction indicated the formation of 4-acetylaminoazobenzene, and either product was identified by t.l.c. Standard incubates contained 1 mM N-hydroxy-4AABP, 0.1 mM 4-aminoazobenzene, and rat liver cytosol from 90mg of tissue in 2.5ml, pyrophosphate buffer, pH 7.0. Addition of 30 mM cysteine increased enzyme activity, indicating that acetyltransferase is an SH-dependent enzyme. Addition of other aromatic amines, such as 2-AF, 4-ABP, 2-NA or benzidine inhibited acetyl transfer to 4-aminoazobenzene by competition.

Bartsch et al.(1972) measured transacetylase activity i) by the rate of acetyl transfer from N-hydroxy-2AAF or N-hydroxy-4AABP to 4-aminoazobenzene and ii) by the rate of arylamination either of N-acetyl methionine to produce 3-methylmercapto-2-aminofluorene or 3-methylmercapto-4-aminobiphenyl, or of [8-^{14}C]-guanosine to produce [8-^{14}C]-guanosinyl-2-aminofluorene. Standard incubation mixture I contained 0.8 mM N-hydroxy-4AABP, 0.1 mM N-hydroxy-2AF, 0.8 mM NAD^{+} , either 10 mM N-acetyl methionine or 2.1 mM [8-^{14}C]-guanosine in 2.5 ml Sorensen phosphate buffer, pH 6.8, and rat liver cytosol from 60 mg liver. Standard mixture II contained 0.2 mM N-hydroxy-2AF or N-hydroxy-4ABP, 0.2 mM acetic anhydride, 22.7 mM N-acetylmethionine, and cytosol from 60 mg wet rat liver in 2.5 ml Sorensen phosphate buffer, pH 7.0. Acetic anhydride served as acetyl donor for the formation of N-hydroxy-2AAF or N-acetoxy-2AF.

King(1974) measured rat liver arylhydroxamic acid acyltransferase activity by the rate of incorporation of the 2-AF residue into [8-^{14}C]-guanosine or of the [9-^{14}C]-2AF residue into t-RNA; in addition, acetyl transfer to 4-aminoazobenzene was measured spectrophotometrically, and 4-acetylaminoazobenzene was identified.

Yeh & Hanna(1982) and Mangold & Hanna(1982) measured N-acylhydroxamic acid N,O-acyltransferase activity (AHAT) i) spectrophotometrically at 497 nm by the rate of acyl transfer to 4-aminoazobenzene and ii) by trapping the generated arylnitrenium ion with N-acetyl methionine or mercaptoethanol.

Booth(1966) has identified either product of acetyl transfer, the N-acetyl derivatives of various aromatic amines, and N-hydroxy-4ABP. King(1974) has identified the product of acetyl transfer from N-hydroxy-2AAF to 4-aminoazobenzene as 4-acetylaminoazobenzene. But in the later experiments with various N-acyl-N-2-fluorenylhydroxylamines, the products of acyl transfer were not identified.

STRUCTURAL REQUIREMENTS FOR N,O-TRANSACYLATION

N-Acyl-arylhydroxylamines with different aryl and acyl residues and a substituted N-hydroxy group were tested as substrates for acyl transfer to 4-aminoazobenzene in the spectroscopic transacylase assay of Booth(1966) and for arylamine transfer to N-acetyl methionine, mercaptoethanol, guanosine, and t-RNA in the N,O-transacylase assay (Booth 1966; Bartsch et al. 1972; King 1974; King et al. 1978; Mangold & Hanna 1982; Yeh & Hanna 1982; Elfarra et al.,1982; Banks et al.,1983; Marhevka et al.,1985; Elfarra & Hanna 1985).

Among the N-arylacetohydroxamic acids tested, the rate of acetyl donation in the transferase reaction with rat liver enzyme decreased in the order: N-hydroxy-4AABP > N-hydroxy-2AAN > N-hydroxy-2AAF > N-hydroxy-acetanilide (Booth 1966). Also with rat liver cytosol, activity of arylamine transfer to N-acetyl methionine decreased in a similar order: N-hydroxy-4AABP > N-hydroxy-2AAF > N-hydroxy-2AAN > N-hydroxy-1AAN (Bartsch et al.,1972). Among the N-2-fluorenyl hydroxamic acids tested with hamster liver enzyme, the activity of acyl donation to 4-aminoazobenzene in the transferase reaction decreased in the order: acetyl $\gg$ propionyl > benzoyl; formyl was not tested, and butyryl lacked any activity; the activity of arylamine transfer to N-acetyl methionine was of the same order (Yeh & Hanna 1982). Beland et al.(1980) found that with rat liver enzyme, the activity of arylamine binding to t-RNA decreased in the order: acetyl > propionyl > formyl, but with human liver enzyme in the order: formyl $\gg$

acetyl > propionyl.

These experiments indicated that not so much the size, but mainly the electronic properties of the aryl residue determine the transition state at the N-atom and the efficacy of an N-arylacetohydroxamic acid for transacylation and arylamination. Only limited structural variations in the acyl group are permissible without loss of substrate activity.

ENZYMOLOGY

Acetyltransferase activity in the soluble fraction of rat tissues decreased in the order: liver > adrenal > kidney > lung > spleen > testis > heart (Booth 1966). Bartsch et al. (1972) found that transacetylase activity in the cytosolic fraction of rat liver homogenate obtained at 105 000 x g was 6 times higher than the activity of the original homogenate, that p-chloromercuribenzoate, iodoacetamide, and N-ethylmaleinimide inhibited activity, and E 600 was without effect; transacetylase activity in liver cytosol from various species decreased in the order: male hamster > male rabbit > male rat > female rat; little or no activity was detected in the liver of male mice, male guinea pigs, male dogs, and humans. Enzyme activity in liver decreased on administration of N-hydroxy-2AAF and was not affected on phenobarbitone administration to rats.

Since both, N-hydroxy-2AAF and N-hydroxy-4AABP are mammary carcinogens for the female rat, the mammary gland was tested for N,O-acyltransferase activity. Bartsch et al.(1973) found that mammary cytosol from 16-21 day pregnant rats had 20% of the enzyme activity of rat liver cytosol at pH 7.5, and that it utilized N-hydroxy-4AABP, but not N-hydroxy-2AAF. King et al.(1979) found that the cytosol of lactating mammary glands contained an enzyme, which had a m.w. of 28 000 and catalysed the arylamination of t-RNA with both substrates, N-hydroxy-2AAF and N-hydroxy-4AABP.

King(1974) established the identity of the transacetylase (Booth 1966) with the N,O-acetyltransferase activity(Bartsch et al.,1972, 1973), when he recovered the two enzyme activities from rat liver cytosol in the same yield by use of precipitation and chromatographic methods. But formyl kynurenine formamidase (Santti & Hopsu-Havu,1968) from rat liver cytosol was precipitated and eluted earlier than N,O-acyltransferase. Since arylhydroxamic acid N,O-acyltransferase and CoASAc-dependent N-acetyl transferase activity from rabbit liver cytosol could not be resolved by various methods, they are apparently properties of the same enzyme, indicating that they are under common genetic control (Glowinski et al.,1980).

N-Hydroxy-2AAF and N-hydroxy-4AABP are irreversible inhibitors of rat and hamster hepatic N,O-acyltransferase (Banks & Hanna, 1979), and the inhibition was shown to fulfill the kinetic criteria for suicide inactivation (Hanna et al., 1982). App. dissociation constants K_I of 89 and 430 μM and limiting rates of inactivation k_i of 1.95 and 0.43 min^{-1} for N-hydroxy-2AAF and N-hydroxy-4AABP, respectively, were determined. Thus, kinetics of enzyme inhibition proved to be a valuable technique for probing the mechanism of arylamine transfer and selective inactivation of N,O-acyltransferase.

BIOLOGICAL SIGNIFICANCE

In order to explain the strong carcinogenicity of N-hydroxy-2AAF in mammals, the hypothesis was tested that, after biochemical N-oxygenation of 2-AAF, the much stronger carcinogen N-hydroxy-2AAF might react with RNA and DNA after enzymic N-deacetylation through the very reactive N-hydroxy-2AF. However, reaction of N-hydroxy-2AF with methionine (Miller et al., 1968) and t-RNA or DNA (Kriek 1965) at pH 7 was low. A secondary activation step was searched for, which might explain arylamination of the guanine residues of RNA or DNA at physiological pH. Enzymic esterification of N-hydroxy-2AAF with sulphuric acid was one of the postulated mechanisms, which could explain, why the N-acetylated 2-aminofluorene moiety was incorporated into guanine. N,O-Transacylation of N-hydroxy-2AAF was the other, which could explain, why 2-aminofluorene residues were incorporated into guanine, since the putative acyloxy arylamines reacted with guanine with loss of the acyl moiety.

The effect of five acyl substituents of N-acyl-N-2-fluorenylhydroxylamines on <u>N-deacylase</u>, <u>N,O-acyltransferase</u>, and <u>sulphotransferase</u> activity, and on mutations in Salmonella typhimurium were tested with rat liver arylhydroxamic acid N,O-acyltransferase (King et al., 1978; Weeks et al., 1980). Microsomal deacylase activity decreased in the order: monochloroacetyl > formyl ≃ acetyl > propionyl ≃ trifluoroacetyl. N,O-Acyltransferase activity decreased in the order: acetyl > propionyl > formyl ≫ monochloroacetyl ≃ trifluoroacetyl, and sulphotransferase, determined by the rate of adduct formation of t-RNA with 2-acylaminofluorenes, decreased in the order: acetyl ≃ formyl > monochloroacetyl ≃ propionyl. Direct mutagenicity decreased in the order: trifluoroacetyl > formyl > monochloroacetyl > acetyl ≃ propionyl, and mutagenicity in the presence of N,O-acyltransferase decreased in the order: monochloroacetyl > formyl > acetyl > propionyl > trifluoroacetyl. These results indicated that the mutagenicity of the five N-acyl-N-2-fluorenylhydroxylamines was consistent with the formation of N-hydroxy-2AF by enzymic hydrolysis, and that bacterial pathways of metabolism may play a role in N-acyl-arylhydroxylamine-induced mutations.

FORMYLATION

In 1966, Boyland & Manson described 2-formamido-1-naphthyl hydrogen sulphate as a urinary metabolite of 2-naphthylamine in the rat and dog. Its formation from the primary metabolite, 2-amino-1-naphthyl hydrogen sulphate, by N-formylation or alternatively, by N-methylation of 2-amino-1-naphthyl hydrogen sulphate and subsequent oxidation of the N-methyl group *in situ*, was envisaged.

4-Formylaminoantipyrine was found as a metabolite in the urine of man, rats, guinea pigs, and rabbits after oral dosing with aminopyrine. Noda et al.(1976) who studied the metabolic fate of 4-[^{13}C-dimethylamino]-antipyrine in man, isolated 4-[^{13}C-formylamino]-antipyrine besides 4-[^{13}C-methylamino]-antipyrine from the urine, indicating oxidation *in situ* of the methyl group to the formyl group.

Lenk & Sterzl(1978) isolated a 5:1 mixture of the N-acetyl and N-formyl derivatives of 4-chloroaniline and 3.4-dichloroaniline after incubation of 4-chloropropionanilide and 3.4-dichloropropionanilide as well as 4-chloroaniline and 3.4-dichloroaniline with microsomal suspensions of rabbit liver microsomes. They used ethyl acetate for extraction. Subsequent studies revealed, that the N-acetyl derivatives were formed by acetyl transfer from ethyl acetate to the arylamines, catalysed by microsomal acetyl transferases, whereas the source for formyl transfer remained obscure. Franz & Krisch(1968) have described N-acetylation of aromatic amines by acetyl transfer from ethyl acetate, catalysed by purified carboxylesterases from pig and bovine liver.

Gothoskar et al.(1979)isolated 2-formylaminoanthraquinone from the kidneys and urine of rats after oral administration of 2-aminoanthraquinone; in addition, the N-acetyl derivative was also found.

Rao et al.(1973) isolated a polar metabolite, 1,3,7-trimethyl-dihydro uric acid, from the urine of rats dosed with caffeine which in solution was in equilibrium with its open form, 4-amino-5-(formylmethylamino)-1.3-dimethyl uracil. In the meantime 6 different 4-amino-5-(formylamino)-methyl uracils were detected as metabolites of caffeine, theobromine, or theophylline which differed in respect to methyl substitution at the position N-1, N-3, and N-5 of 4-amino-5-(formylamino) uracil. Caffeine was converted in vivo into 1,3,7-trimethyl uric acid by xanthine oxidase and reduced to the dihydro uric acid, which, being an unstable hemiaminal, underwent ring cleavage to give the uracil.

Remberg et al.(1980) found trace amounts of two N-formylamino derivatives of verapamil in the urine of man after oral administration of ^{14}C-DL-verapamil, namely N-[4-cyano-4-(3.4-dimethoxyphenyl)-5-methyl hexyl]-formamide(1) and N-[4-cyano-4-(3.4-dimethoxyphenyl)-5-methyl hexyl]-N-methylformamide(2). Since also the corresponding N-methyl derivative of (1) was isolated in substantial amounts (22%), the two formylamino metabolites might also have arisen by oxidation <u>in situ</u> of the corresponding N-methyl compounds.

Coombes et al.(1982) detected N-formylaminoglutethimide and nitroglutethimide as minor urinary metabolites of aminoglutethimide after oral administration to humans. Besides, N-acetylaminoglutethimide was found as the major metabolite. This finding implicates N-acetylation, N-formylation, and N-hydroxylation as relevant pathways of aminoglutethimide metabolism in man.

Koeppel & Tenczer (1985) determined by mass spectrometry two N-formyl derivatives of amantadine (tricyclo[3.3.1.1.^{3,7}] decan-1-amine) as urinary metabolites of man, namely N-formyl-amantadine and N-formyl-N-methyl-amantadine, besides N-acetyl-amantadine as the major metabolite of amantadine.

Bird et al.(1986) isolated N-formylpenicillamine in 15% yield from nonenzymatic degradation of benzylpenicillin at pH 5. Depending on the electronegativity of the acyl residue forming the amide bond of the side chain of the penicillins, the yield of N-formylpenicillamine varied between 0.1 and 46%.

Santti & Hopsu-Havu (1968) have described the characteristics of kynurenine formamidase, a cytosolic enzyme isolated from the liver of guinea pigs and rats. This enzyme, which catalysed the deformylation of N-formyl-L-kynurenine, was shown to deacylate not only the N-formyl-, but also the N-acetyl- and N-monochloroacetyl derivatives of various xenobiotics and to transfer the formyl group to aniline, 1- and 2-naphthylamine, and to anthranilic acid. Whether or not the formamidase of guinea pig or rat liver cytosol is responsible for the N-formylation and N acetylation of aromatic amines, is still an open question.

REFERENCES

TRANS ACETYLATION

Banks, R.B. & Hanna, P.E., 1979, Biochemical Biophysical Research Communications, 91, 1423.

Banks, R.B., Smith, T.J. & Hanna, P.E., 1983, Journal of Medicinal Chemistry, 26, 1780.

Bartsch, H., Dworkin, M., Miller, J.A. & Miller, E.C., 1972, Biochimica Biophysica Acta, 286, 272.

Bartsch, H., Dworkin, C., Miller, E.C. & Miller, J.A., 1973, Biochimica Biophysica Acta, 304, 42.

Beland, F.A., Allaben, W.T. & Evans, F.E., 1980, Cancer Research, 40, 834.

Booth, J., 1966, Biochemical Journal, 100, 745.

Elfarra, A.A. & Hanna, P.E., 1985, Journal of Medicinal Chemistry, 28, 1453.

Elfarra, A.A., Yeh, H.M. & Hanna, P.E., 1982, Journal of Medicinal Chemistry, 25, 1189.

Glowinski, I.B., Weber, W.W., Fysh, J.M., Vaught, J.B. & King, C.M., 1980, Journal of Biological Chemistry, 255, 7883.

Hanna, P.E., Banks, R.B. & Marhevka, V.C., 1982, Molecular Pharmacology, 21, 159.

King, C.M., 1974, Cancer Research, 34, 1503.

King, C.M., Allaben, W.T., Lazear, E.J., Louie, S.C. & Weeks, C.E., 1978, Influence of the acyl group on arylhydroxamic acid N-O-acyltransferase-catalyzed mutagenicity and metabolic activation of N-acyl-N-2-fluorenylhydroxylamines. In Biological Oxidation of Nitrogen, edited by J.W.Gorrod (Elsevier/North Holland Biomedical Press) (Amsterdam, The Netherlands), p.335.

King, C.M., Traub, N.R., Lortz, Z.M. & Thissen, M.R., 1979, Cancer Research, 39, 3369.

Kriek, E., 1965, Biochemical Biophysical Research Communications, 20, 793.

Mangold, B.L.K. & Hanna, P.E., 1982, Journal of Medicinal Chemistry, 25, 630.

Marhevka, V.C., Ebner, N.A., Sehon, R.D. & Hanna, P.E., 1985, Journal of Medicinal Chemistry, 28, 18.

Miller, E.C., Lotlikar, P.D., Miller, J.A., Butler, B.W., Irving, C.C. & Hill, T.J., 1968, Molecular Pharmacology, 4, 147.

Weeks, C.E., Allaben, W.T., Tresp, N.M., Louie, S.C., Lazear, E.J. & King, C.M., 1980, Cancer Research, 40, 1204.

Yeh, H.M. & Hanna, P.E., 1982, Journal of Medicinal Chemistry, 25, 842.

FORMYLATION

Bird, A.E., Jennings, K.R. & Marshall, A.C., 1986, Journal of Pharmacy and Pharmacology, 38, 913.

Boyland, E. & Manson, D., 1966, Biochemical Journal, 99, 189.

Coombes, R.C., Foster, A.B., Harland, S.J., Jarman, M. & Nice, E.C., 1982, The British Journal of Cancer, 46, 340.

Franz, W. & Krisch, K., 1968, Hoppe-Seyler's Zeitschrift für Physiologische Chemie, 349, 1413.

Gothoskar, S.V., Benjamin, T., Roller, P.P. & Weisburger, E.K., 1979, Xenobiotica, 9, 533.

Koeppel, C. & Tenczer, J., 1985, Biomedical Mass Spectrometry, 12, 499.

Lenk, W. & Sterzl, H., 1978, Biotransformation in vitro of the herbicide propanil by rabbit liver microsomes. In Industrial and Environmental Xenobiotics, edited by J.R. Fouts and I.Gut (Excerpta Medica) (Amsterdam, Oxford), p.213.

Noda, A., Goromaru, T., Tsubone, N., Matsuyama, K. & Iguchi, S., 1976, Chemical and Pharmaceutical Bulletin, 24, 1502.

Rao, G.S., Khanna, K.L. & Cornish, H.H., 1973, Experientia, 29, 953.

Remberg, G., Ende, M., Eichelbaum, M. & Schomerus, M., 1980, Drug Research, 30, 398.

Santti, R.S.S. & Hopsu-Havu, V.K., 1968, Biochemical Pharmacology, 17, 1110.

THE PHARMACOGENETICS OF ACYL TRANSFER

W. W. Weber & G. N. Levy
Pharmacology Department, University of Michigan
Ann Arbor, Michigan 48109, USA

INTRODUCTION

Individual differences in the pharmacologic and toxicologic profiles of many amines and hydrazines, whether they be drugs used in medical therapy, or chemicals encountered in the workplace and elsewhere in the environment occur because of the acetylator genes. Phenotypically, individuals are either "slow" or "rapid" acetylators, and "slow" acetylators are homozygous for a slow acetylator gene while "rapid" acetylators are either heterozygous or homozygous for a rapid gene. The difference in two acetylator phenotypes is ascribed to differences in the activities of the drug acetylating enzymes of liver, intestinal mucosa, and probably of other tissues of the gastrointestinal tract such as the pancreas that are encoded by these genes.

MODIFIED RESPONSES ASSOCIATED WITH THE ACETYLATOR PHENOTYPE

Whenever a difference in the disposition of amine drugs, or of chemicals that are biotransformed to amines, is due to the acetylator phenotype, a difference in the response(s) of rapid and slow recipients of the drug should be anticipated. Slow acetylators are more prone to toxicities from numerous drugs, whereas rapid acetylators are more prone to experience a relative lack of therapeutic effectiveness of such drugs. These effects are probably explained by the higher serum concentrations of drugs attained in slow acetylators compared to rapid acetylators at any time after drug ingestion. Examples of both types have been amply discussed elsewhere (Weber,1987). Here, a few examples of sporadic disorders associated with the acetylator phenotype serve to illustrate the diversity of these effects (Table 1).

Table 1. Test of the association between the acetylator phenotype and various sporadic disorders

Sporadic disorder	Number of studies	Relative risk	X^2_1
INH hepatitis	6	S/R: 2.21	14.50 ($p<0.001$)
Bladder cancer			
All studies	11	S/R: 1.36	10.45 ($p<0.01$)
High risk of exposure	3	S/R: 1.70	7.82 ($p<0.01$)
Type I diabetes (Europeans)	4	R/S: 1.62	21.82 ($p<0.001$)

Source: The Acetylator Genes and Drug Response, Weber, 1987. (Oxford University Press, New York)

Cancer induced by aromatic amines is a disorder for which the human acetylator trait has important implications. Urinary bladder cancer in persons occupationally exposed to aromatic amines such as benzidine is the most notable of these. A significant excess of slow acetylators occurs among those affected, and the slowest of the slow acetylators are especially susceptible to this disorder (Cartwright et al., 1982). Slow acetylators are believed to be relatively more susceptible to this disorder because they transport higher concentrations of benzidine to the bladder where it is activated to DNA-reactive metabolites which initiate the malignancy.

In contrast, rapid acetylation may be more

prevalent in association with certain other cancers, specifically among men with a history of colo-rectal cancer (Lang et al., 1986) and among women with breast cancer (Cartwright, 1984). There is evidence from investigation of the acetylator trait in animals (McQueen et al., 1982; 1983) and in tissues obtained from human subjects (Flammang & Kadlubar, 1986; Flammang et al, 1985) suggesting that rapid acetylation enhances mutagenesis and carcinogenesis induced by aromatic amines. Several aromatic amine pyrolysis products formed during cooking of food, which are biotransformed by acetylation, (Sugimura & Sato, 1983) are highly mutagenic and carcinogenic in experimental animals (Takayama et al, 1984a & b). Circumstantial evidence suggests that the genesis of human colo-rectal cancer in some instances, may involve aromatic amine carcinogens of this type and that rapid acetylator genes may favor the susceptibility of individuals to this disorder. The reason for an association between breast cancer in women and rapid acetylation is less clear.

ACETYLATOR STATUS AND METABOLIC ACTIVATION

Most pharmacogenetic traits are due to genetically conditioned differences in the metabolism of the environmental chemical, or to a distinctive pattern of its metabolites (LaDu, 1983). The concept of metabolic activation is consistent with this generalization, but it adds the notion that for some traits, the distinction may depend upon the extent or kind of <u>reactive</u> metabolites that are generated. Often, the molecular mechanisms of these effects are incompletely understood because the distinctive reactive metabolite has not been identified.

Aromatic amines and hydrazines and their acetylated derivatives are seldom directly injurious to tissues, but they can be biotransformed into highly reactive substances that are cytotoxic, mutagenic and can initiate carcinogenesis. The concept of metabolic activation, which originated with the discovery that N-oxidation transforms 2-acetylaminofluorene into reactive electrophiles capable of binding DNA covalently and forming DNA adducts (Cramer et al, 1960), has been widely adopted as an explanation of the carcinogenic and cytotoxic actions of aromatic amines and numerous other environmental chemicals.

For all well studied aromatic amine carcinogens, adducts of the carcinogen to DNA have been identified (Beland & Kadlubar, 1985; Neumann, 1986). The adducts are generated by reaction of DNA with either N-hydroxylamine or N-hydroxyarylacetamide (arylhydroxamic acid) derivatives of the amine, and form adducts with or without the acetyl group. These intermediate metabolites are produced by enzymatic N-oxidation, catalyzed by Phase I oxidation enzymes, i.e. cytochrome P-448, flavin containing monoxygenases, or peroxidases. Further activation of the arylhydroxamic acids involves either deacetylation to the hydroxylamine, N,O-acyltransfer to the N-acetoxyarylhydroxylamine, or conjugation with activated sulfate by sulfotransferase to the N-sulfoxyacetamide. O-Acetylation of the N-hydroxylamine has recently been proposed as another reaction of importance to the metabolic activation of aromatic amine carcinogens (Flammang et al., 1986; Shinohara et al., 1986).

The adducts and their effects are unevenly distributed in tissues. Kriek et al.(1984) attribute this heterogeneity in part to differences in the concentration of the reactive metabolites that are generated in tissues by 1) pharmacokinetic differences between tissues, and to 2) differences in capacity for metabolic activation. Our recent observations suggest that a similar explanation accounts for the difference in the amount of 2-AF-DNA adducts formed in the livers of rapid and slow acetylator mice (Levy & Weber, 1987).

DIFFERENCES IN DNA-AMINOFLUORENE ADDUCTS IN RAPID AND SLOW ACETYLATOR MICE

Our studies of the biochemical differences in 2-aminofluorene (2-AF) metabolism between rapid (C57BL/6J) and slow (A/J) acetylator inbred mouse strains have been extended to include DNA-carcinogen adduct formation as a measure of

DNA damage. Using an HPLC modification of the recently developed ^{32}P-postlabeling assay for carcinogen-DNA adducts (Gupta et al, 1982), we have found that rapid acetylator mice have greater 2-AF adduct formation in hepatic DNA. The ratio of hepatic DNA adduct formation between rapid and slow acetylators approximates the differences seen with other measures of 2-AF metabolism in these strains.

The biochemical characteristics of the hereditary acetylation polymorphism of C57BL/6J and A/J mice with 2-aminofluorene are summarized in Table 2.

Table 2. The acetylation pharmacogenetics of 2-aminofluorene (2-AF) in C57BL/6J and A/J mice

	B6	A
Liver NAT activity		
nmols/min/mg pro	2.64 + 0.22(6)	0.91 + 0.05(10)
Blood 2-AF disappearance		
hr^{-1} 30 mg/kg	0.83 + 0.04(3)	0.35 + 0.07(4)
hr^{-1} 50 mg/kg	0.86 + 0.11(4)	0.21 + 0.04(4)
hr^{-1} 100 mg/kg	0.36 + 0.02(10)	0.12 + 0.02(9)
Hepatocyte 2-AF disappearance		
hr^{-1}	0.76 + 0.13(5)	0.29 + 0.02(5)
Hepatocyte 2-AAF formation		
hr^{-1}	1.60 + 0.21(3)	0.92 + 0.06(2)
Hepatocyte 2-AAF formation		
nmol/10^6 cells/4hr	1.17 + 0.17(3)	0.47 + 0.02(3)
2-AF-liver DNA adduct formation		
pmol adduct/mg DNA	2.85 + 0.89(3)	0.49 + 0.36(3)

CONCLUSIONS

These preliminary observations in rapid and slow acetylator mice suggest that the difference in extent of mutagenesis and tumorigenesis induced by aromatic amine carcinogens in rapid and slow acetylator individuals is due to a difference in the concentrations of reactive metabolites in their tissues. These tissue differences appear to be secondary to both the pharmacokinetic differences in disposition of these amines and to pharmacogenetic differences in enzymatic capacity for metabolic activation that are determined by the acetylator genes.

REFERENCES

Beland, F. & Kadlubar, F., 1985, Environmental Health Perspectives, 62, 19.

Cartwright, R., Glashan, R., Rogers, H., Ahmed, R., Hall, D., Higgins,E. & Kahn, M. 1982, The Lancet, 2, 842.

Cartwright, R., 1984, Epidemiological studies of N-acetylation and C-center ring oxidation in neoplasia. In Banbury Report No. 16, Genetic Variability in Responses to Chemical Exposure, edited by G.S. Omenn and H.V. Gelboin (Cold Spring Harbor Laboratory), p 359.

Cramer, J., Miller, J. & Miller, E., 1960, Journal of Biological Chemistry, 235, 885.

Flammang, T., Yamazoe, Y., & Guengerich, F., 1985, Proceedings of the American Association of Cancer Research, 26, 425.

Flammang, T. & Kadlubar, F., 1986, Carcinogenesis, 7, 919.

Gupta, R., Reddy, M. & Randerath, K., 1982, Carcinogenesis, 3, 1081.

Kriek, E., Der Englese, L., Scherer, E. & Westra, G., 1984, Biochimica Biophysica Acta, 738, 181.

LaDu, B., 1983, Drug Metabolism & Disposition, 11, 283.

Lang,N., Chu, D., Hunter, C., Kendall, D., Flammang, T. & Kadlubar, F., 1986, Archives of Surgery, 121, 1259.

Levy, G. & Weber, W., 1987, The Toxicologist, 7, 213.

McQueen, C., Maslansky, C., Glowinski, I., Crescenzi, S., Weber, W. & Williams, G., 1982, Proceedings of the National Academy of Science (USA), 79, 1269.

McQueen, C., Maslansky, C. & Williams, G., 1983, Cancer Research, 43, 3120.

Neumann, H., 1986, Journal of Cancer Research and Clinical Oncology, 112, 100.

Shinohara, A., Saito, K., Yamazoe, Y., Kamataki, T. & Kato R., 1986, Cancer Research, 46, 4362.

Sugimura, T. & Sato, S., 1983, Cancer Research (Suppl.) 43, 2415s.

Takayama, S., Nakatsura, Y. & Masuda, M., 1984, Gann, 75, 467.

Takayama, S., Masuda, M., & Mogami, M., 1984, Gann, 75, 207.

Weber, W., 1987, The Acetylator Genes and Drug Response (Oxford University Press).

ACYLATION OF AMINO ACIDS AND OTHER ENDOBIOTICS BY XENOBIOTIC CARBOXYLIC ACIDS

John Caldwell, Keith Sinclair and Andre Weil

Department of Pharmacology, St. Mary's Hospital Medical School, London W2 1PG, England

The carboxyl (-COOH) group, present as such or as simple esters, is an important structural feature of a wide range of drugs (analgesics, antiinflammatory agents, diuretics, hypolipidaemics, aldose reductase inhibitors), agricultural chemicals (herbicides and pesticides) and plasticizers. There thus occurs a considerable human exposure to xenobiotic carboxylic acids and in recent years there has been a resurgence of interest in the toxicology of such agents. Some 150 years ago, studies of carboxylic acids were the foundation of what we now call "drug metabolism" (Conti & Bickel, 1977) and since then there have been regular additions to our knowledge of their fate.

The metabolism of the carboxyl group of xenobiotic carboxylic acids in the animal body involves a series of acylation reactions, in which an acyl (R-CO-) group is transferred to one of four types of functionalities present in endogenous conjugating agents, *viz.* the esterification of hydroxyl groups, amide formation at primary amine centres, thioesterification of -SH groups, and the special case of acylation of a methyl group, as occurs during fatty acid chain elongation. Examples of each of these are listed in Table 1, from which it seen that these acylations involve a wide variety of endogenous conjugating agents, including sugars, sterols, glycerol, amino acids, carnitine, proteins, protein and non-protein thiols and fatty acids.

This simple chemical classification of the metabolic reactions of the carboxyl group is unfortunately not especially useful when we come to consider their biochemical mechanisms, since different acylations may be involved at different stages of metabolism. The acylation potential of most carboxylic acids and their simple esters is low, and thus, to carry out these biosyntheses, energy must be supplied.

Table 1. Acylation of endobiotics by xenobiotic carboxylic acids

(for references see Caldwell, 1982; Caldwell & Marsh, 1983; Quistad, 1986; Quistad & Hutson, 1986; Van Breemen & Fenselau, 1985)

<u>Esterifications of -OH groups of</u> :

Carbohydrates	-	glucuronic acid glucose xylose	
Carnitine			
Glycerol			
Sterols	-	bile salts and acids cholesterol	

<u>Amide formation with -NH$_2$ groups of</u> :

Amino acids	-	glycine taurine	glutamine ornithine *etc.*
Protein side chains			
Ammonia (-CONH$_2$ formation)			

<u>Thioesterification of -SH groups of</u> :

Coenzyme A
Glutathione, leading to acylmercapturates
Protein side chains

<u>Acylation of -CH$_3$ groups in</u> :

Fatty acid chain elongation (ω-acylation)

At the present time, three mechanisms are recognised to operate in the acylation of endobiotics:

(i) The high energy intermediates in most examples of acylation by endogenous carboxylic acids are Coenzyme A thioesters, and these are known to be the obligatory intermediates in the amino acid conjugations (N-acylations). Analogy with intermediary metabolism suggests their likely participation in the chain elongation of fatty acids (C-acylation), carnitine conjugation (N-acylation) and esterification of glycerol and of sterols.

(ii) The carboxyl group is esterified by a variety of UDP-sugars, notably UDP-glucuronic acid, under the influence of a transferase specific for the UDP-sugar in question.

(iii) Acylation can occur by transesterification, involving either a xenobiotic which is a simple carboxylate ester, as occurs in the formation of the cholesterol esters of prednimustine (under the influence of lecithin:cholesterol acyl transferase) and fenvalerate, or a xenobiotic acyl glucuronide acting as an acyl donor (Van Breemen & Fenselau, 1985), as is thought to occur in the formation of thiomercapturates, protein adducts and in the artefactual formation of amides by the reaction of the acyl glucuronide with ammonium ions in urine. Thus the formation of those conjugates which are the ultimate excretion products of xenobiotic carboxylic acids may be the result of two or more sequential reactions at the -COOH group, sometimes involving different bond types.

The newer aspects of the interrelationships between the metabolism of xenobiotic carboxylic acids and lipid biochemistry are mentioned elsewhere in this volume by Dr. Hutson (for reviews, see Caldwell & Marsh (1983) and Quistad & Hutson (1986)), and the present coverage will deal with the classical drug metabolism pathways of amino acid conjugation and ester glucuronidation, which are complementary reactions in the fate of many acids.

The amino acid conjugations

A considerable number of xenobiotic carboxylic acids undergo amino acid conjugation, via a three-step reaction sequence as follows (Killenberg & Webster, 1980):

(i) R.COOH + ATP ⟶ R.CO~AMP + PPi

(ii) R.CO~AMP + CoA.SH ⟶ R.CO~S.CoA + AMP

(iii) R.CO~S.CoA + H_2N.R′.COOH ⟶ R.CONH.R′.COOH + CoA.SH

The formation of acyl CoAs is seemingly a general process of carboxylic acids which enter the cell, since many which do not give rise to amino acid conjugates have the ability to reduce free CoA.SH levels within the cell. It has long been recognized that the amino acid conjugations exhibit a very marked substrate specificity, which is exerted at the third step of the sequence, acyl transfer to the amino group of the amino acid. The nature and extent of amino acid conjugation which a given acid will undergo is a feature of its pKa, lipid solubility, the size and shape of the aryl or alkyl moiety, the steric environment around the carboxyl group, and the animal species in question (Caldwell, 1982; Caldwell *et al.*, 1980). With simple aromatic acids, the extent of amino acid conjugation is clearly structure-dependent, with its extent falling with increasing bulk of substituents ortho- to the -COOH group

(Caldwell, 1982). There occurs an analogous effect with the arylacetic acids, where substitution upon the α-carbon similarly inhibits amino acid conjugation (Caldwell, 1982). The nature of the structure-activity relationships of the aryloxy-acetates, propionates and isobutyrates remain obscure at present (Van der Waterbeemd *et al.*, 1986).

The principle amino acid conjugation mechanism is the glycine conjugation, which operates with most acids in most species (Caldwell, 1982). The major exceptions are certain birds and reptiles, where it is replaced by ornithine, and, in the case of the arylacetic acids, primate species where it is replaced by glutamine (Caldwell, 1982). Although the glutamine conjugation has been thought of as a biochemical marker of primate species, it is now clear that it can occur very rarely in non-primates, especially with 2-naphthylacetic acid (Emudianughe *et al.*, 1978). In addition, there are odd examples of "deficiencies" of glycine conjugation, for example the formation of benzoylglutamic acid in place of hippuric acid by various fruit bats. The taurine conjugation involves principally arylacetic acids (Caldwell *et al.*, 1980), but some aromatic acids (benzoic, 3-phenoxybenzoic) can undergo this reaction. Its species occurrence is sporadic, but it is especially well developed in carnivorous mammals and aquatic life, both fish and crustaceans (James, 1986).

In addition to these four major amino acid conjugations, there occur a wide variety of other reactions, at present viewed as restricted to particular combinations of species and acid (Caldwell *et al.*, 1980; Quistad, 1986). These include aspartic acid, glutamic acid, alanine, histidine, arginine, and certain dipeptides, glycylglycine, glycyltaurine and glycylvaline. There is no reason not to suppose that all 22 amino acids will at some time be found to be involved in the conjugation of xenobiotic carboxylic acids.

The functional significance of the amino acid conjugations is hard to delineate. Although the products are less acutely toxic than the parent acids, the advantage gained is small in comparison with the complexity of the reaction sequence involved (Caldwell *et al.*, 1980). It is perhaps more interesting to consider the possibility that these reactions may serve to protect the cell against the harmful effects of the obligatory acyl CoA intermediates - many acyl CoAs have enzyme inhibitory activity (Caldwell, 1984). In this context, the ability of exogenous glycine to protect against toxic acids given exogenously *e.g.* hypoglycin A, or excess endogenous acids, as occurs in the amino acidurias, is noteworthy.

Glucuronidation

The formation of glucuronic acid conjugates is a general fate of carboxylic acids of virtually all chemical types (Caldwell, 1985). Its occurrence is less sensitive to changes in chemical structure than in the case for the amino acid conjugates, but curious examples of its absence do occur *e.g.* the aryloxypropionates (Van der Waterbeemd *et al.*, 1986). The glucuronic acid mechanism has a very widespread distribution amongst animal species, but its absence in the domestic cat and other Felidae is noteworthy. This metabolic defect has taxonomic significance as a "cat" characteristic, and occurs in other felines (lion, lynx) and related species (civet, genet, hyena), thus distinguishing them from the dog-like carnivores, where the reaction is extant (Caldwell *et al.*, 1978).

Glucuronic acid conjugation of xenobiotics with UDP-glucuronic acid is catalysed by the enzyme UDP-glucuronyl transferase. This exists as a family of isoenzymes, and carboxylic acids are amongst the substrates for at least three of the known forms (Dutton, 1980). The species differences observed are perhaps a consequence of the differential distribution of these various isoenzymes.

The last 10 years have seen a resurgence of interest in the formation of ester glucuronides, triggered by a reappraisal of their chemical properties. Acyl glucuronides undergo facile hydrolysis in mild alkali and may be characterised by their lability to β-glucuronidase (Caldwell & Hutt, 1986). In the 1960s and 70s, it became clear that the extent of enzyme cleavage is often less than obtained with alkali, and this was particularly noted in studies with the hypolipidaemic drug clofibrate (see Faed, 1984). This paradox was resolved in 1978 by Ellen Faed, working in New Zealand, who by analogy with the known behaviour of the ester glucuronides of bilirubin IXα, proposed that there occurs a pH-dependent migration of the clofibryl moiety from C-1 of glucuronic acid to the other hydroxyl groups of the sugar ring (Faed & McQueen, 1978). Only the 1-O-acyl β-D-glucopyranosiduronates are labile to β-glucuronidase, but the rearrangement products are all cleaved by mild alkali (Caldwell & Hutt, 1986). Following this proposal, Caldwell & Emudianughe (1979) isolated a sample of 1-O-clofibryl β-D-glucopyranosiduronate from rabbit urine and characterized it by MS and NMR. Incubation of this at mild alkaline pH produced a variety of products all containing glucuronic acid but with a free anomeric carbon atom (C-1) (Sinclair & Caldwell, 1982). Subsequently, a considerable number of acyl glucuronides have been shown to undergo the same phenomenon of intramolecular rearrangement (Table 2). Indeed, it seems that this is a general reaction of acyl glucuronides, the only such conjugate known not to undergo rearrangement being salicyl acyl glucuronide (Hutt *et al.*, 1982).

The detailed structural elucidation of these products is difficult (see Caldwell & Hutt, 1986). MS presents problems as the molecules are polar and non-volatile, and either undergo excessive fragmentation or, with soft ionization techniques, give little information other than molecular weight. In either case, it is virtually impossible to determine the position of acylation. The application of NMR is hampered by the large quantities required and the fact that, even in HPLC, it is likely that a number of products may co-elute. The number of possible isomers is very great: there are 4 hydroxyls for acylation, and, for all except C-1, there could occur furanose, pyranose (both as α and β anomers) and open chain forms, while lactonization could also occur (Sinclair & Caldwell, 1982).

This demonstration of the intramolecular reactivity of acyl glucuronides leads logically to the possibility that they could act as acyl donors towards appropriate centres on other molecules (Stogniew & Fenselau, 1982). Interest has focussed particularly on the -SH of glutathione and -SH and $-NH_2$ centres of proteins. The chemical reactivity of ester glucuronides as acylating agents towards model nucleophiles is low in comparison with classical reactive xenobiotics (Van Breemen & Fenselau, 1986), but there is a correlation between acylation potential and ease of hydrolysis and rearrangement. The thioester conjugate clofibryl mercapturic acid, a very minor excretion product of clofibrate, is proposed to arise from the acylation of glutathione by clofibryl glucuronide (Stogniew & Fenselau, 1982). Additionally, various authors have shown the reactivity of acyl glucuronides towards proteins, although the reaction mechanism(s) are problematical at present (Van Breemen & Fenselau, 1985).

To what extent, then, should we regard acyl glucuronides as a new class of reactive intermediate, with toxicological sequelae to be expected from their formation? It seems that there is a correlation between the various reactivities outlined above, *viz.* ease of spontaneous hydrolysis, intramolecular acyl migration and acylation of protein and non-protein nucleophiles, so an assessment of their chemical properties will indicate their reactivity and potential for toxicity. Assembly of the available data (Table 3) serves to show that this class of metabolite varies very widely in reactivity, by a factor of at least 100, from highly labile glucuronides like that of isoxepac, to the very stable fenofibric acid glucuronide. The full biological consequences of this reactivity of ester glucuronides remain to be explored - thus far, a

Table 2. Xenobiotic carboxylic acids whose acyl glucuronides undergo intramolecular acyl migration

Clofibric acid
Diflumisal
Fenclofenac
Isoxepac
Probenecid
Valproic acid
Wy 18251
Zomepirac
Indomethacin
Benzoic acid
Flufenamic acid
Wy 41770
Fenofibric acid

(for references see Caldwell & Hutt, 1986)

Table 3. Stability of xenobiotic acyl glucuronides

Aglycone	Half-life for intramolecular rearrangement* (h)
Isoxepac	0.23
Wy 18251	0.48
Zomepirac	0.98
Indomethacin	1.4**
Benzoic acid	4.9
Clofibric acid	6.7
Flufenamic acid	7.0**
Wy 41770	9.1
Fenofibric acid	34.0

* determined at pH 7.0 at 37°
** determined at pH 7.4 at 37°

(for references see Weil, 1987)

role in the allergenicity of zomepirac has been proposed - but it seems unreasonable to condemn them as a class on the present evidence. Furthermore, the relationship between aglycone structure and glucuronide reactivity is obscure at present, further hindering "predictive toxicology". Like other potential reactive metabolites, *e.g.* epoxides, ester glucuronides vary very widely in reactivity and must be considered on a case-by-case basis.

Comments

The exposure of human and animal populations to xenobiotic acids and their simple esters is very widespread, and will remain so. The present renewal of interest in the toxicity of acidic compounds may reasonably be expected to lead to both increased use of presently available information and to act as a stimulus for further experimentation.

REFERENCES

Caldwell, J. (1982) in 'Metabolic Basis of Detoxication' (ed. W.B. Jakoby, J.R. Bend & J. Caldwell) Academic Press, New York, p.271.
Caldwell, J. (1984) Biochemical Society Transactions, 12, 9.
Caldwell, J. (1985) in 'Advances in Glucuronide Conjugation' (ed. S. Matern, K.W. Bock & W. Gerok) MTP Press, Lancaster, p.7.
Caldwell, J. & Hutt, A.J. (1986) Progress in Drug Metabolism, 9, 11.
Caldwell, J. & Marsh, M.V. (1983) Biochemical Pharmacology, 32, 1667.
Caldwell, J., Idle, J.R. & Smith, R.L. (1980) in 'Extrahepatic Metabolic of Drugs and Other Foreign Compounds' (ed. T.E. Gram) S.P. Medical, New York, p.435.
Caldwell, J., Williams, R.T., French, M.R. & Bassir, O. (1978) European Journal of Drug Metabolism & Pharmacokinetics, 3, 61.
Conti, A. & Bickel, M.H. (1977) Drug Metabolism Reviews, 6 (1), 1-50.
Dutton, G.J. (1980) 'Glucuronidation of Drugs and Other Xenobiotics', CRC Press, Boca Raton, FL.
Emudianughe, T.S., Caldwell, J., Dixon, P.A.F. & Smith, R.L. (1978) Xenobiotica, 8, 525.
Faed, E.M. (1984) Drug Metabolism Reviews, 15, 1213.
Faed, E.M. & McQueen, D.S. (1978) Clinical and Experimental Pharmacology and Physiology, 5, 195.
Hutt, A.J., Caldwell, J. & Smith, R.L. (1982) Xenobiotica, 12, 601.
James, M.O. (1986) in 'Xenobiotic Conjugation Chemistry', ACS Symposium Series No. 299, p.29.
Killenberg, P.G. & Webster, L.T., Jr. (1980) in 'Enzymic Basis of Detoxication, Vol. II' (ed. W.B. Jakoby), Academic Press, New York, p.141.
Quistad, G.B. (1986) in 'Xenobiotic Conjugation Chemistry', ACS Symposium Series No. 299, p.221.
Quistad, G.B. & Hutson, D.H. (1986) in 'Xenobiotic Conjugation Chemistry', ACS Symposium Series No. 299, p.204.
Sinclair, K.A. & Caldwell, J. (1982) Biochemical Pharmacology, 31, 953.
Stogniew, M. & Fenselau, C. (1982) Drug Metabolism and Disposition, 10, 609.
Van Breemen, R.B. & Fenselau, C. (1985) Drug Metabolism and Disposition, 13, 318.
Van Breemen, R.B. & Fenselau, C. (1986) Drug Metabolism and Disposition, 14, 197.
Van der Waterbeemd, H., Testa, B. & Caldwell, J. (1986) Journal of Pharmacy and Pharmacology, 38, 14.
Weil, A. (1987) Ph.D. Thesis, University of Paris 6.

METABOLIC CLEAVAGE OF AMIDE BONDS

N.N. Sertkaya and J.W. Gorrod

Chelsea Department of Pharmacy,
Kings College London (KQC),
Chelsea Campus, Manresa Road,
London SW3 6LX, U.K.

Amide bonds occur in a number of drugs and other xenobiotics. In some cases, the pharmacological or toxicological properties of the molecule are associated with this function. In other cases, acylation of an amino, imino, or hydrazino group may be considered a detoxication reaction. Deacetylases are key enzymes in the conversion of amide carcinogens into amine carcinogens (Booth & Boyland, 1964; Miller et al., 1964; Kadlubar, 1987). Acetylation of aromatic amines often alters the site of metabolic hydroxylation of the ring system compared to the parent amine (Gorrod & Manson, 1986). Cleavage of these amide bonds can clearly alter the above situations and therefore this process is important in any study of the metabolism and toxicology of nitrogenous foreign compounds. Amide bonds can occur in a variety of chemical environments; they can be part of an aliphatic system as in mercapturic acids or the nitrogen can be adjacent to an aromatic ring system as in acetanilide, or part of a sulphonamide or hydrazide group. The acyl group can vary both in the chain length and in the degree of branching. The commonest acyl group utilized in a phase 2 process is the acetyl, although formylation and succinylation have been reported.

Carboxyl groups also form amide bonds during conjugation with amino acids (Killenberg & Webster, 1980) and cyclic amides can occur as the result of metabolic oxidation of cyclic amines (Gorrod, 1987). In the following paper, we comment upon the cleavage of these amide bonds.

The enzymes involved in the deacetylation of arylamides are classified as carboxylesterases (Krisch, 1971; Heymann 1980; Mentlein et al., 1987). These enzymes in addition to catalysing the hydrolysis of endogenous esters, also hydrolyse drug or xenobiotic esters. Of the carboxylesterases exhibiting arylamide deacetylating activity, the non-specific acetanilide/phenacetin hydrolysing enzyme [ES-3, lysophospholipase (PI 5.6); Mentlein et al., 1987] appears to be the most active. However, other carboxylesterases such as ES-4, ES8/10 and ES-15 (Mentlein et al., 1987) may also participate in arylamide deacetylation. To complicate matters further, some carboxylesterases are reported to occur as several isozymes (Krisch, 1971; Heymann & Junge, 1979; Mentlein & Heymann, 1984) each of which may exhibit slightly different substrate specificities. Inhibitors can facilitate the characterisation of the multiple forms of carboxylesterases (amidases) and a number of agents have been used for this purpose, including inorganic fluoride (Irving, 1966; Jarvinen et al., 1971) and SKF-525A (Bernhammer & Krisch 1965; Benohr and Krisch, 1967; Gorrod, 1979). Clearly these agents cannot be regarded as inhibitors of any specific carboxylesterases. The organophosphate esters are regularly used as inhibitors of N-deacetylation, however, these compounds are non-selective in terms of substrate specificity. Paraoxon has been used to classify esterases into two classes (A and B) by their sensitivity to this agent (Aldridge, 1952; Brandt et al., 1980). This organophosphate is extensively used as an inhibitor of all serine esterases including carboxylesterases (Brandt et al., 1980). Bis-p-(nitrophenyl) phosphate (BNPP) is reported to be a selective inhibitor of acetanilide deacetylase in rat liver (Baumann et al., 1984) but it is also a potent inhibitor of AAF deacetylase in rabbit liver (Aune et al., 1985). One esterase inhibitor that appears to selectively inhibit a specific enzyme is bis(4-cyanophenyl)phosphate. This inhibitor was found to completely inhibit <u>in vivo</u> and <u>in vitro</u> the rat acetanilide-cleaving esterase [ES-3, PI 5.6; Mentlein & Heymann, 1984]. Bis (4-cyanophenyl)phosphate may therefore prove useful in characterising the esterase(s) involved in arylamide deacetylation.

Gorrod (1971) and Sertkaya & Gorrod (1987) investigated the effects of isomeric arylamide configuration on the rate of N-deacetylation in a number of mammalian species. The data obtained with the positional isomers of acetamidobiphenyl clearly demonstrated that the hepatic microsomal deacetylation rate (in addition to species differences) is influenced by the substrate structure. The deacetylation rates were generally in the order of 2-AABP>3-AABP>4-AABP. In a recent investigation into the hepatic deacetylation of ortho-, meta- and para-substituted acetophenetidines and acetamidophenols, the o-substituted compounds were deacetylated more rapidly than m-analogues, whereas p-structures were also only poor to moderate substrates (Baumann et al., 1984). Estus & Mieyal (1983) investigated the rate of N-deacetylation of a homologous series of alkoxy acetanilides and their N-hydroxy derivatives. The deacetylation rates increased with increasing chain length of the alkoxy group; the deacetylation of the N-hydroxy derivatives proceeded at approximately one hundred times the rate of hydrolysis of the parent amides.

It is clear that deacetylation of arylamides is influenced by the physico-chemical properties of the amide. Increasing deacetylation rates have been observed for the hydrolysis of substituted acylanilides with increasing lipophilicity of the acyl function (Echert et al., 1970; Heymann, 1982). This in turn may depend upon the intracellular distribution of the enzyme, with membrane associated enzymes being only accessible to lipophilic substrates. Although the acetanilide/phenacetin hydrolysing enzyme was early obtained in a highly purified form (Krisch, 1963), it was only recently that this enzyme was positively characterised as a ES-3 carboxylesterase (Mentlein & Heymann, 1984). Kiese & Renner (1966) extensively studied the hydrolysis of acetanilide, phenacetin and several other compounds using hepatic microsomes and cytoplasm obtained from rabbit, guinea pig, dog and cat. The ratio of activities towards different amide substrates varied considerably depending on the animal species. Simple anilides are considered poor substrates (Arndt et al., 1978) for the carboxylesterases. Heymann and Krisch (1969) reported that acetanilide and phenacetin induced methaemoglobinemia was greatly reduced by concomitant

I.P. administration of BNPP. More recently Grossman and Jollow (1986) reported that deacetylation plays a significant role in the disposition of acetanilide, as pretreating rats with BNPP prior to acetanilide administration, greatly reduced the formation of aniline from acetanilide. The marked species differences observed in phenacetin mutagenicity was reported to be due to the differences in deacetylating activity between rat and hamster liver microsomes (Nohmi et al., 1983).

Recently, Newton et al., (1985) proposed that deacetylase dependent activation was an essential step in the pathogenesis of acetaminophen induced renal cortical necrosis. A mammalian liver N-deacetylase enzyme has been investigated in mouse, rat, hamster, guinea pig and dog (Irving, 1966; Jarvinen et al., 1971; Gorrod, 1971). This enzyme(s) is reported to be responsible for N-deacetylation of various arylacetamides such as 4-AABP, 2-AAF and 2-AAN (Lower & Bryan, 1973; Brodie & Axelrod, 1948). Deacetylase activity is not confined to the liver as significant levels of microsomal deacetylase activity have been identified in Syrian hamster intestine, lung, kidney but not bladder tissue (Hein et al., 1986). Intestinal microflora are also capable of effecting the N-deacetylation of a number of compounds structurally related to phenacetin *in vitro* (Smith & Griffith, 1974) and this process may be significant *in vivo*.

It is apparent that most mammalian species have multiple forms of carboxylesterases. There appears to be 10-15 carboxylesterases in each mammal (Mentlein et al, 1987) with some enzymes expressed as several isozymes. Two N-deacetylase enzyme systems have been proposed for the mouse, a microsomal N-deacetylase which is more specific for monoarylamides and a cytosolic N-deacetylase which is more specific for diarylamides (Glinsukon et al., 1980). Recently, Hein et al. (1986) reported acetylator-related genetic control of both microsomal AAF and N-OH-AAF deacetylase activity in the mouse. Jarvinen et al., (1971) reported two guinea pig N-deacetylase enzymes: the larger of the two enzymes was more effective in the deacetylation of N-hydroxy-and the smaller enzyme was more effective at hydrolysing AAF. One enzyme also hydrolysed 2-acetylaminonaphthalene at twice the rate of hydrolysis of the 1-isomer, whereas the other enzyme hydrolysed the 1-isomer five times faster than the 2-isomer. The larger enzyme is absent in the rat (Glowinski et al., 1983) and this species only hydrolyses N-OH-AAF slowly. Heymann et al., (1972) and Junge & Heymann (1979) have suggested that the pig liver enzymes in their native forms are mixtures of numerous hybrids of at least three protein subunits which have slightly different primary sequences. It is possible that Jarvinen et al., (1971) isolated both a monomeric and polymeric form of guinea pig carboxylesterase (Steward & Floyd, 1980).

N-Deacetylation of arylamides is not confined to mammals; it has been reported for plants (Brooks 1984), avians (Mull & Giri, 1972), cestodes (Douch & Gahagan, 1976) and nematodes. The nematode Ascaris lumbricoides var suum deacetylates acetanilide; this process is inhibited by organophosphates and p-chloro mercuribenzoate (Douch & Gahagan, 1977). This enzyme was predominately present in the cytoplasmic fraction and contrary to the mammalian enzymes hydrolysed para substituted acetanilides faster than the corresponding ortho analogues.

The malathion derivative dimethoate (Brooks, 1984) possesses an N-methylcarboxamide group (Uchida & O'Brien, 1967) which facilitates rapid amidase hydrolysis in vertebrates, thereby offering the non-target organism an opportunity to detoxify the molecule. The N-demethylation of dimethoate gives the primary amide with a relatively greater increase in toxicity towards houseflies than to mice and consequently an improvement in mammalian selectivity ratio (Lucier & Menzer, 1970). Inhibitors of carboxylesterases which may be present as contaminants in preparations of these organophosphates (Toia et al., 1980; Ali & Fukuto, 1982) can present a serious hazard to mammals.

An enzyme isolated from sheep hepatic microsomes and classified as an "alkylamidase", catalysed the in vitro hydrolysis of dimethoate (Chen & Dauterman, 1971). It is evident that this enzyme is a B-type serine carboxylesterase/amidase isozyme (Heymann, 1982). The hydrolytic metabolism of dimethoate has been reviewed by Ecobichon (1977). The herbicide propanil is believed to be activated in vivo by α-hydroxylation of the side-chain ethyl group. This reaction competes with hydrolytic attack by an arylacylamidase to give the corresponding non-herbicidal aniline derivative (Still & Herrett, 1975). Propanil is reported to be hydrolysed by liver carboxylesterase (Singleton & Murphy, 1973) with the formation of a toxic product. The phosphorothiolate fungicides such as kitazin-P inhibit the propanil hydrolysing amidases of rice (Uesugi et al, 1974) and it may be useful to investigate the effects of phosphorothiolates on mammalian amidases as an aid in their differentiation.

Hydrolysis of an N-formyl xenobiotic has been observed with 4'-chloro-o-methylformanilide (Ahmad & Fargash, 1976) and may be mediated via the enzyme that hydrolyses N-formylkynurenine in the tryptophan to niacin pathway. A relatively specific serine hydrolase (formamidase) from the soluble fraction of rat hepatocytes has been implicated in the hydrolytic metabolism of chlordimeform and formatenate (Ahmad & Forgash, 1976; Arndt et al., 1973). Herbicides of the carbanilate type are believed to be hydrolysed by B-type carboxylesterases in rat liver and plasma of various mammals including man (Sonaware & Knowles, 1972). The miticide N-methyl-N-(1-naphthyl)-monofluoroacetamide (MNFA; Hashimoto et al., 1968) is hydrolysed to form N-methyl-1-naphthylamine and fluroacetate (Noguchi et al., 1968). Liver homogenate prepared from the guinea pig was found to hydrolyse MNFA thirty five times faster than similar rat or mouse preparations. It is suggested that the hydrolysis of MNFA may be carried out principally by the smaller N-deacetylase isozyme described for the guinea pig by Jarvinen et al., 1971.

Hydrolysis of the side-chain amide bond or the lactam bond of penicillins has been observed with bacterial enzymes (Balasingham et al., 1972; Findlater & Orsi, 1974). Penicillin acylase not only hydrolyses the amide side-chain of penicillins but also hydrolyses certain cephalosporins (Cole, 1969) and a variety of acylamino acids, amides and esters. Combination therapy with β-lactam antibiotics and β-lactamase inhibitors such as clavulanic acid is useful as a means of combating bacterial resistance to β-lactam antibiotics (Parker & Eggleston, 1987; Campoli-Richards & Brogden, 1987). An enzyme capable of cleaving some penicillins and isocarboxazide has been isolated from guinea pig liver microsomes (Satoh & Moroi, 1972).

A major chloramphenicol metabolite excreted in the urine, is the corresponding free amine. Hydrolysis of the amide bond in chloramphenicol has been demonstrated in a number of organisms including man, bacteria (Vining, 1975) and mice (Hill & Struck, 1973). The chloramphenicol hydrolysing enzyme has been reported to be sensitive to organophosphates (Junge & Krisch, 1975) and more recently the enzyme obtained from guinea pig liver was characterised as a B-type carboxylesterase isozyme (Heymann, 1982). Chloramphenicol contains a dichloracetyl moiety as part of the amide group; previously Nimmo-Smith (1960) had shown that mono or dichloro substitution of an acetyl group greatly influences the rate of hydrolysis of the compound compared to that of the parent acetamide.

The in vivo deacylation of a number of N-acylated sulphonamides has been reported (Krebs et al., 1947; Bridges & Williams, 1963; Webber, 1971). A deacetylase present in the chicken kidney that hydrolyses N^4-acetylated sulfonamides has been described (Shaffer & Beiter, 1950). This enzyme is present in various birds (Mill & Giri, 1972). Franklin et al., (1969) found that the soluble fraction from rat kidney deacetylated p-acetamido benzoic acid to a greater extent than acetanilide, but did not deacetylate N^4-acetylsulphonilamide. This data suggests that N^4-acetysulphonilamide is hydrolysed by an isozyme or enzyme distinct from the B-carboxylesterase/amidase reported for acetanilide (Mentlein & Heymann, 1984).

Isocarboxazid is hydrolysed to form benzylhydrazine by a mammalian liver amidase. This enzyme was isolated from the guinea pig (Satoh & Moroi, 1972) and, in vitro was found to preferentially hydrolyse isocarboxazid. Other amides such as phenathicillin, propicillin and L-alanyl-β-naphthylamine are also hydrolysed. The enzyme is inhibited by both p-chloromercuribenzoate and organophosphates (Satoh & Moroi, 1973) and is reported to be induced by phenobarbitone in rats and mice but not in guinea pigs or rabbits (Kaur & Ali, 1983). Mentlein et al., (1987) have proposed that this enzyme is the ES-8/ES-10 serine carboxylesterase. Isoniazid (isonicotinic acid hydrazide) which is acetylated, has been extensively studied, due to the widespread use of this anti-tubercular drug and the genetic control of its acetylation (Weber, 1967). It is now recognised that hydrolysis of this metobalite to yield N-acetylhydrazine is a major determinant of its hepatic toxicity of (Nelson et al., 1975). The sedative/hypnotic N-acetylbromodiethylacetylurea (N-acetylcarbromal) has been reported to be hydrolysed in rabbit liver microsomes by a serine hydrolase that is inhibited by paraoxon (Kaeferstein et al., 1974). Hollunger (1960) reported that lidocaine is hydrolysed by a microsomal amidase that showed greater activity towards the monodeethylated derivative of lidocaine. Lidocaine proved to be a competitive inhibitor of the monoethylglycine-2,6-xylidide- cleaving enzyme. The membrane-bound microsomal enzyme was less strongly inhibited by SKF-525A than the solubilized form (Hollunger, 1960). The local anaesthetic butanilicain is a very good substrate for the highly purified carboxylesterase isolated from pig liver microsomes (Junge & Heymann, 1979). The amide bond of butanilicain is also cleaved by isoenzymes from rat liver (Arndt et al., 1973; 1978), and human liver (Junge & Krisch, 1975) at high rates.

The benzodiazepines are today amongst the most widely used drugs in the world. As a chemical group a large number undergo hydrolytic cleavage to form ring opened metabolites. Lorazepam undergoes ring opening to form 2-amino-2,5-dichlorobenzophenone in dogs, pigs, and cats (Schillings et al., 1971). Rat urinary metabolites of oxazepam include the ring opened 2-amino-5-chloro-benzophenone and 2-amino-5-chloro-4'-hydroxy-benzophenone (Yasumura et al, 1971). Chlordiazepoxide undergoes hydrolytic cleavage in dogs and man to form the ring-opened metabolite N-(2- amino-5-chloro-phenyl-benzylidine)-glycine-N-oxide, which was excreted as such or as alkali-labile conjugates (Koechlin et al, 1965). Conversely, the benzodiazepine "450191-S" was developed as a ring-opened derivative of a triazolobenzodiazepine (Hirai & Sugimoto, 1979). In experimental animals, this compound has strong sleep-inducing, anxiolytic and anticonvulsant effects. The active metabolites are ring closed compounds (Fujimoto et al., 1984; Koike et al, 1987).

Bray and co-workers reported (1949) that many primary amides of aliphatic and aromatic carboxylic acids underwent hydrolysis in the presence of crude liver extracts. Amidases which hydrolyse 2-3 carbon amides have been reported in microorganisms (Jakoby & Fredericks, 1964). Chen and Dauterman (1971) purified a carboxylesterase from sheep liver microsomes that hydrolysed the lower members of a series of N-methyl-substituted amides, reaching a maximum activity with N-methylcaproamide. The amidase, purified to homogeneity by Hersh (1971), is reported to catalyse the hydrolysis of the amides of glutamate and succinate. Mercapturic acids have been reported to be mutagenic in bacterial tester systems (Inskeep & Guengerich, 1984; Vamvakas et al., 1987). The mutagenicity of S-pentachlorobutadienyl-N-acetylcysteine was reported by Wild et al., (1986). It is apparent that this mercapturic acid is hydrolysed by a bacterial amidase (Jakoby & Fredericks, 1964) to form the corresponding cysteine conjugate; this is then cleaved by β-lyase to form mutagenic metabolites (Wild et al., 1986, Elfarra & Anders, 1984). Mammals are also capable of hydrolysing the amide bond of mercapturic acids. Enzymes carrying out this reaction have been reported in a number of species and tissues (Tateishi, 1983) including rat liver and kidney (Suzuki & Tateishi, 1981). The enzyme identified in rat liver exhibits a high specificity for aromatic mercapturic acids and is largely inactive against aliphatic substituents. The rat renal enzyme hydrolyses both aliphatic and aromatic mercapturic acids. An enzyme which hydrolyses S-alkyl mercapturic acids with low activity towards S-aralkyl and S-aryl conjugates has been identified in rat liver and isolated from hog liver (Tateishi, 1983). Recently, Vamvakas et al., (1987) demonstrated that mercapturic acids can be deacetylated by rat renal and hepatic enzymes.

The heterocyclic ring of a number of cyclic amides can be cleaved hydrolytically by dihydropyramidase (Maguire & Dudley 1977; Dudley et al., 1974). The cyclic amides succinimide, glutarimide and adipimide are ring opened by this enzyme to give the corresponding acid (Maguire & Dudley, 1978). Succinimide was found to be a poor but definite substrate, but the introduction of a phenyl group in the α-position (α-phenylsuccinimide) enhanced the ability of the enzyme to cleave this ring system. Ring opening of some 5-alkylhydantoins was reported by Dudley & Roberts (1978), who demonstrated that only the (R)-isomer of 5-methylhydantoin or 5-isopropylhydantoin were substrates (Maguire et al., 1982). The enzyme is also reported to catalyse the ring opening of hydantoin (Walach & Grisolia, 1957), 5-phenylhydantoin (Dudley et al., 1974) and dihydro-5-fluorouracil (Mukherjee & Heidelberger, 1960). The antiepileptic drug phensuximide undergoes N-dealkylation, para-hydroxylation of the phenyl ring and cleavage of the succinimide ring (Dudley et al., 1972).

The analgesic propiram (N-1-methyl-2-piperidinoethyl)-N-(2-pyridylpropionamide gives as a ring opened major metabolite N-2-(2-pyridylamino)propyl-N-propionyl-5-aminovaleric acid in rats (Duhm et al., 1974). The imidazolidine ring of clonidine is reported to be hydrolytically cleaved (Darda et al., 1978).

Indeloxazine, a potential antidepressant, undergoes degradation of the morpholine ring (Kamimura et al., 1987). It has been suggested that this may occur via the formation of a carbinolamine. Cotinine, which is formed via a carbinolamine, has been shown to be an early primary metabolite of nicotine in a number of animal species (Gorrod & Jenner, 1975). Castro et al., (1980) reported that cotinine undergoes ring opening of the pyrrolidine ring to give 4-(3-pyridyl)-4-methylaminobutyric acid. The hypotensive agent guanethidine was found to undergo ring opening in humans to form 2-(6-carboxyhexylamino)-ethylguanidine (McMartin & Simpson, 1971). This process may very well involve hydrolysis of a cyclic amide bond formed by the metabolic oxidation of the cyclic tertiary amine.

It can be seen that a number of enzymes are capable of cleaving the -CONH-bond. This bond may be part of an original xenobiotic or be formed during the metabolism of a compound. At the present time, it is not possible to present an authoritative statement as to the substrate specificity of any one enzyme in different species. It is clear that the situation is complex and that amide forming and cleaving enzymes both play a role in the overall metabolic pattern of many foreign compounds. In this review we have tried to indicate the wide variety of chemical structures which are known substrates for these hydrolytic processes but have not, in the space available, given every example. Many of the processes are involved in either initiating or terminating pharmacological and toxicological responses and are well worthy of further study.

Lastly, it should be recalled that amide bond cleavage can be used in the prodrug approach, but until the complete structure activity relationships of amide hydrolysing enzymes are established the risk of undesirable effects remain.

Nevertheless, certain compounds have been administered as the inactive, more soluble N-acylated form which are subsequently hydrolysed to give the active drug, for example, bis (N-n-propylaminoacetyl)-4,4'-diaminodiphenyl sulphone is hydrolyzed to 4,4'-diaminodiphenylsulphone which is used in the treatment of leprosy (Eckert et al., 1970).

Acknowledgement: Dr. N.N. Sertkaya is currently supported by a Sigma Tau Career Development Fellowship tenable in the Chelsea Department of Pharmacy.

REFERENCES:

Ahmad, S. & Forgash, A.J., 1976, Drug Metabolism Reviews, 5, 141.

Aldridge, W.N., 1953, Biochemical Journal, 53, 110.

Ali, F.A.F. & Fukuto, T.R., 1982, Journal of Agricultural & Food Chemistry, 30, 126.

Allahyari, R. & Fukuto, T.R., 1980, Journal of Agricultural & Food Chemistry, 28, 599.

Arndt, R., Junge, W., Michelsen, K. & Krisch, K., 1973, Hoppe Seylers Zeitschrift fur Physiologische Chemie, 354, 1583.

Arndt, R, Schlaak, H.E., Uschtrin, D. & Sudi, D., Michelssen, K., & Junge, W., 1978, Hoppe Seylers Zeitschrift fur Phsyiologische Chemie, 359, 644.

Aune, T., Vanderslice, R.R., Croft, J.E., Dybing, E., Bend, J.R. & Philpot, R. M., 1985, Cancer Research, 45, 5859.

Balasingham, K., Warburton, D., Dunnill, P. & Lilly, M. D., 1972, Biochimica et Biophysica Acta, 276, 250.

Baumann, J., Bruchhausen, F. & Wurm, G., 1984, Arzneimittel Forschung, 34, 1278.

Sertkaya, N.N. & Gorrod, J.W., 1987, Anti-Cancer Research, (in the press).

Benohr, H.C. & Krisch, K., 1967, Zeitschrift fur Physiologische Chemie, 348, 1102.

Bernhammer, E. & Krisch, K., 1965, Biochemical Pharmacology, 14, 863.

Brant, E., Heymann, E. & Mentlein, R., 1980, Biochemical Pharmacology, 29, 1927.

Bridges, J.W. & Williams, R.T., 1963, Biochemical Journal, 87, 19.

Brodie, B.B. & Axelrod, J., 1948, The Journal of Pharmacology and Experimental Therapeutics, 94,22.

Brooks, G.T., 1984, Metabolism and Pesticide Design, Vol. 8, edited by J.W. Bridges & L.F. Chasseaud, Taylor & Francis Ltd., P. 101, In Progress in Drug Metabolism.

Campoli-Richards, D.M. & Brogden, R.N., 1987, Drugs, 33, 577.

Castro, A., Monji, N., Ali, H., Y.I., J.I., Bowman, E.R. & McKennis, H., 1980, European Journal of Biochemistry, 104, 331.

Cher, P.R.S. & Dauterman, W.C., 1971, Biochimica et Biophysica Acta, 250, 216.

Cole, M., 1969a, Biochemical Journal, 115, 33.

Cole, M., 1969b, Biochemical Journal, 115, 47.

Cundy, K.C. & Crooks, P.A., 1987, Xenobiotica, 17, 785.

Darda, S., Forster, H.J., & Stahle, H., 1978, Arzneimittel Forschung, 28, 255.

Dudley, K.H., Bius, D.L. & Grace, M.E., 1972, The Journal of Pharmacology and Experimental Therapeutics, 180, 167.

Dudley, K.H. Butler, T.C. & Bius, D.L., 1974, Drug Metabolism and Disposition, 2, 103.

Dudley, K.H. & Roberts, S.B., 1978, Drug Metabolism and Disposition, 6, 133.

Dudley, K.H. & Buis, D.L., 1976, Drug Metabolism and Disposition, 4, 340.

Douch, P.G.C. & Gahagan, H. M., 1976, Xenobiotica, 6, 769.

Douch, P.G.C. & Gahagan, H.M., 1977, Xenobiotica, 7, 309.

Duhm, B., Maul, W., Medenwald, H., Patzschke, K. & Wegner, L.A., 1974, Arzneimittel Forschung, 24, 632.

Eckert, T., Reimann, I. & Krisch, K., 1970, Arzneimittel Forschung, 20, 487.

Ecobichon, D.J., 1977, Hydrolytic transformation of environmental pollutants. In Handbook of Physiology. Section 1: Reactions to Environmental Agents, Edited by D.H.K. Lee, Williams & Wilkins, Baltimore, Maryland, P.441.

Estus, G.S. & Mieyal, J.J., 1983, Drug Metabolism & Disposition 11, 471.

Elfarra, A.A., Jakobson, I. & Anders, M.W., 1986, Biochemical Pharmacology, 35, 283.

Findlater, J.D. & Orsi, B.A., 1974, Analytical Biochemistry, 58, 294.

Franklin, M.R., Bridges, J.W. & Williams, R.T., 1969, Biochemical Journal, 114, 6.

Franklin, M.R., Bridges, J.W. & Williams, R.T., 1971, Xenobiotica, 1, 121.

Fujiimoto, M., Hashimoto, S., Takahashi, S., Hirose, K., Hatakeyama, H. & Okabayashi, T., 1984, Biochemical pharmacology, 33, 145.

Glinsukon, T., Lookyee, A., Toskulkao, C. & Shank, R.C., 1980, Biochemical Pharmacology, 29, 1189.

Glowinski, I.B., Savage, L., Lee, M. & King, C.M., 1983, Carcinogenesis, 4, 67.

Gorrod, J.W., 1971, Biochemical Journal, 123, 10p.

Gorrod, J.W. & Jenner, P., 1975, The Metabolism of tobacco alkaloids In Essays in Toxicology. Vol. 6, edited by W.J. Hayes, Academic Press, New York p.35.

Gorrod, J.W., 1979 PhD Thesis, University of London, P.138.

Gorrod, J.W., 1987, This Volume.

Gorrod, J.W. & Manson, D., 1986, Xenobiotica, 16, 933.

Grossman, S.J. & Jollow, D.J., 1986, Drug Metabolism & Disposition, 14, 689.

Hashimoto, Y. Makita, T., Miyata, H., Noguchi , T. & Ohta, G., 1968, Toxicology and Applied Pharmacology, 12,536.

Hashimoto, Y., Noguchi, T., Mori, T. & Kitagawa, H., 1968, Toxicology and Applied Pharmacology, 13, 174.

Hatakeyama, H. & Okabayashi, T., 1984, Biochemical Pharmacology, 33,145.

Hein, D.W., Kirlin, W.G., Ogolla, F., Trinidad, A., Thompson, L.K. & Ferguson, R.J., 1986, Drug Metabolism & Disposition, 14, 566.

Hersh, L.B., 1971, Biochemistry, 10, 2884.

Heymann, E. & Krisch, K., 1969, Biochemical Pharmacology, 18, 801.

Heymann, E. & Junge, W., 1979, European Journal of Biochemistry, 95, 509.

Heymann, E., 1980, Carboxylesterases and amidases. In Enzymatic Basis of Detoxication, Vol. 2, edited by W.B. Jakoby, Academic Press, New York. p.291.

Heymann, E., 1982, Metabolic basis of Detoxication, In Hydrolysis of Carboxylic Ester and Amides, Chapter 12, edited by W.B. Jakoby, J.R. Bend & J. Caldwell, Academic Press, New York p.229.

Hill, D.F. & Struck, R.F. 1973, Biochemical Pharmacology, 22, 127.

Hirai, K. & Sugimoto, H., 1979, U.S. Patent, 4, 159, 374.

Hollunger, G., 1960, *Acta Pharmacologica et Toxicologica*, 17, 374.

Irving, C.C., 1966, *Cancer Research*, 26, 1390.

Inskeep, P.B. & Guengerich, F.P., 1984, *Carcinogenesis*, 5, 805.

Jakoby, W.B. & Fredericks, J., 1964, *Journal of Biological Chemistry*, 239, 1978.

Jarvinen, M., Santti, R.S.S. & Hopsu-Havu, V.K., 1971, *Biochemical Pharmacology*, 20, 2971.

Junge, W. & Krisch, K., 1975, *CRC Critical Reviews in Toxicology*, 3, 371.

Junge, W. & Heymann, E., 1979, *European Journal of Biochemistry*, 95, 519.

Kadlubar, F.F., 1987, *ISI Atlas of Science*, 129.

Kaferstein, H. & Sticht, G., 1974, *Arzneimittel Forschung*, 24, 1619.

Kamimura, H., Enjoji, Y., Sasaki, H., Kawai, R., Kaniwa, H., Niigata, K. & Kageyama, S., 1987, *Xenobiotica*, 17, 645. Kaur, S. & Ali, B., 1983, *Biochemical Pharmacology*, 32, 3479.

Kellenberg, P.G. & Webster L.T., 1980, Conjugation by Peptide Bond Formation In *Enzymatic Basis of Detoxification*, Vol.2, edited by W.B. Jakoby, Academic Press, U.S.A., p.141.

Kiese, M. & Renner, G., 1966, *Archive der Pharmakologie de Experimental Pathologie*, 252, 480.

Krebs, H.A., Sykes, W.O. & Bartley, W.C., 1947, *Biochemistry*, 41, 622.

Koechlin, B.A., Schwartz, M.A., Krol, G. & Oberhansli, W., 1965, *Journal Pharmacology*, 148, 399.

Koike, M., Norikura, R., Futaguchi, S., Yamaguchi, T., Sugeno, K., Iwatani, K., Ikenishi, Y. & Nakagawa, Y., 1987, *Drug Metabolism & Disposition*, 15, 426.

Krisch, K., 1971, In *The Enzymes, 3rd ed.*, Vol. 5, edited by P.D. Boyer, Academic Press, New York, p.43.

Lower, G.M. & Bryan, G.T., 1973, *Biochemical Pharmacology*, 22, 1581.

Lower, G.M. & Bryan, G.T. 1976, *Journal of Toxicology and Environmental Health*, 1, 421.

Lucier, G.W. & Menzer, R.E., 1970, *Journal of Agricultural & Food Chemistry*, 18, 698.

Maguire, J.H. & Dudley, K.H., 1977, *Analytical Chemistry*, 49, 292.

Maguire, J.H. & Dudley, K.H., 1978, *Drug Metabolism & Disposition*, 6, 140.

Maguire, J.H., Butler, T.C. & Dudley, K.H., 1982, Drug Metabolism & Disposition, 10, 595.
McMartin, C. & Simpson, P., 1971, Clinical Pharmacology & Therapeutics, 12, 73.
Mentlein, R. & Heymann, E., 1984, Biochemical Pharmacology, 33, 1243.
Mentlein, R., Reuter, G. & Heymann, E., 1985, Archives of Biochemistry & Biophysics, 240, 801.
Mentlein, R. & Heymann, E., 1987, Biochemical Journal, (in the press).
Miller, E.C., Miller, J.A. & Enomoto, M., 1964, Cancer Research, 24, 2018.
Mull, R.L. & Giri, S.N., 1972, Biochimica et Biophysica Acta, 273, 222.
Mukherjee, K.L. & Heidelberger, C., 1960, Journal of Biological Chemistry, 235, 433.
Nakagawa, Y., 1987, Drug Metabolism and Disposition, 15, 426.
Newton, J.F., Pasino, D.A. & Hook, J.B., 1985, Toxicology and Applied Phamacology, 78, 39.
Nelson, S.D., Snodgrass, W.R. & Mitchell, J.R., 1975, Federation Proceedings, 34, 784.
Nimmo-Smith, R.H., 1960, Biochemical Journal, 75, 284.
Noguchi, T., Yashinobu, H. & Miyata, H., 1968, Toxicology & Applied Pharmacology, 13, 189.
Parker, R.H. & Eggleston, M., 1987, Infection Control, 8, 36.
Satoh, T. & Moroi, K., 1972, Biochemical Pharmacology, 21, 3111.
Satoh, T. & Moroi, K., 1973, Life Sciences, 12, 169.
Satoh, T., 1973, Life Sciences, 13, 1181.
Schillings, R.T., Shrader, S.R. & Ruelius, H.W., 1971, Arzneimittel Forschung, 21, 1059.
Schut, H.A.J., Wirth, P.J. & Thorgeirsson, S.S., 1978, Molecular Pharmacology, 14, 682.
Shaffer, J.M. & Bieter, R.N., 1950, Journal Pharmacology, 100, 192.
Singleton, S.D. & Murphy, S.D., 1973, Toxicology & Applied Pharmacology, 25, 20.
Smith, G.E. & Griffiths, L.A., 1976, Xenobiotica, 6, 217.
Sonawane, B.R. & Knowles, C.O., 1972, Pesticide Biochemical Physiology, 1, 472.
Steward, J.E. & Floyd, R.A., 1980, Cancer Biochemistry and Biophysics, 5, 47.

Stil, G.G. & Herrett, R.A., 1975, In Herbicide Chemistry , Degradation and Mode of Action, Vol. 2, edited by P.C. Kearney & D.D. Kaufman, Marcel Dekker, New York P. 609.

Suzuki, S. & Tateishi, M., 1981, Drug Metabolism & Disposition, 9, 573.

Tateishi, M., 1983, Drug Metabolism Reviews, 14, 1207.

Toia, R.F., March, R.B., Umetsu, M, Mallipudi, N.M., Allahydri, R. & Fukuto, T.R., 1980, Journal of Agricultural & Food Chemistry 28, 599.

Uchida, T. & O'Brien, R.D., 1967, Toxicology and Applied Pharmacology, 10, 89.

Uesugi, Y., Katagiri, M. & Noda, O., 1974, Agricultural & Biochemical Chemistry, 38,907.

Vamvakas, S., Dekant, W., Berthold, K., Schmidt, S., Wild, D. & Henschler, D., 1987, Biochemical Pharmacology, 36, 2741.

Vining, L.C., 1975, Methods in Enzymology, 43, 734.

Wallach, D.P. & Grisolia, S., 1957, Journal of Biological Chemistry, 226, 277.

Weber, W.W. & Cohen, S.N., 1967, Molecular Pharmacology, 3, 266.

Weber, W.W., 1971, In Handbook of Experimental Pharmacology, Acetylating, Deacetylating and Amino Acid Conjugating Enzymes, Vol. 28, edited by B.B. Brodie & J. Gillette, Springer-Verlag, Berlin, p.565.

Wild, D., Schutz, S. & Reichert, D., 1986, Carcinogenesis, 7, 431.

Yasumura, A., Muratta, H., Hattori, K. & Matsuda, K., 1971, Chemical & Pharmaceutical Bulletin, (Japan) 19, 1929.

6. Phase 2 processes as toxication reactions

THE GENERATION OF REACTIVE INTERMEDIATES FROM XENOBIOTICS BY SULFATE CONJUGATION, AND THEIR ROLE IN DRUG TOXICITY

GERARD J. MULDER, E. DINANT KROESE AND JOHN H.N. MEERMAN

Division of Toxicology, Center for Bio-Pharmaceutical Sciences, University of Leiden, Leiden, The Netherlands.

For many types of substrates, sulfation means the generation of conjugates that have lost the pharmacological and toxic properties of the parent compound. The reason for this most likely is that a highly hydrophilic, anionic sulfate group has been introduced into the molecule, so that the resulting conjugate does not fit any more in the binding site of the receptor for the parent compound.

In certain cases, however, the position of the sulfate group is apparently far away from the receptor-bound part of the molecule, so that sulfation does not have any effect on the biological activities of the compound. Thus, sulfate conjugates of some cholestatic bile salts are as cholestatic as the unconjugated form (Vonk et al, 1981).

GENERATION OF REACTIVE INTERMEDIATES BY SULFATION: N-HYDROXY-2-ACETYLAMINOFLUORENE (NOHAAF)

For an increasing number of compounds, however, it has been established in recent years that their sulfation leads to more toxic conjugates, that may cause cell necrosis or chemical carcinogenesis (Mulder et al, 1986). The best studied example of such a compound is NOHAAF. This is a metabolite of the carcinogen, 2-acetylaminofluorene (2AAF), that causes tumors in the liver and at some other sites (Miller, 1978). It is, for instance in the liver, converted to NOHAAF, which subsequently may be sulfated (Fig. 1). It was shown by de Baun et al. (1970) and King & Phillips (1968) that this sulfation leads to a reactive intermediate that binds covalently to protein, RNA or DNA. A reactive nitrenium ion has been postulated as the breakdown product of the sulfate conjugate. It could be shown that the necrosis in the liver that is caused by NOHAAF is due to its sulfation, since the selective sulfation inhibitor, pentachlorophenol (PCP), completely prevented this necrosis in the periportal zone of the liver (Meerman & Mulder, 1981).

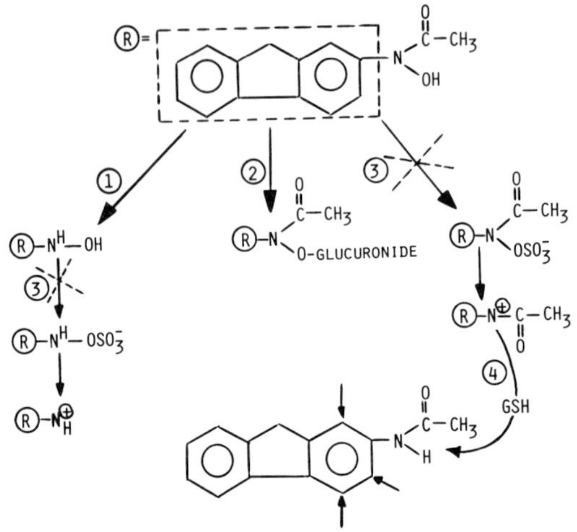

Fig. 1. Some pathways of metabolism of NOHAAF
1 De-acetylation; 2 Glucuronidation; 3 Sulfation;
4 Glutathione conjugates (in 1, 3 or 4 Position:→)
X Pentachlorophenol inhibition.

This confirmed earlier suggestions that the sex difference in hepatotoxicity and hepatocarcinogenicity of 2AAF was due to a much lower sulfation activity in the liver of female than of male rats (Irving, 1971). This is illustrated in Table 1: the metabolism of NOHAAF to the glucuronide and the two glutathione conjugates (the 1- and 3-glutathione conjugates) has been determined in male and female rats in vivo. The glutathione conjugates are derived from the ni-

Table 1. Sex differences in sulfation and glucuronidation in the rat in vivo

Substrate	Glucuronide excreted in males (% of dose ± SEM)	Ratio S/G or GS/G	males	females
NOHAAF	25.9 ± 2.1	GS/G:[a)]	0.51	0.07
p-Nitrophenol	39.4 ± 5.6	S/G:	0.84	0.91
Phenol	46.2 ± 2.8	S/G:	1.15	1.04

[a]S/G = ratio sulfate over glucuronide; GS/G = ratio glutathione conjugates over glucuronide (See Fig. 1). Data from Meerman, et al., (1987).

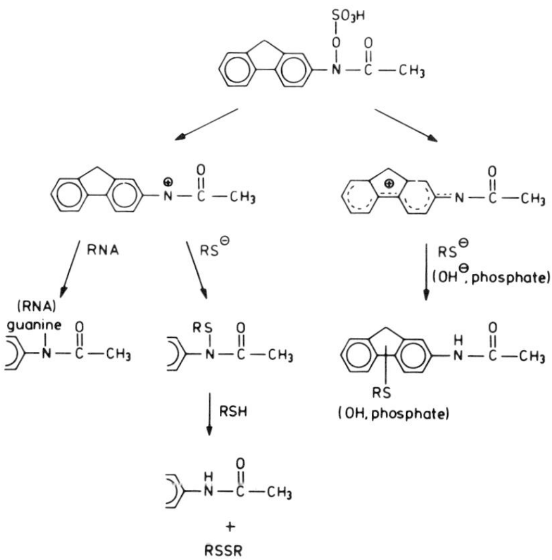

Fig.2 Postulated mechanism of the reaction of AAFSO4 in vitro. The sulfate desintegrates into a delocalized singlet state nitrenium ion and into a localized triplet state nitrenium ion. The "hard" triplet state nitrenium ion prefers to react with "hard" nucleotides, as G in RNA. Besides in the presence of a thiol an N-SR-AAF conjugate will be formed, which is reduced by a second RS^- ion to afford AAF and a disulfide. The "soft" singlet state nitrenium ion will prefer to react with the "softer" RS^- ions to form RS-ring-AAF conjugates. Other negative ions as OH^- or phosphate will compete with the RS^-.
Taken from van den Goorbergh et al (1985), with permission from Carcinogenesis (IRL press).

trenium ion that is formed from the sulfate conjugate (Fig. 1). The results show also that this sex difference is not a general phenomenon for sulfation of all substrates in the rat (Meerman et al, 1987).

The metabolism of NOHAAF is rather complex. Several routes of metabolism have been identified and compete with each other. Even the breakdown of the sulfate conjugate seems to result in more than one reactive form of the nitrenium ion (van den Goorbergh et al, 1985), as shown in Fig 2. This is based on the observation that there is no competition between RNA on one hand, and protein or glutathione on the other hand, for adduct formation from the sulfate conjugate (van den Goorbergh et al, 1985, 1987a). Prevention of RNA adduct formation by glutathione or protein (Table 2) does not result in increased adduct formation to glutathione or protein, but rather to increased formation of 2AAF by some as yet unknown mechanism. To account for these observations we have postulated the scheme as shown in Fig. 2. The sulfate conjugate is assumed to break down to two separate reactive nitrenium ions, possibly one the singlet state, and the other the triplet state. Before these can equilibrate, they react with available nucleophiles to form either adducts or 2AAF. Because of the way RNA and protein/glutathione influence each others reaction it seems unavoidable that two reactive forms have to be postulated. An alternative may be that one form is the nitrenium ion, while the other may be a direct attack of the intact sulfate conjugate of NOHAAF by glutathione.

Table 2. Effect of RNA and bovine serum albumin (BSA) on adduct formation with the sulfate ester of NOHAAF (AAFSO4)

RNA (2.7 mg/ml)	BSA (12 mg/ml)	% of added ^{14}C-AAFSO4 bound to RNA	to BSA
+	-	47 ± 1	-
+	+	23 ± 0	7.6 ± 0.1
-	+	-	8.1 ± 0.2

Data taken from van den Goorbergh et al, 1987b

TRAPPING OF A REACTIVE NITRENIUM ION BY NUCLEOPHILES.

The scheme of Fig. 2 suggests that glutathione would be protective against adduct formation by NOHAAF in vivo, so that depletion of glutathione would increase the covalent binding to protein, RNA and DNA. However, when this hypothesis was tested by pretreatment of rats with diethyl maleate to deplete glutathione, surprisingly no such effect was found: the level of covalent binding was unaffected (Meerman & Tijdens, 1985) in spite of the fact that glutathione had been depleted in these animals.

A tentative explanation for this unexpected phenomenon may be found in the following. When we determined the extent of covalent binding of the chemically synthesized sulfate conjugate of NOHAAF, AAF-SO4, to increasing concentrations of RNA and bovine serum albumin (BSA), we observed a pronounced difference. For RNA the extent of covalent binding of AAF-SO4 increased as expected to 90% of the added amount at 54 mg/ml RNA. However, for protein covalent binding was much lower, and showed a maximum of only 9.5 % bound at 12 mg/ml BSA; at higher BSA concentration a lower binding was found, e.g. 4 % at 120 mg/ml BSA. An explanation for these findings (van den Goorbergh et al., 1987b) may be that at the higher BSA concentration the viscosity of the solution is so high that the reactive nitrenium ion derived from AAF-SO4 can not readily reach a reaction site (-SH or SCH_3 group) on the surface of a neighbouring BSA molecule. Although increasing concentrations of RNA also result in more viscous solutions, yet on the "surface" of the RNA molecule there are sites for reaction available at a much higher density than in BSA (where only one free -SH and possibly a $-SCH_3$ group are exposed). The most relevant finding, however was that a number of compounds that prevent covalent binding of AAF-SO4 to BSA in vitro, are much less protective at high than at low BSA concentration (Table 3). The protein concentration in liver cytosol in situ is approx. 125 mg/ml. Therefore, it is highly likely that under such conditions in vivo glutathione similarly is little protective against covalent binding of the nitrenium ion generated in situ by sulfation, so that depletion of glutathione will not result in a major increase in toxicity.

Necrosis by NOHAAF in the liver is thought to be due to sulfation. The resulting nitrenium ion binds to proteins (enzymes etc.) and would disturb cell homoeostasis. However, recent work with a number of thioethers has shown that adduct formation to DNA rather than to protein may be res-

Table 3 Inhibition by various thioethers of covalent binding of AAFSO4 to two concentrations of bovine serum albumine .

	BSA binding (% of control)	
	Low BSA concn (12 mg/ml)	High BSA conc (60 mg/ml)
Control	100	100
Thiazolidine	26	76
2-Methylthio-benzimidazole	15	57
Methyl 4-Methyl-thiobenzoate	16	67

Incubations of BSA (12 or 60 mg/ml) and thioethers (5 mM) with [9-^{14}C]-AAF-N-sulfate were carried out at 20°C in 50 mM Tris-HCl buffer, pH 7.4, for 30 min. Data taken from van den Goorbergh et al (1987b)

ponsible for cell death (van den Goorbergh et al, 1987a). These agents were tested in vitro and in vivo as to their ability to prevent covalent binding of AAFSO4 to RNA in the test tube, to prevent NOHAAF-induced hepatotoxicity in vivo and to affect adduct formation to DNA and protein in vivo in the liver. Interestingly, the compounds that prevented RNA binding of AAFSO4 and in vivo hepatotoxicity, turned out to decrease DNA binding in vivo, but had no effect on protein adduct formation in vivo. Thus, DNA adducts may cause cell death in the liver by NOHAAF.

AAFSO4 can bind to DNA in the cell nucleus, as demonstrated by the fact that in isolated rat liver nuclei it bound at a high level to DNA (Meerman et al., 1986). Methionine effectively prevented covalent binding of AAFSO4 to both DNA and protein in the isolated nuclei. This shows that AAFSO4 formed outside the nucleus can reach nuclear DNA.

ROLE OF SULFATION IN INITIATION OF CARCINOGENESIS

As yet it is unclear how sulfation of NOHAAF is involved in carcinogenesis by 2AAF. Meerman (1986), using the Salt & Farber model for the generation of preneoplastic foci in the liver of the rat, showed that the number of these foci initiated by NOHAAF was actually increased by inhibition of sulfation at the time of initiation. This might indicate that sulfation leads to a nitrenium ion that is not involved in initiation so that inhibition of sulfation makes more of the substrate available for another initiating pathway (forming de-acetylated adducts?). Another explanation is that sulfation of NOHAAF kills a number of initiated cells, that otherwise would have grown out to form foci, so that inhibition of sulfation makes more initiated cells survive.

Inside the preneoplastic foci the sulfation activity for NOHAAF seems to have decreased (Kroese et al., 1987). When NOHAAF (1.14 mCi/kg) was injected in the rat with and without PCP pretreatment, and the liver was taken out 4 hours later, autoradiography of liver slices showed that over the preneoplastic foci less radioactivity could be measured than over the surrounding, normal liver tissue. Moreover, PCP pretreatment decreased the radioactivity in the surrounding tissue, while in the foci no change was found. This suggests that sulfation plays no role in the generation of covalently bound AAF-adducts to (mainly) protein in the foci.

Although the exact role of sulfation in carcinogenesis by 2AAF is not yet completely clear, recent work by the group of the Millers has shown that sulfation most likely is involved in the initiation phase of carcinogenesis by NOHAAF. They treated new-born mice with a single dose of NOHAAF (Lai et al., 1985). The mice got liver tumors after 9 months. PCP treatment just before the injection of NOHAAF decreased the tumor incidence markedly. Similarly, in mice which were deficient in the biosynthesis of "active sulfate" (brachymorphic mice), and therefore can not conjugate xenobiotics with sulfate, a much reduced liver tumor incidence of NOHAAF was found. These data, in combination with identification of NOHAAF-derived DNA adducts (and the effect of PCP thereon), indicated that in the newborn mice NOHAAF is converted to N-hydroxy-2-aminofluorene, which subsequently needs sulfation for activation to an ultimate carcinogen.

Very similar results were obtained with 1'-hydroxy safrole by Boberg et al., 1983. They found pronounced reduction in liver tumor incidence of this compound after pretreatment with PCP or in the brachymorphic mice. Similarly, PCP decreased DNA adduct formation of 1'-hydroxysafrole. These results indicate that sulfation is the activating reaction of 1'-hydroxysafrole to its ultimate carcinogenic metabolite. The above work has recently been reviewed (Miller et al., 1985).

The above data show that sulfation can activate both through the formation of N-sulfate and C-sulfate esters to form nitrenium and carbonium ions respectively. At the same time they illustrate how complicated the mechanisms involved are, because even for such an extensively studied compound like NOHAAF, the precise chemical mechanism of, and the role of the various metabolites in carcinogenesis can not yet be identified with certainty. There is, however, no question that sulfation is involved in the toxicity of several armatic amines and benzylic alcohols.

REFERENCES

Boberg, E.W., Miller, E.C., Miller, J.A., Poland, A. & Liem, A., 1983, _Cancer Research_ 43, 5163.

DeBaun, J.R., Miller, E.C. & Miller, J.A., 1970, _Cancer Research_ 30, 577.

Irving, C.C., 1971, _Xenobiotica_ 1, 387.

King, C.M. & Phillips, B., 1968, _Science_ 159, 1351.

Kroese, E.D., Tijdens, R.B., Mulder, G.J. & Meerman, J.H.N. 1987, _Carcinogenesis_, 8, in press.

Lai, C.C., Miller, J.A., Miller, E.C. & Liem, A., 1985, _Carcinogenesis_, 6, 1037.

Meerman, J.H.N., 1985, _Carcinogenesis_, 6, 893.

Meerman, J.H.N. & Mulder, G.J., 1981, _Life Sciences_ 28, 2361.

Meerman, J.H.N. & Tijdens, R.B., 1985, Cancer Research, 45, 1132.
Meerman, J.H.N., Tijdens, R.B. & Mulder, G.J., 1986, Journal of Biochemical Toxicology, 1 (2), 1
Meerman, J.H.N., Nijland, C. & Mulder, G.J., 1987, Biochemical Pharmacology, in press.
Miller, E.C., 1978, Cancer Research 38, 1479.
Miller, E.C. Miller, J.A., Boberg, E.W., Delclos, K.B., Lai C.C., Fennell, T.R., Wiseman, R.W., Liem, A., 1985, Sulfuric acid esters as ultimate electrophilic and carcinogenic metabolites of some alkenylbenzenes and aromatic amines in mouse liver. In Carcinogenesis, edited by E. Huberman & S.H. Barr. Raven Press, New York, p. 93.
Mulder, G.J., Meerman, J.H.N. & Van den Goorbergh, A.M., 1986, Bioactivation of xenobiotics by Conjugation. In Xenobiotic Conjugation Chemistry, edited by G.D. Paulsen J. Caldwell, D.H. Hutson & J.J. Menn, American Chemical Society (ACS Symposium series No 299), p. 282.
Van den Goorbergh, J.A.M., Meerman, J.H.N., de Wit, H. & Mulder, G.J., 1985, Carcinogenesis, 6, 1635.
Van den Goorbergh, J.A.M., de Wit, H., Tijdens, R.B., Mulder, G.J. & Meerman, J.H.N. 1987a, Carcinogenesis, 8, 275.
Van den Goorbergh, J.A.M., Mulder, G.J. & Meerman, J.H.N., 1987b, submitted.
Vonk, R.J., Tuchweber, B., Masse, D., Perea, A., Audet, M., Roy, C.C. & Yousef, I., 1981, Gastroenterology, 81, 242.

GLUCURONIDATION AND ITS TOXICOLOGICAL SIGNIFICANCE

K.W. Bock

Department of Pharmacology and Toxicology
University of Göttingen, Robert-Koch-Str. 40,
D-3400 Göttingen, F.R.G.

ABSTRACT

(1) Glucuronidation, catalyzed by glucuronyltransferase, is a major pathway in the detoxication and elimination of nucleophilic endo- and xenobiotics. However, some glucuronides may be hydrolyzed for example in the urinary bladder or the colon and in this way determine the target of toxicity. (2) Glucuronyltransferase represents a family of differentially inducible isozymes with different but overlapping substrate specificity. (3) Examples are given in which the isozyme pattern of glucuronyltransferases and enzyme saturation are major factors controlling toxicity.

INTRODUCTION

Glucuronides determining the target of toxicity

Glucuronidation is quantitatively the major pathway in the detoxication and elimination of nucleophilic endo- and xenobiotics (Dutton, 1980). In most instances electrophilic metabolites are the ultimate reactants initiating toxicity (Miller & Miller, 1981). However the more abundant nucleophilic metabolites can also be converted to electrophiles. For example, phenols can be oxidized to toxic polyphenols, semiquinones and quinones. Quinones may undergo quinone/quinol redox-cycles with the generation of reactive oxygen species (Lorentzen & Ts'o, 1977). Hence the control of both electrophilic and nucleophilic metabolites is important in drug metabolism.

Glucuronides may determine the target of toxicity. For example, (a) the bladder carcinogen ß-naphthylamine is oxidized in the liver to N-hydroxy-2-naphthylamine and then glucuronidated to a N-glucuronide (Miller & Miller, 1981). The conjugate is transported to the kidney and actively secreted. In slightly acidic urine the glucuronide decomposes and the resulting hydroxylamine is protonated to a reactive nitrenium ion which may be an ultimate carcinogen. (b) High molecular weight glucuronides are actively secreted by anionic carriers in the canalicular membrane of the hepatocyte via the bile into the intestine. Most glucuronides are hydrolyzed by bacterial ß-glucuronidase in the colon where the aglycone is liberated. In the case of the colon carcinogen 3,2'-dimethyl-4-aminobiphenyl the compound is oxidized to the hydroxylamine in the liver and a N-glucuronide is formed (Weisburger, 1971). The conjugate is secreted into the intestine where the ultimate carcinogen, the hydroxylamine, is liberated by ß-glucuronidase. In the above instances the glucuronides represent stable transport forms of proximate carcinogens.

RESULTS AND DISCUSSION

Isozymes of glucuronyltransferase in rat liver

In intact cells, organs and the whole organism an increasing complexity of factors determines the formation and disposition of glucuronides. Nevertheless the level of a particular isozyme may become the rate limiting step in the overall process. Evidence for multiple isozymes has accumulated in the past in studies on genetic defects, on ontogenic development and on differential induction of glucuronyltransferase (GT) activities. Recently the existence of several isozymes has been clearly established in rat liver (Table 1). Isolation has been accomplished by anionic exchange chromatography or chromatofocusing and subsequent affinity chromatography on UDP-hexanolamine Sepharose. Some isozymes are more specific for endogenous substrates such as bilirubin (Scragg et al., 1985) and various steroids (Falany et al., 1986). For many isozymes no typical endogenous substrate has yet been found. They have been termed according to a generally accepted substrate and to their inducibility; for example p-nitrophenol GT (Falany et al., 1986) or phenol GT_{MC} (Bock et al., 1979; Bock et al., 1984a). The isozymes show different monomeric molecular weights in the range of M_r 50000 to 56000. In the case of 3α-OH-steroid GT (3α-hydroxysteroid GT) or androsterone GT the complete amino acid sequence of the protein has been deduced from complementary DNA (Jackson & Burchell, 1986; Mackenzie, 1986). Many isozymes are differentially inducible by xenobiotics whereas steroid GTs appear not to be markedly inducible. MC-inducible phenol GTs appear to be almost ubiquitously distributed in extrahepatic tissues (Dutton, 1980). However, more work is needed to characterize these extrahepatic GT isozymes.

Table 1. Isozymes of glucuronyltransferase (GT) in rat liver microsomes. * BP, benzo(a)pyrene; ** von Meyerinck et al. (1985). Other references in the text.

Isozyme	Inducer	M_r
a) Bilirubin GT	Clofibrate Phenobarbital	54000
b) 3α-OH-steroid GT (Androsterone GT)	-	52000
17ß-OH-steroid GT (Testosterone GT)	-	50000
Aromatic steroid GT (Estrone GT)	-	?
c) Phenol GT_{MC} (GT_1) (BP-3,6-quinol GT)*	3-Methylcholanthrene	54000 (56000)
Morphine GT (GT_2)	Phenobarbital	54000 (56000)
Digitoxigenin monodigitoxoside GT	Pregnenolone-16α-carbonitrile **	?

Table 2. Substrate specificity of glucuronyltransferase (GT). * BP, benzo(a)pyrene; ** Wolf et al. (1986). Other references in the text.

Phenol	Substrate
Phenol GT_{MC}	BP-3,6-quinol * (mono- and diglucuronide formation) 3-OH-BP* Mitoxantrone ** N-OH-2-naphthylamine 4-Methylumbelliferone 1-Naphthol 4-Nitrophenol
3α-OH-steroid GT	Androsterone Etiocholanolone Lithocholic acid 4-Aminobiphenyl
17ß-OH-steroid GT	Testosterone Estradiol (at C_{17}) 1-Naphthol 4-Nitrophenol

The various steroid GTs clearly recognize the shape of their respective substrates and are remarkably stereo- and regioselective (Table 2). For example, 17ß-OH-steroid GT or testosterone GT attaches the glucuronic acid moiety only to the C_{17} of estradiol whereas aromatic steroid GT only conjugates estradiol at the C_3 of the aromatic ring (Falany et al., 1986). On the other hand testosterone GT unspecifically conjugates a number of simple phenols such as 1-naphthol and 4-nitrophenol. Similarly, androsterone GT unspecifically glucuronidates 4-aminobiphenyl (Green et al., 1985). Phenol GT_{MC} or GT_1 unspecifically conjugates a number of phenols provided they are planar in shape (Bock et al., 1979; Bock et al., 1984b; Okulicz-Kozaryn et al., 1981). Bulky phenols such as morphine are conjugated by GT_2. However, GT_{MC} also appears to be regioselective. For example, a recent study on the inducibility of a variety of phenols of polycyclic aromatic hydrocarbons (PAHs) suggests that GT_{MC} prefers planar substrates with distinct dimensions. When viewed from the phenolic group to the plane of PAHs the substrates of GT_{MC} appear to be shorter than 1.3 nm whereas longer PAH phenols are conjugated by phenobarbital-inducible phenol GTs (Lilienblum, Platt, Schirmer, Oesch & Bock, submitted).

BP-3,6-quinol appears to be a particularly interesting substrate of GT_{MC}. The quinol is conjugated sequentially to the mono- and diglucuronide (Lilienblum et al., 1985; Segura-Aquilar et al., 1986). Mono- and diglucuronide formation is markedly induced by MC-treatment in rat liver microsomes (10- and 40-fold, respectively). The different induction factors for the two reactions have been interpreted as evidence for the existence of more than one phenol GT_{MC} in rat liver. The reaction may be of toxicological interest since conjugation of the quinol reduces cytotoxicity due to quinone/quinol redox-cycles. Co-induction of this isozyme with other drug metabolizing enzymes such as P_1-450 and quinone reductase or DT-diaphorase may represent an adaptive program which has evolved to efficiently detoxify dietary PAHs (Bock and Schirmer, 1987; Nebert and Jensen, 1979).

Differential induction of glucuronyltransferase activities in human liver

Establishment of liver banks from kidney transplant donors has been a major advance to obtain meaningful enzyme data from human individuals (von Bahr et al., 1980). Some patients have been treated with high doses of antiepileptic phenobarbital-type inducers. Determination of GT activities

Fig. 1. Differential induction of human liver glucuronyltransferase activities by phenobarbital-type inducers.
* $p < 0.05$; ** Ratio of liver microsomal enzyme activities from induced patients (n = 4) and untreated controls (n = 7).

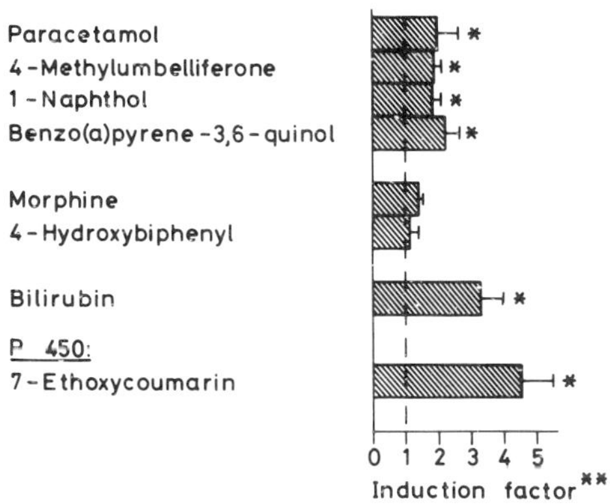

in microsomal samples from such a liver bank suggest differential induction of GT activities in human liver (Fig. 1), extending previous findings (Bock et al., 1984b). Enzyme activities from induced patients could be clearly distinguished from those of individuals who did not receive inducing drugs. GT_1 activities, as classified in rat liver, were found to be moderately but significantly increased, whereas GT_2 activities appeared not to be induced. The latter finding is in contrast to the marked induction of GT_2 activities by phenobarbital-type inducers in rats (Bock et al., 1979). These observations suggest the existence of multiple GT isozymes in human liver. But they also add to a number of reports on species differences in the inducibility of GT isozymes.

Recently a simple, non-invasive test has been developed to monitor glucuronidation in patients using paracetamol as test drug (Bock et al., 1987). Using this test it was found that paracetamol glucuronidation was significantly increased in patients treated with the phenobarbital-type inducers phenytoin or rifampicin, in agreement with metabolic clearance data (Prescott et al., 1981). Paracetamol glucuronidation was also shown to be increased in heavy smokers (Bock et al., 1987). These findings suggest that paracetamol glucuronidation is induced in human liver by both phenobarbital- and MC-type inducers.

GT isozymes as major factors controlling toxicity

Several examples illustrate that GT isozymes may be key factors controlling toxicity. It has been shown, that 4-ipomeanol, the poison of moldy sweet potatoes, leads to selective necrosis of the Clara cells in bronchial epithelium (Statham & Boyd, 1982). Phenobarbital-treatment of rats protects the animals from ipomeanol toxicity. This is probably due to the induction of a phenobarbital-inducible GT isozyme in liver conjugating ipomeanol. In this way the concentration of the toxin is efficiently reduced in the organism.

An example for the role of MC-inducible GT isozymes has been reported by Greenlee and Irons (1981). Bone marrow toxicity due to benzene exposure is probably caused by benzene oxidation in liver and bone marrow whereby mainly phenol is formed. Saturation of phenol glucuronidation and sulfation allows further oxidation to hydroquinone and semiquinone radicals which may be the ultimate bone marrow toxins. Induction of phenol GT by the MC-type inducer 3,4,3',4'-tetrachlorobiphenyl protected against benzene toxicity in the bone marrow and lymphoid organs. In a similar way saturation of 2-OH-biphenyl glucuronidation and sulfation may explain its dose-dependent toxicity in the urinary bladder epithelium (Fig. 2). At low doses 2-OH-biphenyl is mostly excreted as the glucuronide and sulfate ester, and no toxicity is observed. At high doses conjugating pathways are saturated and the compound is further oxidized to the corresponding hydroquinone and semiquinones which are probably responsible for covalent binding, genotoxicity and initiation of bladder carcinogenicity (Reitz et al., 1983). 2-OH-biphenyl is widely used as an antimicrobial agent to protect edible crops, and hence the human population may be exposed. It is assumed that this human exposure does not lead to a significant health hazard. The disproportionate increase in covalent protein binding of 2-OH-biphenyl metabolites with increasing dose may have some bearing on the ungoing discussion of threshold levels. In summary these examples emphasize that a balance between activating and inactivating reactions, including glucuronidation, may be a major determinant of tissue toxicity.

Fig. 2. Scheme of 2-OH-biphenyl metabolism in relation to its toxicity
(Reitz et al., 1983).

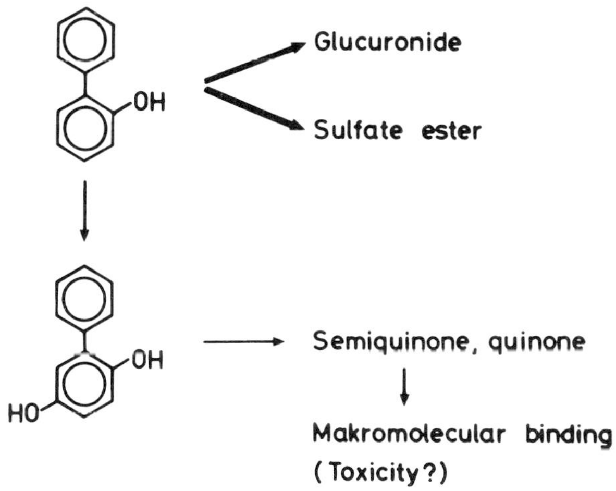

ACKNOWLEDGEMENTS

This work was supported by the Deutsche Forschungsgemeinschaft.

REFERENCES

Bahr von, C., Groth, C.G., Jansson, H., Lundgren, G., Lind, M. & Glaumann, H., 1980, Clinical Pharmacology and Experimental Therapeutics, 27, 711.

Bock, K.W., Josting, D., Lilienblum, W. & Pfeil, H., 1979, European Journal of Biochemistry, 98, 19.

Bock, K.W., Lilienblum, W., Ullrich, D. & Fischer, G., 1984a, Biochemical Society Transactions 12, 55.

Bock, K.W., Lilienblum, W. & Bahr von, C., 1984b, Drug Metabolism and Disposition, 12, 93.

Bock, K.W. & Schirmer, G., 1987, Archives of Toxicology, Suppl. 10, 125.

Bock, K.W., Wiltfang, J., Blume, R., Ullrich, D. & Bircher, J., 1987, European Journal of Clinical Pharmacology, 31, 677.

Dutton, G.J., 1980, Glucuronidation of Drugs and Other Compounds, (CRC Press, Boca Raton, Florida).

Falany, C.N., Green, M.D., Swain, E. & Tephly, T.R., 1986, Biochemical Journal, 238, 65.
Green, M.D., Irshaid, Y. & Tephly, T.R., 1985 the formation of N-glucuronides catalyzed by purified hepatic 17ß-hydroxysteroid and 3α-hydroxysteroid UDP-glucuronyltransferases. In Advances in Experimental Medicine and Biology, 197, 399.
Greenlee, W.F. & Irons, R.D., 1981, Chemico-Biological Interactions, 33, 345.
Jackson, M.R. & Burchell, B., 1986, Nucleic Acids Research, 14, 779.
Lilienblum, W., Bock-Hennig, B.S. & Bock, K.W., 1985, Molecular Pharmacology, 27, 451.
Lorentzen, R.J. & Ts'o, P.O.P., 1977, Biochemistry, 16, 1467.
Mackenzie, P.I., 1986, Journal of Biological Chemistry, 261, 14112.
Meyerinck von, L., Coffman, B.L., Green, M.D., Kirkpatrick, R.B., Schmoldt, A. & Tephly, T.R., 1985, Drug Metabolism and Disposition, 13, 700.
Miller, E.C. & Miller, J.A., 1981, Cancer, 47, 2327.
Nebert, D.W. & Jensen, N.M., 1979, CRC Critical Reviews in Biochemistry, 6, 401.
Okulicz-Kozaryn, I., Schaefer, M., Batt, A.M., Siest, G. & Loppinet, V., 1981, Biochemical Pharmacology, 30, 1457.
Prescott, L.F., Critchley, J.A.J.H., Balali-Mood, M. & Pentland, B., 1981, British Journal of Clinical Pharmacology, 12, 149.
Reitz, R.H., Fox, T.R., Quast, J.F., Hermann, E.A. & Watanabe, P.G., 1983, Chemico-Biological Interactions, 43, 99.
Scragg, I., Celier, C. & Burchell, B., 1985, FEBS Letters, 183, 37.
Segura-Aquilar, J.W., Barreiro, V & Lind. C., 1986, Archives of Biochemistry and Biophysics, 251, 266.
Statham, C. & Boyd, M.R., 1982, Biochemical Pharmacology, 31, 3973.
Weisburger, J.H., 1971, Cancer, 27, 60.
Wolf, C.R., Macpherson, J.S. & Smyth, J.F., 1986, Biochemical Pharmacology, 35, 1577.

ACETYLATION AND ITS TOXICOLOGICAL SIGNIFICANCE

John A Timbrell

Toxicology Unit, The School of Pharmacy,
University of London, U.K.

The acetylation of amine, hydrazine and sulphonamide groups in foreign compounds is an important phase II reaction. In man acetylation shows a genetic polymorphism for some substrates and is usually regarded as a detoxication reaction. For example the antihypertensive drug hydralazine causes a significant incidence of lupus erythematosus, as high as 10.4% in patients taking 200 mg daily doses (Cameron and Ramsay, 1984). This syndrome, believed to have an immunological basis, occurs almost exclusively in patients of the slow acetylator phenotype (Perry et al., 1970). The drug is metabolised by acetylation but in slow acetylators more is metabolised by the alternative oxidative pathway to phthalazinone which may be involved in the toxic effect (Timbrell et al., 1984).

It has recently been shown that the acetylated metabolite of hydralazine (methyltriazolophthalazine) and the acetylated metabolites of other lupus inducing drugs are less active in an *in vitro* system which measures binding of the C4 component of the complement system (Sim et al, 1984). These results suggest that acetylation reduces the activity of the reactive hydrazine moiety.

The neurotoxicity of isoniazid is another example of acetylation as an important detoxication reaction. In man it was found that the slow acetylators of isoniazid were more susceptible to the peripheral neuropathy induced by the drug (Devadatta et al., 1960). Similarly in rabbits phenotyped as rapid or slow acetylators, survival time after doses of isoniazid or acetylhydrazine was shorter in slow acetylators than rapid acetylators, (Hein and Weber, 1984).

However in a few cases the acetylation reaction gives

rise to toxicity and a simple example of this is the acetylation of certain sulphonamides which produces metabolites which are less water soluble from the parent drug. The crystallisation of the acetylated metabolites in the kidney tubules may give rise to kidney damage (Weinstein, 1970).

Another example is the hepatotoxicity of isoniazid. Isoniazid is a widely used anti-tubercular drug which causes a significant incidence (12%+) of liver damage (Mitchell et al, 1976). The metabolism involves an initial acetylation step (Fig. 1) which has long been known to show a genetic polymorphism (Evans et al, 1960). Epidemiological studies have variously suggested that the slow (Musch et al, 1982) rapid (Mitchell et al, 1975) or neither acetylator phenotype (Riska, 1976) is more susceptible to the hepatotoxic effects. The report by Mitchell et al (1975) prompted a study of the mechanism underlying the hepatotoxicity and the role of acetylation. The major metabolic differences between rapid and slow acetylators were well established: rapid acetylators produced more acetylisoniazid and isonicotinic acid than slow acetylators. It was predicted that rapid acetylators would produce more acetylhydrazine (Mitchell et al, 1976). However when this was investigated in volunteers it was found that although acetylhydrazine was indeed a metabolite (Table 1) there was no difference between rapid and slow acetylators in the amount excreted because it was further acetylated to diacetylhydrazine (Timbrell et al, 1977) Fig. 1, Table 1. Recent data in man (Lauterburg et al, 1985) has shown that although the peak plasma concentration of acetylhydrazine after a dose of isoniazid may be slightly higher in some rapid acetylator individuals the area under the plasma concentration time curve is greater for slow acetylators. That is the slow acetylators have a greater exposure to acetylhydrazine than rapid acetylators. This would explain the most recent epidemiological data which clearly indicated that slow acetylators were more at risk from the severe isoniazid hepatotoxicity (Musch et al, 1982).

Animal studies however revealed that acetylisoniazid and particularly acetylhydrazine were acutely hepatotoxic in rats whereas diacetylhydrazine was relatively non toxic. So acetylation of the remaining nitrogen reduced the toxicity. The toxicity of acetylhydrazine could be modified by pretreatment of the animals with phenobarbital (increased) or with cobalt chloride (decreased). The toxicity of acetylisoniazid could be reduced by treatment with bis-p-nitro phenyl phosphate (Mitchell et al, 1976), an acetylamidase inhibitor which blocked hydrolysis to acetylhydrazine (Timbrell et al., 1980)(Fig. 1).

The effects of microsomal enzyme inducers and inhibitors indicated that monooxygenase mediated metabolism was involved. Using radiolabelled acetylisoniazid and acetylhydrazine it was found that the acetyl moiety was bound to liver protein and that there was a correlation between the extent of binding and the hepatotoxicity (Mitchell et al., 1976; Timbrell et al., 1980). More recent studies have shown that extensive binding occurs in many tissues but that only that in the liver is increased by phenobarbital

Table 1. Urinary excretion of acetylated metabolites of isoniazid by human volunteers.

Acetylator Phenotype	% Dose in 0-24 hr Urine AcINH	AcHz	DiAcHz
Rapid (5)	46.3±2.4*	1.8±0.4	23.0±2.0*
Slow (4)	28.9±1.7	2.5±0.5	4.9±0.9

*p<0.001
Data of Timbrell et al., 1977.

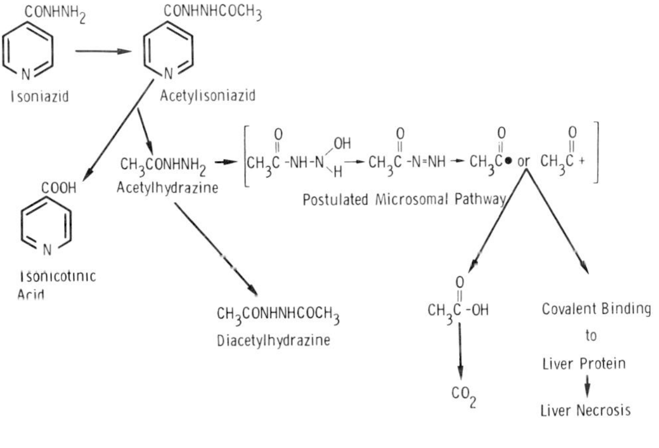

Figure 1. Metabolism of isoniazid

treatment. Mitochondrial and microsomal proteins seem to be particular targets for this binding (Woodward and Timbrell, 1984).

Further in vitro studies indicated that the metabolic activation was mediated by cytochrome P450 (Nelson et al., 1976a) and probably involved oxidation of the nitrogen, dehydration and breakdown of the diazene to either a carbon centred radical or a carbonium ion, Fig. 1 (Nelson et al., 1976b). A radical was favoured by analogy with isopropyl hydrazine which yields propane as a metabolite via a free radical mechanism (Nelson et al, 1976b; 1978). More recent ESR studies have shown that acetylhydrazine will produce a carbon centred free radical in microsomal incubations although the trapped product did not correspond to that for acetyl radical (Augusto and Ortiz de Montellano, 1981). Acetylhydrazine was found to be only hepatotoxic in animals induced with phenobarbital and also to lead to a loss of cytochrome P450 but only in induced animals (Woodward and Timbrell, 1984; Fleet and Timbrell, unpublished observations).

Comparing various microsomal enzyme inducers and using various inhibitors has suggested that a phenobarbital inducible form of cytochrome P450 is responsible for the induction of the hepatotoxic pathway for acetylhydrazine. However after induction with 3-methylcholanthrene, acetylhydrazine treatment also gives rise to loss of cytochrome P450 (Fleet & Timbrell, unpublished observations). This suggests that the hepatic necrosis and loss of cytochrome P450 are separate events. It is conceivable that the metabolism of acetylhydrazine involves another oxidation pathway which may be involved in the destruction of cytochrome P450.

Isoniazid hepatotoxicity clearly involves the acetylation reaction in two ways: a) it gives rise indirectly to a toxic metabolite, acetylhydrazine; b) this metabolite may then be detoxified by a further acetylation reaction to diacetylhydrazine. In man this is under genetic control. It is clear that the susceptibility may depend on complex factors, in particular the relative rates of metabolism by the various pathways (Fig. 1). However it should also be noted that the role of hydrazine itself in the hepatotoxicity of isoniazid has not yet been fully explored.

Another example of toxicity due to acetylation concerns the carcinogenicity of certain aromatic amines. Acetylation may feature in the carcinogenicity of aromatic amines in at least two ways. For bladder cancer which may be caused by aromatic amines such as 2-naphthylamine and benzidine, acetylation may be an important detoxication reaction. For example the dog which is unable to acetylate aromatic amines, develops tumours of the bladder after certain arylamines are administered and tumours of the liver and bladder after the acetylated arylamines are given (Poirier et al., 1963). In rabbit bladder explant cultures acetyl and diacetylbenzidine caused less DNA damage than benzidine itself (McQueen et al.,1987). Several epidemiological studies have shown that the slow acetylator phenotype is significantly more common in patients with bladder cancer (Mommsen et al., 1985) and studies examining workers in the dye industry who are exposed to aromatic amines have found a greater incidence of the slow acetylator phenotype in bladder cancer patients (Cartwright et al., 1982).

However for other types of aromatic amine-induced cancer acetylation seems to be a requirement. The aromatic amine aminofluorene and its acetylated derivative have been extensively studied by many groups. It has long been known that N-hydroxyarylacetamides (arylhydroxamic acids) are more potent carcinogens than the parent arylacetamides (Cramer et al.,1960) and that conjugation of these arylhydroxamic acids with sulphate or acetate yielded very reactive electrophiles (King et al., 1969). The conjugation with acetate occurred by transacetylation (Bartsch et al., 1972) and was catalysed by the enzyme, N,O-arylhydroxamic acid acyltransferase (AHAT) (King et al., 1979). The product was a highly reactive acetoxy compound capable of reacting with macromolecules spontaneously. Therefore it seems that metabolic activation by acetyl transfer occurs and that this accounts for the formation of some of the adducts with nucleic acids (Fig. 2). Production of the acetoxy derivative by transacetylation utilises the transferase enzyme but is independent of acetyl CoA. More recently it has been suggested that microsomal deacetylation of N-hydroxy-acetylaminofluorene followed by direct O-acetylation of the N-hydroxyaminofluorene in an acetyl CoA dependent O-acetyltransferase catalysed reaction may occur (Fig. 2) (Lai et al.,1985, 1987).

In vitro and in vivo studies have indicated that N-acetoxyaminofluorene gives rise to DNA adducts and that the major derivative is N-(deoxyguanosin-8-yl)-2-aminofluorene. The acetoxy derivative which may arise either by transacetylation or O-acetylation yields a reactive nitrenium ion following loss of the acetoxy group (Fig. 2). However a direct causative role for the DNA adduct or N-acetoxy aminofluorene has not been clearly demonstrated. A recent study however suggests that sulphate conjugation of the

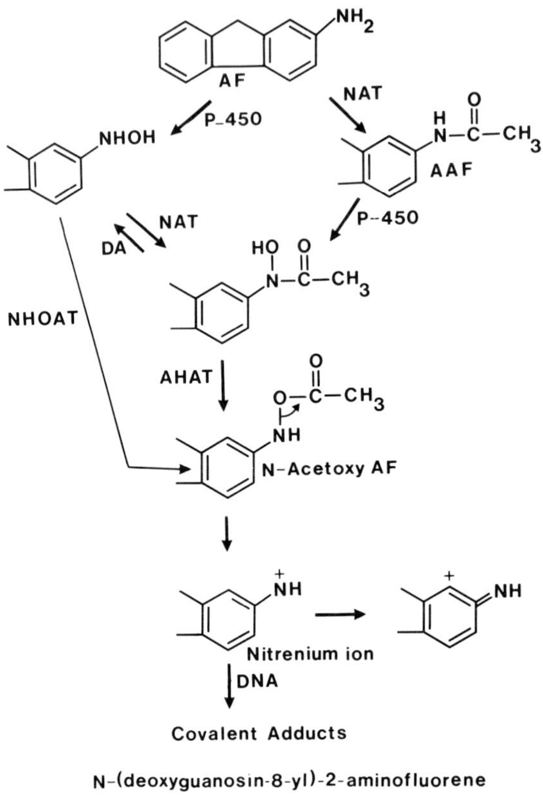

Figure 2. Metabolic activation of aminofluorene.

N-hydroxyaminofluorene may be involved in the formation of the same DNA adduct and hepatocarcinogenesis, in mice (Lai et al., 1987). However a correlation has been shown between acetylator phenotype and DNA damage in rabbit hepatocytes exposed to aminofluorene and benzidine, with rapid acetylators being more susceptible (McQueen et al., 1982; 1983).

It is clear from the literature that there are numerous intraspecies and interorgan differences in the activation of arylamines, such as aminofluorene, to carcinogens. For example the mammary gland has no deacetylase and does not carry out sulphate conjugation. A single application of N-hydroxyacetylaminofluorene (Fig. 2) gives tumours at the site of application (Malejka-Giganti et al., 1973). The N,O-acetyltransferase (AHAT) catalysed reaction may therefore be involved in the induction of mammary tumours (Fig. 2). However not all tissues with AHAT activity respond to carcinogenic arylhydroxamic acids with tumours and dogs which have no AHAT activity still get liver tumours when exposed to acetylaminofluorene. Some species and tissues may have high levels of deacetylase which gives rise to N-hydroxyaminofluorene which may then undergo O-acetylation or sulphation. Lower (1982) has suggested that there are several parallel routes of activation: acetylation, sulphation and glucuronidation which produce the tumours at various sites.

Therefore as with isoniazid metabolism enzymatic acetyl transfer occurs twice in the metabolic activation of arylamines such as 2-aminofluorene: acetyl-CoA dependent acetylation of the amino group followed either by intra-molecular transfer of the acetyl group to the N-hydroxyl group (independent of acetyl CoA) or de-acetylation followed by O-acetylation (acetyl CoA dependent).

REFERENCES

Augusto, O. & Ortiz de Montellano, P.R., 1981, Biochemical and Biophysical Research Communications, 101, 1324.

Bartsch, H., Dworkin, M., Miller, J.A. & Miller, E.C., 1972, Biochimical Biophysica Acta, 286, 272.

Cameron, H.A. & Ramsay, L.E., 1984, British Medical Journal, 289, 410.

Cartwright, R.A., Glashan, R.W., Rogers, H.J., Ahmad, R.A., Hall, D.B., Higgins, E. & Kahn, M.A., 1982, Lancet, 2, 842.

Cramer, J.W., Miller, J.A. & Miller, E.C., 1960, Journal of Biological Chemistry, 235, 885.

Devadatta, S., Gangadharam, P.R.J., Andrews, R.H., Fow, W., Ramakrishnan, C.V., Selkin, J.B. & Velu, S., 1960, Bulletin of the World Health Organisation, 23, 587.

Evans, D.A.P., Manley, K.A. & McKusick, V.A., 1960, British Medical Journal, 2, 485.

Hein, D.W. & Weber, W.W., 1984, Journal of Pharmacology and Experimental Therapeutics, 228, 588.

King, C.M. & Phillips, B., 1969, Journal of Biological Chemistry, 233, 6209.

King, C.M., Traub, N.R., Lortz, Z.M. & Thissen, M.R., 1979, Cancer Research, 39, 3369.

Lai, C.C., Miller, J.A., Miller E.C. & Liem, A., 1985, Carcinogenesis, 6, 1037.

Lai, C.C., Miller, E.C., Miller, J.A. & Liem, A., 1987, Carcinogenesis, 8, 471.

Lauterburg, B.H., Smith, C.V., Todd, E.L. & Mitchell, J.R., 1985, The Journal of Pharmacology and Experimental Therapeutics, 235, 566.
Lower, G.M., 1982, Cancer, 49, 1056.
Malejka-Giganti, D., Rydell, R.E., & Guttman, H.R., 1977, Cancer Research, 37, 111.
McQueen, C.A., Maslansky, C.J., Glowinski, I.B., Crescenzi, S.B., Weber, W.W. & Williams, G.M., 1982, Proceedings of the National Academy of Sciences (USA), 79, 1269.
McQueen, C.A., Way, B.M. & Williams, G.M., 1983, Carcinogenesis, 8, 401.
Mitchell, J.R., Thorgiersson, U.P., Black, M., Timbrell, J.A., Snodgrass, W.R., Potter, W.Z., Jollow, D.J. & Keiser, H.R., 1975, Clinical Pharmacology and Therapeutics, 18, 70.
Mitchell, J.R., Zimmerman, H.J., Ishak, K.G., Thorgiersson, U.P., Timbrell, J.A., Snodgrass, W.R. & Nelson, S.D., 1976, Annals of Internal Medicine, 84, 181.
Mommsen, S., Barfod, N.M. & Aagaard, J., 1985, Carcinogenesis, 6, 199.
Musch, E., Eichelbaum, M., Wang, J.K., Sassen, W.V., Wochenschrift, 60, 513.
Nelson, S.D., Mitchell, J.R., Timbrell, J.A., Snodgrass, W.R. & Corcoran, G.B., 1976a, Science, 193, 901.
Nelson, S.D., Hinson, J.A. & Mitchell, J.R., 1976b, Biochemical Biophysical Research Communications, 69, 900.
Perry, H.M., Tan, E.M., Carmody, S. & Sakamoto, A., 1970, Journal of Laboratory and Clinical Medicine, 76, 114.
Poirier, L.A., Miller, J.A. & Miller, E.C., 1963, Cancer Research, 23, 790.
Riska, N., 1976, Bull. of the International Union against Tuberculosis, 51, 203.
Sim, E., Gill, E.W. & Sim, R.B., 1984, The Lancet, 421.
Timbrell, J.A., Wright, J.M. & Baillie, T.A., 1977, Clinical Pharmacology and Therapeutics, 22, 602.
Timbrell, J.A., Mitchell, J.R., Snodgrass, W.R. & Nelson, S.D., 1980, The Journal of Pharmacology and Experimental Therapeutics, 213, 364.
Timbrell, J.A., Facchini, V., Harland, S.J. & Mansilla-Tinoco, R., 1984, European Journal of Clinical Pharmacology, 27, 555.
Weinstein, L., 1970, The Sulphonamides. In The Pharmacological basis of Therapeutics, 4th ed, edited by L.S. Goodman and A. Gilman (The Macmillan Company), 1184.
Woodward, K.N. & Timbrell, J.A., 1984, Toxicology, 30, 65.

Glutathione conjugation as a toxication reaction

PETER J. VAN BLADEREN, CATHALINA DEN BESTEN, IRENE M. BRUGGEMAN, JOS J.W.M. MERTENS, BEN VAN OMMEN, BERT SPENKELINK, ANGELO L.M. RUTTEN, JOHAN H.M. TEMMINK AND RIA M.E. VOS.

Department of Toxicology,
Agricultural University, Wageningen, The Netherlands

INTRODUCTION

Glutathione conjugation is one of the major pathways for the detoxification of electrophilic compounds in the body. In general, the reaction is catalyzed by the glutathione S-transferases, a ubiquitous class of enzymes that is found in almost every species of animal, and in most organs of mammals (Mannervik, 1985). However, a number of substrates have been recognized where conjugation leads to the formation of more toxic products. In principle two modes of action can be distinguished: **i)** the effect arises by interaction with a specific receptor, or **ii)** a relatively unreactive compound is transformed into an electrophilic species that will bind covalently to cell macromolecules. This review will deal only with the second group, where toxicity is mediated by the formation of reactive intermediates. According to their mode of action, such activating conjugations with glutathione can be divided in a number of groups. The earliest example is the increased DNA methylation by methylnitronitrosoguanidine found in the presence of glutathione (Lawley and Thatcher, 1970). A recent example of the same type, i.e. enhanced formation of the toxic species, was described for trialkyl phosphorothioates and -dithioates, impurities found in insecticides such as malathion. These compounds are substrates for the glutathione S-transferases (Aldridge et al., 1985), and appear to exert their toxic effect only after one of the O-methyl groups has been removed by conjugation (Thomas et al., 1986).

In addition three groups of toxic glutathione conjugates can be distinguished. The best example of the first group, where the conjugate is reactive by itself is 2-bromoethylglutathione, formed from 1,2-dibromoethane (Van Bladeren et al., 1980). The second group is formed by compounds like hexachlorobutadiene: these give rise to glutathione conjugates which still need metabolic activation (e.g. Wolf et al., 1984). Lastly the reaction with glutathione may be reversible: as a consequence, the glutathione conjugate derived from e.g. benzyl isothiocyanate displays a toxicity similar to the parent compound (Bruggeman et al., 1986).

REACTIVE GLUTATHIONE CONJUGATES

Numerous reports have appeared on the role of glutathione in the toxic action of vicinal dihalogenoalkanes. Most attention has been given to the known carcinogen 1,2-dibromoethane. The primary product of the conjugation of this compound with glutathione is S-2-bromoethylglutathione (see figure 1). Reactions of such β-halothioethers take place via an intermediate thiiranium ion: the lone electron pair of the sulfur substituent attacks the carbon bearing the halogen substituent. Thus, the mutagenicity of 1,2-dibromoethane can be enhanced considerably by the addition of rat liver cytosol to the incubation mixture, and in agreement with this result, S-2-bromoethyl-N-acetyl-L-cysteine methyl ester was shown to be a potent mutagen (Van Bladeren et al., 1980). Since that time the glutathione pathway has been shown to be involved in e.g. the induction of DNA repair in rat spermatocytes and hepatocytes (Working et al., 1986) and induction of DNA single strand breaks in rat hepatocytes (White et al., 1984). The same type of genotoxicity was found <u>in vivo</u> (Storer and Conolly, 1983).

The binding of 1,2-dibromoethane to DNA in isolated hepatocytes was decreased by the glutathione depleting agent diethylmaleate, and not influenced by the cytochrome P450 inhibitor SKF 525A (Sundheimer et al., 1982). Subsequently Ozawa and Guengerich (1983) demonstrated very elegantly that a near-stoichiometric binding of labels to DNA in rat hepatocytes occurred when both ^{14}C-1,2-dibromoethane and ^{35}S-labelled glutathione were used. Recently the structure of the major DNA adduct both <u>in vivo</u> and in isolated hepatocytes was elucidated conclusively (Koga et al., 1986; Inskeep et al., 1986) (fig. 1). Interestingly, the full glutathione moiety is still present in the adduct.

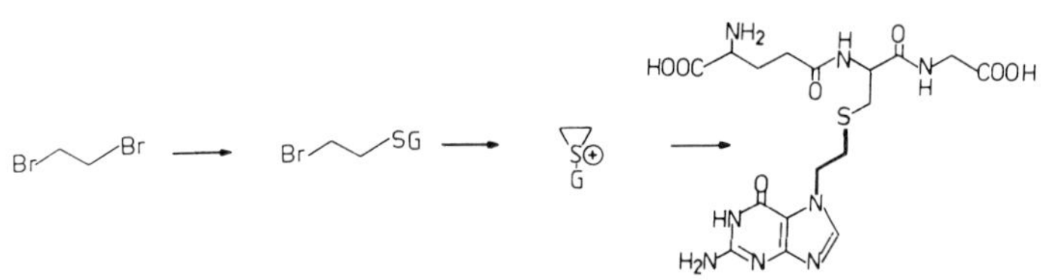

Fig. 1: The biotransformation of 1,2-dibromoethane (Van Bladeren, 1980). The glutathione conjugate is responsible for the major part of the DNA binding (Koga et al., 1986).

In addition to the β-halothioethers, other types of reactive conjugates can be envisaged. For instance, Saito et al., in a study on the metabolism of 3-amino-1-methyl-5H-pyrido 4,3-b indole, a carcinogen formed during the pyrolysis of food-stuffs, discovered a glutathione conjugate that was a more potent mutagen than the N-hydroxy metabolite. However the chemical structure of this conjugate is still unknown (Saito et al., 1983). Recently we isolated a glutathione conjugate of tetra-chlorobenzoquinone that still possesses powerful alkylating properties, as witnessed by its efficient binding to protein and the formation of polyconjugates (Van Ommen et al., 1986) (see figure 2). Quinones are well-known substrates for glutathione conjugation. Usually however, the resulting compounds are in the hydroquinone form (e.g. Monks et al., 1985). A second oxidation step might activate such conjugates.

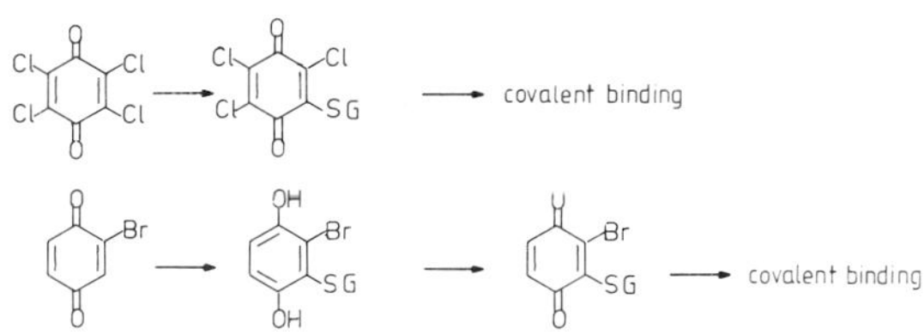

Fig. 2: Comparison of the glutathione conjugates derived from bromobenzoquinone (Monks et al., 1985) and tetrachlorobenzo-quinone (Van Ommen et al., 1987).

REACTIVE METABOLITES FORMED FROM GLUTATHIONE CONJUGATES

The nephrotoxicity of S-(1,2-dichlorovinyl)-L-cysteine has been known for almost thirty years (e.g. Derr and Schulze, 1963). However, in recent years it was found that such conjugates might also be formed metabolically from a number of poly-halogenovinyl compounds. Chlorotrifluoro ethylene and hexachlorobutadiene are the best studied examples to date. Interestingly for both compounds the microsomal glutathione S-transferase is important in catalyzing the conjugation reaction: hexachlorobutadiene is exclusively conjugated via the microsomal enzyme (Wolf et al., 1984), while chlorotrifluoroethylene is a substrate for both cytosolic and microsomal enzymes (Dohn and Anders, 1982). In the first case an addition/elimination reaction occurs resulting in a vinyl-glutathione adduct, while for the fluorinated compounds an addition takes place.

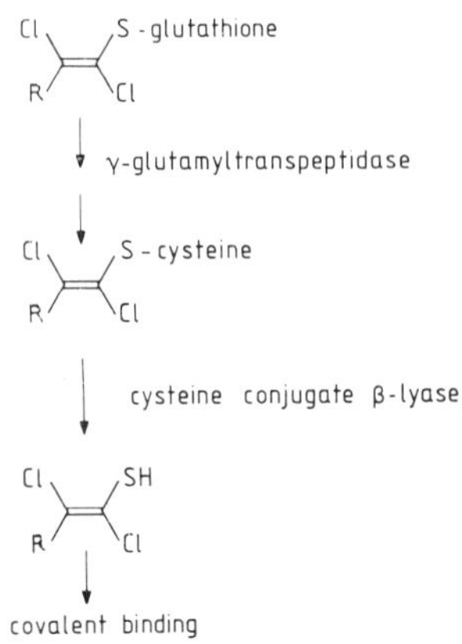

Fig. 3: The metabolism of glutathione conjugates derived from halogenovinyl compounds (R = e.g. H, F, etc.).

The pathway for activation of these conjugates is depicted in figure 3. Two enzymes are critical. Firstly γ-glutamyl transpeptidase, responsible for removing the γ-glutamic acid moiety and secondly cysteine conjugate β-lyase (Stevens and Jacoby, 1983; Stevens, 1985), an enzyme that catalyzes the β-elimination of an electrophilic sulfur-containing fragment from the cysteine derivative. These two enzymes combine in targetting these conjugates to the kidney, thus explaining the selective nephrotoxicity observed (e.g. Jones et al., 1986; Gandolfi et al., 1981). The vinyl-thiol ultimately formed (fig. 3) is electrophilic and can react covalently with cellular macromolecules (Stevens et al., 1986). As depicted in fig. 4, when inhibitors of either the γ-glutamyltranspeptidase or the β-lyase are present, the glutathione conjugate derived from hexachlorobutadiene does not cause any cytotoxic effects towards LLC-PK1 cells.

In addition to vinylderivatives, several glutathione conjugates derived from 2-bromobenzoquinone are activated via a similar route. They display a substantial nephrotoxicity in vivo that can be inhibited to a large extent by acivicin, an inhibitor of γ-glutamyl-transpeptidase (Monks et al., 1985).

A final example was found recently in a study on the mutagenicity of chlorodinitrobenzene in strains of Salmonella typhimurium derived from TA100. In strain NG57, possessing only 10% of the amount of intracellular glutathione, mutagenicity was decreased, indicating a role for glutathione in the mutagenic effect. An attractive hypothesis is the conversion of the S-dinitrophenylglutathione conjugate into a reactive intermediate by nitro reduction, since S-dinitrophenylcysteine did induce mutations in the GSH-strain NG57, but not in TA100NR, a nitroreductase deficient strain (Kerklaan et al., 1987).

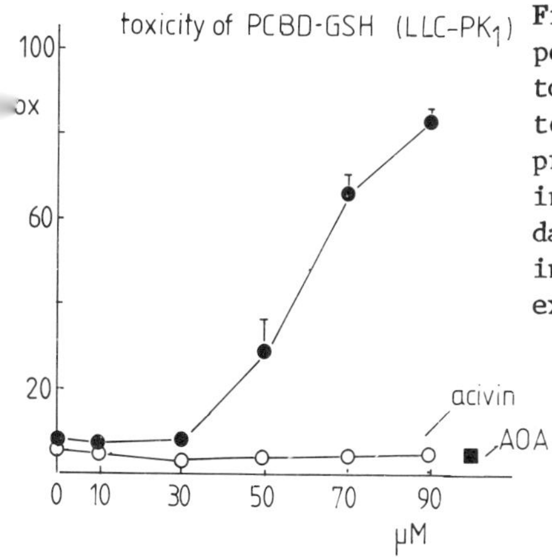

Fig. 4: In situ cytotoxicity of S-pentachlorobutadienyl glutathione towards the cell line LLC-PK1. No toxicity is observed in the presence of acivicin (0.5 mM), an inhibitor of γ-glutamyltranspeptidase or 0.3 mM oxyacetic acid, an inhibitor of β-lyase. Cells were exposed for 16 hours.

GLUTATHIONE CONJUGATES THAT ARE IN EQUILIBRIUM WITH THE PARENT COMPOUNDS

Isothiocyanates are known to react reversibly with thiols. When equimolar amounts of glutathione and allyl or benzyl isothiocyanate are dissolved in water 10-15 minutes, an equilibrium situation is reached where 15-20% of the isothiocyanates is still present in the unconjugated form. The position of this equilibrium can be influenced by conditions of pH and the concentration of the reactants (Bruggeman et al., 1986). In agreement with these results it was shown that the conjugates of these isothiocyanates display toxicities very similar to the parent compounds (Bruggeman et al., 1986; Temmink et al., 1986). In table 1 results are shown of a cytotoxicity assay. Although toxicity is diminished considerably, when 5 mM of glutathione is added to the incubation medium, enough free isothiocyanate is available to cause some effect. On the other hand increasing or decreasing the intracellular glutathione levels does not have an effect on cytotoxicity. Perhaps the isothiocyanate reacts with the cell membrane, and does not come into contact with the intracellular glutathione. On the other hand even a low level of glutathione may be sufficient to act as a transporting agent. The implications of this equilibrium for the in vivo situation are not easy to estimate, but it seems very possible that the isothiocyanates are detoxified at first, but can be released at some other site, where e.g. glutathione concentrations are lower or conditions of pH are different. In this respect it is interesting that allyl isothiocyanate exerts its carcinogenic effect in the bladder of the rat (Dunnick et al., 1982), where the pH is usually basic, thus favouring release of the isothiocyanate.

Table 1. Cytotoxic effect of allyl isothiocyanate (AITC) in Chang liver cells determined as % cloning efficiency.

μM AITC	% intracellular GSH			
	100%	100% + 5 mM extracellular	± 200%[a)]	± 40%[b)]
25	38 ± 8	86 ± 2	41 ± 5	42 ± 8
50	20 ± 4	75 ± 1	22 ± 5	24 ± 3

all compounds were added in 10 μl DMSO (n ≥ 3) AITC exposure 2 hr

a) pretreatment with 20 mM monoethylester of glutathione for 18 h.

b) pretreatment with 155 μM diethylmaleate for 2 h.

Thusfar the isothiocyanates are the only examples of this type of toxic glutathione conjugate. Based on chemical considerations, one might envisage other classes of chemicals showing this type of behaviour, e.g. α,β-unsaturated ketones, where a reversible Michael addition might occur. It is certainly possible that more examples will come to light in the near future.

INTERACTION OF REACTIVE GLUTATHIONE CONJUGATES WITH GLUTATHIONE S-TRANSFERASES

When reactive glutathione conjugates are formed enzymatically the glutathione S-transferases seem natural targets for these conjugates. Although relatively large amounts of these enzymes are present in most cells (e.g. up to 10% of the cytosolic protein in rat liver cells; Mannervik, 1985) and covalent binding to the transferases has been suggested to be a way of detoxifying reactive electrophiles (Ketterer et al., 1976), not very many instances are known where such an interaction has been observed. Of course only the conjugates of the first and third groups discussed above are candidates for such binding. 1,2-Dibromoethane has been found to inhibit the transferases to a certain extent: up to 44% inhibition through covalent binding (Iranetich et al., 1984), but this binding was apparently not due to the glutathione conjugate.

A similar effect has been observed for benzyl isothiocyanate, but not for allyl isothiocyanate (Van Bladeren et al., 1987): 0.5 mM of the glutathione conjugate derived from benzyl isothiocyanate inhibited a mixture of cytosolic rat liver transferases to the extent of 20%. Increasing the concentration did not result in a higher inhibition. Inhibition appeared to be selective: isozymes 3-3 and 3-4 were inhibited for 80 and 70%

respectively, all others for no more than 20-30%.

Recently a similar interaction was discovered for the glutathione conjugate derived from tetrachlorobenzoquinone. Covalent binding resulting in inhibition of the transferases was observed at relatively low (μM) concentrations, as depicted in table 2. In spite of the ubiquitous nature of the glutathione S-transferases, their inhibition by reactive conjugates might still have toxicological implications.

Table 2. Inhibition of rat liver glutathione S-transferases by the S-3,5,6-trichlorobenzoquinone-glutathione (CAN-GSH)

ratio CAN-GSH/enzyme	% binding (nmol/nmol monomer)	inhibition %
1	0.28	27
5	0.58	44
10	0.75	66
20	0.83	69

a) binding was determined using ^3H CAN-GSH. The conjugate was separated from the transferases using a Biogel P-6DG column.
b) inhibition was determined using chlorodinitrobenzene as substrate (Habig and Jacob, 1981) after gel filtration.
The inhibitor was incubated with 4 μM of the transferases for 5 min.

REFERENCES

Aldridge, W.N., Grasdalen H., Aarstad, K., Street, B.W. and Norkor, T. (1985). Chemico Biological Interactions **54**, 243.

Van Bladeren, P.J., Breimer, D.D., Rotteveel-Smijs, G.M.T. De Jong, R.A.W., Buijs, W. and Van der Gen, A. (1980). Biochemical Pharmacology **29**, 2975.

Van Bladeren, P.J., Breimer, D.D., Rotteveel-Smijs, G.M.T., De Mnijff, P., Mohn, G.R., Van Meeteren-Wälchli, B., Buijs, W. and Van der Gen, A. (1981). Carcinogenesis **2**, 499.

Van Bladeren, P.J. (1987). Proceedings Workshop glutathione S-transferases and carcinogenesis, Dublin 1986, in press.

Bruggeman, I.M., Temmink, J.H.M. and Van Bladeren, P.J. (1986a). Toxicology Applied Pharmacology **83**, 349.

Derr, R.F. and Schulze, M.O. (1986). Biochemical Pharmacology **12**, 465.

Dohn, D.R. and Anders, M.W. (1982). Biochemical Biophysical Research Communications **109**, 1339.

Dunnick, J.K., Prejean, J.D., Haseman, J., Thompson, R.B., Giles, H.D. and McConnell, E.E. (1982). Fundamental Applied Toxicology 2, 114.

Gandolfi, A.J., Nagle, R.B., Soltis, J.J. and Plescia, F.H. (1981). Research Communications Chemical Pathology Pharmacology **33**, 249.

Inskeep, P.P., Koga, H., Cmarik, J.L. and Guengerich, F.P. (1986). Cancer Research 46, 2839.

Ivanetich, K.M., Ziman, M.R., Mennie, R.E.M., Eidne, K.A., Corrigall, A. and Kirsch, R.E. (1984). Research Communications Chemical Pathology and Pharmacology **45**, 233.

Kerklaan, P.R.M. Bouter, S., te Koppele, J.M., Vermeulen, N.P.E., Van Bladeren, P.J. and Mohn, G.R. (1987). Mutation Research **176**, 171.

Ketterer, B., Tipping, E., Beale, D. and Meuwissen, J.A.T.P. (1976). In "glutathione: Metabolism and Function" eds Arias I.M. and Jacoby W.B., p. 243, Raven Press NY.

Koga, M., Inskeep, P.B., Harris, T.M. and Guengerich, F.P. (1986). Biochemistry **25**, 2192.

Lawley P.D. and Thatcher, C.J. (1970). Biochemical Journal **116**, 693.

Mannervik, B. (1985). Advances Enzymology **57**, 357.

Monks, T.J., Lau, S.S., Higet, R.J. and Gillette, J.R. (1985). Drug Metabolism Disposition **13**, 553.

Van Ommen, B., Adang, A.E.P., Brader, L., Posthumus, F., Müller, F. and Van Bladeren, P.J. (1986). Biochemical Pharmacology **35**, 3233.

Ozawa, H. and Guengerich, F.P. (1983). Proceedings National Academy Sciences USA, **80**, 5266.

Saito, K., Yamazoe, Y., Kamataki, T. and Kato, R. (1983). Carcinogenesis **4**, 1551.

Stevens, J.L. (1985). Journal Biological Chemistry **260**, 7945.

Stevens, J.L., Hayden, P. and Taylor, G. (1986). Journal Biological Chemistry **261**, 3325.

Storer, R.D. and Conolly, R.B. (1983). Carcinogenesis **4**, 1491.

Sundheimer, D.W., White, R.D., Brendel, K. and Sipes, I.G. (1982). Carcinogenesis **3**, 1129.

Temmink, J.H.M., Bruggeman, I.M. and Van Bladeren, P.J. (1986). Archives Toxicology **59**, 103.

Thomas, I.K., Koizumi, A. and Imamura, T. (1986). Journal Toxicology Environmental Health **19**, 465.

White, R.D., Petry, T.W. and Sipes, I.G. (1984). Chemico Biological Interactions **49**, 225.

Wolf, C.R., Berry, P.M., Nash, J.A., Green, T. and Lock, A.E. (1984). Journal Pharmacology Experimental Therapy **228**, 202.

Working, P.K., Smith-Oliver, T., White, R. and Butterworth, B.E. (1986). Carcinogenesis **7**, 467.

7. Alternatives to whole animals in xenobiotic research

ALTERNATIVES TO WHOLE ANIMALS IN XENOBIOTIC RESEARCH

Gillian M. Powell

Department of Biochemistry, University College,
PO Box 78, Cardiff CF1 1XL, Wales, UK

Man has always exploited the rest of the animal kingdom and from earliest times animals have afforded a means of understanding those conditions that affect human health and well-being. It is quite clear that the use of experimental animals has contributed immeasurably to man's health, nutrition and welfare both directly and indirectly, particularly in relation to the production of food. However, therein lies a central and often-debated dilemma, for the moral implications of animal usage are seemingly incompatible with the benefits that accrue. All cultures, irrespective of religious doctrines place upon man specific responsibilities towards the use and treatment of animals. The current climate of opinion urges scientists to take those responsiblities more and more seriously and at the extreme end of the spectrum, opinion is that animal usage is both immoral and unnecessary. The counter argument is equally forceful - it is that the whole animal is indispensable to xenobiotic research and that the complexity of the whole organism cannot be reconstructed by methods *in vitro*.

It should be acknowledged at the outset that in certain areas of xenobiotic research, there are no fully acceptable alternatives to the use of the whole animal. Serious constraints in the use of *in vivo* methods are predicted for the future and it has been suggested that the possibility of these constraints has acted as a spur for the development of additional sophisticated *in vitro* techniques which will contribute to minimising the number of animal experiments. However, the motivation for using alterntive *in vitro* methods relies heavily on confidence in their applicability and reliability.

Many factors, both theoretical and practical may undermine confidence in various *in vitro* methods but the major factor is that most *in vitro* systems are poorly defined biochemically and the facts that have emerged on the use of isolated cell preparations, for example, have not in general been encouraging. Thus it is known that freshly isolated hepatocytes rapidly undergo changes in enzyme complement and that enzyme activities decrease at different rates, the activating enzymes more rapidly than the inactivating ones. Further, toxicological investigations in most mammalian cell lines in culture have doubtful validity because of the limited capacity to activate chemicals metabolically. The recording of false positives and false negatives has persistently dogged the search for *in vitro* methods for toxicity testing and tests such as the Ames test have been subjected to intense scrutiny and evaluation on these grounds. Considerations and implications such as these have meant that many investigators caution the applicability of *in vitro* methodology and question the extent to which results may be extrapolated to the *in vivo* situation.

The problems that surround the transposition of results obtained *in vitro* to the situation *in vivo* should not obscure nor denigrate the immense value of *in vitro* methodology. The history of Biochemistry is generously littered with examples of how experimentation *in vitro* has contributed immeasurably to the advance of knowledge. However, the choice of technique has been undeniably important. For example, Krebs who attributed some of Warburg's major discoveries to perceptive choices of experimental material, said that his own rapid progress in elucidating the urea cycle was partly a result of prior experience with liver slices that, unlike the broken cell proparations then available, retained the ability to produce urea from added ammonium salts or amino acids. This experience is mirrored totally in xenobiotic research. Homogenates and sub-cellular fractions have provided valuable information concerning the biochemical, physiological and pharmacological mechanisms regulating xenobiotic metabolism in many types of metabolic investigation. In particular, sub-fractions have been used to assess the stability of compounds in the presence of liver metabolic enzymes and many studies have been prosecuted in order to verify that a metabolite perhaps already identified in excreta in whole animal studies is in fact generated by liver enzymes.

Comparisons of hepatic xenobiotic metabolizing capacity in different species have been especially valuable (Smith *et al.*, 1984; Watkins and Klaassen, 1986). For example, the greater activation of pyrrolizidine alkaloids in liver microsomes from cattle compared to sheep was used to explain the corresponding greater sensitivity of cattle to those plant toxins (Shull *et al.*, 1976). Methodologically, homogenates and sub-cellular fractions are relatively simple, inexpensive and versatile requiring low quantities of tissue and test compounds. However, for several reasons, sub-cellular fractions may be an unacceptable and inadequate means of approximating *in vivo* metabolism. The loss of compartmentalization, intracellular control mechanisms and essential inter-relationships between various sub-cellular organization may play a prominent role in the regulation of xenobiotic metabolism in the intact animal. Co-factor levels achieved by mitochondria may be important in controlling xenobiotic metabolism in the endoplasmic reticulum and mitochondrial control is of course inoperative in sub-fractions (Erikson and Holtzman 1976).

Co-factors may be added to mimic the whole cell situation but the level of co-factor may be critical and concentrations of co-factor which achieve optimal activity may give rise to the formation of metabolites which may be of minor importance *in vivo*. An additional adverse effect of tissue homogenization is the functional alteration of membrane-bound enzymes (Billings *et al.*, 1977) that result from the liberation of enzymes and inhibitors from sub-cellular organelles (Fry and Bridges, 1977). The loss of natural relationships that exist between Phase I and II enzymes and the regulatory influence of xenobiotic translocation into the intact cells has also been particularly noted by Fry and Bridges (1977).

What emerges from all these considerations is that *in vitro* methods entailing cell disruption have a very valuable function in xenobiotic research but the *in vitro/in vivo* correlation may be far from perfect. Nevertheless, it should not be assumed that correlations are impossible. For example, Ciramadol, a potent analgesic in experimental animals and man is metabolized to form two glucuronides, one resulting from the conjugation of the phenolic hydroxy group, the other from the glucuronidation of the phenolic hydroxy group in the cyclohexanol moiety. The alicyclic glucuronide is the most abundant urinary metabolite in the rhesus monkey whereas it is only a minor metabolite in man. This could have been predicted from *in vitro* experiments which showed that microsomes from rhesus monkey liver produce five times more alicyclic glucuronide than aryl glucuronide. With human microsomes only the aryl glucuronide is formed (Ruelius 1987). Findings such as these have important consequences for, if a good *in vitro/in vivo* correlation is validated, *in vitro* experiments with human tissue could become a predictive tool.

Isolated whole cells provide opportunities to examine a wide range of experimental variables in recent years isolated cells, most notably hepatocytes, have become an increasingly valuable *in vitro* method for studying xenobiotic metabolism and toxicity (Fry and Bridges, 1979,; Moldeus *et al.*, 1983; Smith and Orrenius, 1984). They have the advantage that sub-cellular architecture is maintained, the cellular environment can be manipulated and the relationship between metabolism and toxic manifestation can be assessed. However, there are also immense problems in extrapolating results to the *in vivo* situation for several reasons. It is known that enzymic capacity is altered in some cases and that changes in cell surfaces occur, presumably due to the preparative procedures (Hughes *et al.*, 1985). Perhaps more seriously, putative toxic metabolites normally cleared either via the bile or blood remain in the media with the result that false positive toxicity is generated (Hughes *et al.*, 1985).

Isolated organ perfusion can serve as a useful bridge between other *in vitro* studies and *in vivo* studies but Fry and Bridges (1979) have cited several methodological difficulties with respect to the isolated perfused liver, the most extensively studied system, including interferences from hormones and vasoactive factors, insufficient gas exchange and the difficulties of verifying viability during perfusion. The technique has also been described as inflexible and limiting in that only one set of variables can be studied in a single liver (Shull *et al.*, 1987). However, considerable advances have been made in validating the isolated perfused liver system and viability parameters have been extensively explored. Technical difficulties have been largely overcome and it has been shown that the system is particularly valuable for studies on xenobiotic metabolism and the partitioning of compounds and their metabolites between blood and bile. Furthermore, the system produces hightly reproducible results and is highly versatile rather than inflexible (Al-Quesy *et al.*, 1985; Hughes *et al.*, 1985; Mutni *et al.*, 1986; Roy *et al.*, 1987).

At this stage it is useful to highlight some considerations of *in vitro* techniques:

1. The limitations of *in vitro* model systems certainly require close scrutiny and the results of experiments in relation to *in vivo* work can be assessed only with due regard to those limitations.
2. Much current research is directed towards careful validation of *in vitro* models with detailed investigations of criteria of acceptibility in terms of metabolic and physiological competence.
3. The effectiveness of *in vitro* systems is undeniable for tackling fundamental problems of toxicity, particularly mechanistic problems.

4. The choice of an *in vitro* system must depend upon the experimental goals and the appropriateness of the system to them.
5. The effects of a chemical *in vivo* are never fully explained by studies *in vitro*. Nevertheless, the advance of xenobiotic research is dependent on progress in understanding mechanisms of action of compounds and mechanisms of toxicity at the molecular level. Perceptions of the dangers and benefits of xenobiotics and their usage can be widened only by *in vitro* methodology.

The advances in *in vitro* technology are prodigious but *in vitro* findings cannot yet be used in a predictive manner. It should always be borne in mind that *in vitro* conditions present a number of problems and limitations when results have to be extrapolated to *in vivo* conditions particularly in man. The animal model must remain a basic tool in xenobiotic research. Meaningful studies *in vitro* may depend entirely on suitably designed experiments *in vivo* and particular attention should be given to kinetic studies *in vivo* as necessary preludes to studies *in vitro*. A simple and obvious example is that xenobiotic distribution may be uneven in different organs and there is a real need to measure compound concentrations and flux in all organs. Without these measurement it may be impossible to design meaningful experiments *in vitro* and misleading results may be obtained. Knowledge of the applicability of *in vivo* and *in vitro* systems is advancing rapidly and it is clear that xenobiotic research demands judicious use of the entire spectrum of available methods.

REFERENCES

Al-Quesy, A., Curtis, C.G. and Powell, G.M., 1985, *Biochemical Society Transactions*, 13, 1156.

Billings, R.E., McMahon, R.E., Ashmore, J., and Wagle, S.R., 1977, *Drug Metabolism and Disposition*, 5, 518-526.

Erikson, R.R. and Holtzman, J.L., 1976, *Biochemical Pharmacology*, 25, 1501-1506.

Fry, J.R. and Bridges, J.W., 1977, In *Progress in Drug Metabolism*, edited by J.W. Bridges and L.F. Chasseud (Chichester: John Wiley and Sons), pp.71-118.

Fry, J.R. and Bridges, J.W., 1979, *Reviews in Biochemical Toxicology*, 1, 102-247.

Hughes, H.H., Powell, G.M. and Curtis, C.G., 1985, *Biochemical Society Transactions*, 13, 760-761.

Moldeus, P., Jernstrom, B. and Dawson, J., 1983, *Reviews in Biochemical Toxicology*, 5, 239-265.

Mutni, A., Powell, G.M. and Curtis, C.G., 1985, *Biochemical Society Transactions*, 13, 1191-1192.

Roy, A.B., Curtis, C.G. and Powell, G.M., 1987, *Xenobiotica*, in press.

Ruelius, H.W., 1987, *Xenobiotica*, 17, 255-265.

Shull, L.R., Buckmaster, G.W. and Cheeke, P.R.,1976, *Journal of Animal Science*, 43, 1247-1253.

Shull, L.R., Kirsch, D.G., Lohse, C.L. and Wisniewski, J.A., 1987, *Xenobiotica*, 17, 345-363.

Smith, M.T. and Orrenius, S., 1984. In *Drug Metabolism and Drug Toxicity*, edited by J.R. Mitchell and M.G. Horming (NY: Raven Press), pp.71-98.

Smith, G.S., Watkins, J.B., Thompson, T.N., Rozman, K. and Klasssen, C.D., 1984, *Journal of Animal* Science, 58, 386-395.

Watkins, J.B. and Klaassen, C.D., 1986, *Journal of Animal Science*, 63, 933-942.

THE USE OF HEPATOMA CELLS IN CULTURE AS AN ALTERNATIVE FOR THE STUDY OF DRUG METABOLIZING ENZYMES

G. SIEST[1], D. BAGREL[1], M. LEVY[1], N. FEBVRE[1], S. FOURNEL-GIGLEUX[1], S. ROLIN[2], N. SABOLOVIC[1], M. WELLMAN-BEDNAWSKA[1], M.M. GALTEAU[1] and Y. TOYODA[3]

[1] Centre du Medicament, UA CNRS 597, 30 rue Lionnois, 54000 Nancy, France.
[2] Universite Libre de Bruxelles, Departement de Biologie Moleculaire, 67 rue des Chevaux, 1640 Rhode-St-Genese, Belgium.
[3] Department of Clinical Biochemistry, Faculty of Pharmacy, Meijo University, Nagoya 468, Japan.

Isolated or cultured cell systems are appropriate models for pharmacotoxicological studies. In order to investigate hepatic metabolism, a number of cell systems have been used ranging from freshly isolated hepatocytes to established cell lines. Freshly isolated hepatocytes tend to most resemble in vivo hepatocytes but their useful lifetime is short, generally only a few hours.

In contrast, when put in culture, parenchymal cells survive for several days or weeks depending on experimental conditions. The cultures are made up from either explants or cells isolated using proteolytic enzymes. In conventional cultures, adult hepatocytes retain much of the liver's capability of transforming xenobiotics, but they rapidly exhibit phenotypic alterations leading to decline or loss of the most specific functions - particularly involving drug metabolizing enzymes (Sirica & Pitot, 1980).

The changes in the transformation rates of some xenobiotics are not uniform for the different enzymes. The fact that phase I activities diminish whilst simultaneously, several conjugative activities neither vary nor increase (Croci & Williams, 1985) needs to be considered in using these cells for metabolic studies. Many attempts have been made to maintain xenobiotic transformation rate (improvements in the perfusion technique, use of high quality proteases, culture in enriched media by adding mixtures of hormones, ligands, haem precursors, inducers etc. (Grant et al., 1985).

Human hepatocytes in primary culture seem to be more stable than rat ones.

By co-culturing adult hepatocytes in the presence of another liver epithelial cell type, the maintenance of another liver epithelial cell type, the maintenance of cytochrome P-450 (P-450) and associated activities is greatly enhanced. P-450 content of hepatocytes remains stable up to 9 days and these co-cultured cells are able to synthesize de novo species of P-450 as shown by phenobarbital (PB) induction (Begue et al., 1984).

During the last years, established hepatoma cell lines have also been proposed as a model for pharmacological and toxicological approaches.

DESCRIPTION OF THE HEPATOMA CELL LINES

Many different cell lines derived from rodent hepatoma have now been established in culture. They have been found to differ widely from one to another in the expressed liver functions as well as in their monoxygenase activities. They are mainly of mouse and rat origin; to our knowledge, no rabbit hepatoma cell lines have been established.

Cultured cell lines are usually characterized by different cytological properties such as morphological aspects, serum requirement, doubling times (calculated from growth curves) and plating efficiencies (or colony forming ability); these last two properties are dependent on the culture medium used. They are also characterized by their chromosome number, their differentiated or de-differentiated functions (based on the expression of liver specific functions and depending on growth medium). Lastly, their tumorigenicity (defined as their capacity to produce tumours in nude mice) is also characteristic.

In this paper we describe hepatoma cell lines used for the study of xenobiotic metabolizing enzymes. Two mouse hepatoma cell lines (Hepa-1 and BWT G3) have been independently isolated from the same mouse hepatome (BW7756). Two rat hepatoma cell lines (H5 and Fao) are variants isolated with many others from the line H4IIEC3 of Pitot et al., (1964) derived from the Reuber H35 hepatoma (Reuber, 1961). These cell lines differ both in morphology and in the expression of liver specific functions - in H5 no expression of very specific functions is detectable while Fao secretes albumin, shows alcohol dehydrogenase and aldolase isoenzymes and high basal activities or hormone inducibility of tyrosine aminotransferase.

Until recently few cell lines have been established from human hepatoma. Some of them have been found to retain many of the specific functions which are usually lost upon culturing. Their origin and some of their major properties are summarized in Table I. Three of them (Hep 3B, PLC/PRF/5 and huH-1) contain the hepatitis B virus (HBV) genome integrated into their cellular genome and express the HBV surface antigen (HBsAg).

TABLE I: Hepatoma cell lines: Origin and major properties

Cell lines	Origin	Chromosomes[a]	Functions[b]	Tumorigenicity[c]	Cyt. P-450 PB[d]	Cyt. P-450 BP[e]
Human						
Hep G2	Hepatoblast	54	+++	++	±	+
Hep 3B	Hepatocel. carcin.	60	+++	++	±	+
SK-HEP-1	Liver adeno-carcin.	61	±	++	-	-
PLC/PRF/5	Hepatocel. carcin.	59	+	++	±	+
huH-1	Hepatoblast.	± 60	+++	ND	+	+
HuH-7	Hepatocel. carcin.	60	+++	++	ND	ND
KYN-1	Hepatocel. carcin.	71	+++	++	ND	ND
Mouse						
Hepa-1	BW 7756 Hepatoma	58	++	ND	-	+
BWT G3	BW 7756 Hepatoma	64	++	ND	ND	ND
Rat						
H5	Reuber H35 Hepatoma	47	-	ND	-	+
Fao	Reuber H35 Hepatoma H4IIEC3 deriv.	50	+++	ND	+	+

[a] Chromosome mean number
[b] The hepatoma cell lines have been characterized as differentiated (+) or dedifferentiated (-) based on their expression of some liver specific functions
[c] i.e. producing tumors in nude mice
[d] Cytochrome P-450 inducible by phenobarbital as determined by aldrin epoxidase activity or aflatoxin or N,N dimethylnitrosamine metabolism
[e] Cytochrome P-450 inducible by benzo(a)pyrene as determined by AHH activity or benzo(a)pyrene activation
ND: not determined

Human hepatoma cell lines retain their epitheloid morphology with passage in culture except for SK-HEP-1 which is rather fibroblastic. Hep G2 and Hep 3B at confluence always present vacuoles, perhaps as evidence of their active secetory state. PLC/PRF/5 are always larger and flatter than the other cell lines and their cytoplasm is granular. The chromosome numbers of these human cell lines are stable: few cells are hypertetraploid but the majority of them are hypotriploid. In addition to these human hepatoma cell lines, recent studies reported the establishment of some other human cell lines such as huH-1, HuH-7 or KYN-1.

CELL CULTURE CONDITIONS

Cells are grown as monolayers on plastic vessels at 37°C in a humidified atmosphere of 5% CO_2 in air. For sub-cultivation, cells are harvested by trypsin-EDTA treatment. Usually, the basic medium (Dulbecco's modified Eagle medium, RPMI) is supplemented with 10% serum (foetal or newborn calf serum) and antibiotics (penicillin, tylosin, mycostatin). Until recently the presence of calf serum appeared to be a general requirement for cell viability in vitro. However the presence of serum may modify certain characteristics or properties. Some specific functions like the extent of protein processing could be regulated by the conditions of culture: for instance, the human hepatoma cell line Hep G2 incubated in serum-free medium secretes only pro-apolipoprotein A-I (pro-Apo A-I) whereas in the presence of foetal calf serum both pro- and processed Apo A-I are secreted (Benerjee et al., 1986). Recently chemically defined media which show excellent ability to support growth and colony formation of human hepatoma cell lines have been proposed (Nakabayashi et al., 1984).

ENZYMATIC ACTIVITY MEASUREMENTS

Drug metabolizing inzymes are mostly associated with endoplasmic reticulum but the quantity of cells which can be collected upon culturing is very small and special methods must be developed to prepare these membranes as microsomes. Enzyme activities are therefore usually measured in cell homogenates. This renders these enzyme activities very difficult to measure in hepatoma cell lines and very sensitive techniques have to be used.

CYTOCHROME P-450 AND HEPATOMA CELL LINES

Hepatoma cell lines in clulture may contain certain forms of monooxygenases differing from those prodominating in liver. They preferentially express 3-methylcholanthrene-inducible forms of P-450 which metabolize planar, aromatic and highly lipophilic compounds. These enzymes are present in almost all mammalian and foetal tissues. The PB-inducible P-450 form is present only in a few well-differentiated hepatoma cell lines (Wiebel & Singh, 1980; Wiebel et al., 1984a; Owens & Nebert, 1975). Hepa-1 (mouse) exhibits a very high activity of arylhydrocarbon hydroxylase (AHH) (Hankinson, 1979), highly inducible by 2,3,7,8-tetrachlorodibenzo-p- dioxin (TCDD) and P1-450 appears to be responsible for the total AHH activity present in this cell line (Hankinson et al., 1985).

Rat hepatomas are the best known cells among hepatoma cell lines. P-450 in Reuber cell lines have been widely studied by Wiebel et al. (1984b). They distinguish three types of hepatoma cell lines with respect to their monooxygenase activities:

- lines containing P-450b and other cytochromes P-450 but no detectable P-450c (C2Rev7)
- lines containing only P-450c (H5)
- lines containing both P-450b and P-450c (Fao, 2sFou)

Monooxygenase activities are usually lower than in vivo. The activity of AHH drops from 1.0 nmol/min/mg protein in rat liver (Croci & Williams, 1985) to 0.25 pmol/min/mg protein in H5 (Wiebel et al., 1984b). Sometimes they are not constitutively expressed but can be induced. For example, Fu5-C8 (Reuber hepatoma-derived line) under usual culture conditions does not produce any detectable P-450c after 3-methylcholanthrene (3-MC) treatment (Frey et al., 1984). Moreover, induction in these cell lines may assume particular aspects. PB induces P-450c-dependent monooxygenase activities in some cell lines. In a recent work, McManus et al. (1985) showed that PB induces 2-acetylaminofluorene metabolites in McA-RH7777 to a similar extent as TCDD. These results confirm earlier observations made by others on various liver-derived lines (Wiebel et al., 1984b; Owens & Nebert, 1975; Benedict et al., 1973). This capacity of PB to induce both monooxygenase types (which does not occur in adult rat liver) resembles the findings of Kremers et al. (1981) in cultured foetal hepatocytes. However, some well-differentiated cells may mimic liver with respect to the induction of monooxygenase activities by PB. In C2Rev7, PB increases aldrin epoxidase activity and monoclonal antibodies directed to PB-induced P-450 of rat liver inhibit PB-induced aldrin epoxide activity to the same extent as they do in rat liver microsomes (Wiebel et al., 1984a, b).

Then differentiated hepatoma cell lines may be useful to analyse the mechanism of induction.

Cytochrome P-450 content of human cell lines has been investigated far less. Hap G2 shows an O-deethylation of 7-ethoxycoumarin activity which is slightly increased by PB- (x 1.5) and strongly increased by 3-MC-treatment (x 30). However, attempts to identify the P-450 isozymes in these cells have not been yet successful (Dawson et al., 1985); Sassa et al., 1987). Limbosch (1983) found that Hep G2, Hep 3B and PLC/PRF/5 are able to metabolize benzo(a)pyrene more efficiently than aldrin. SK-HEP-1 seems devoid of both activities. In contrast, huH-1 shows high AHH activity and has retained the capacity to metabolize aflatoxin B1 and N,N dimethylnitrosamine (Huh et al., 1982).

For our part, we found AHH activity much lower in Hap G2 than in the dedifferentiated rat cell line H5.

In conclusion, human as well as rat hepatoma cells display different ranges of monoxygenase activities and efforts must be made to identify cytochrome P-450 isozymes in human cell lines.

EPOXIDE HYDROLASE AND UDP-GLUCURONOSYLTRANSFERASE

Concerning phase II enzymes, microsomal epoxide hydrolase activity (EHm) increases by more than 2-fold in hepatocytes after 24 h in culture and remains elevated in contrast to the cytosolic enzyme (EHc) which drops off rapidly in culture. Hepatoma cells express multiple forms of the microsomal enzyme at various degrees (Razzouk et al., 1985; Duthu and Hankinson, 1983; Raphael et al., 1982).

In the Reuber hepatoma cell line H-4-II-E, Raphael et al. (1982) failed to induce EH whereas monooxygenase activity was increased by a variety of compounds. We obtained the same results by measuring EH levels using an immunoenzymatic method. We could not detect any induction of EHm after PB- or 3-MC-treatments in H5. This lack of induction indicates that EH and monooxygenases are under different controls. As EH of hepatocytes in culture can be induced (Goujon et al., 1980), H5 has probably lost this capacity by dediffenerentiational changes.

UDP-glucuronosyltransferase (UDPGT) and specially UDP-GT1 (preferentially inducible by 3-MC, using planar substrates and distributed in all tissues) is selectively increased in pre-neoplastic liver nodules and in some hepatoma (Bock et al., 1982). In hepatoma cell lines, UDPGT is active and can be induced by different classes of monooxygenase inducers (Malik et al., 1979; Dawson et al., 1985). However no clear correlation appears to exist between the presence and the level of monooxygenase and UDPGT activity. The cultures may express on or both enzymes (Wiebel & Singh, 1980). However, the level of induction of AHH activity is always higher than the level of induction of UDPGT in these cell lines (Malik et al., 1979).

GAMMA-GLUTAMYLTRANSFERASE

Some monooxygenase inducers have been shown to increase in vivo liver GGT. Induction of hepatic GGT by PB has been demonstrated as a possible source of increased GGT in serum (Tazi et al., 1979). These observations led to propose GGT as an index of induction of liver xenobiotic-metabolizing enzymes (Siest et al., 1982). The activitiy of this enzyme is found elevated to foetal pre-neoplastic or neoplastic cells and tissues from several animal species in contrast to its negligible activity in normal rat hepatocytes.

In primary cultures of rat hepatocytes, the initial low GGT activity of freshly isolated hepatocytes is preserved for 2-3 days and thereafter increases progessively from 0-1 nmol/min/mg protein to 10 nmol/min/mg protein after 140 hr in culture. In this system GGT can be induced by PB, dexamethasone or pregnenolone carbonitrile but is not induced by 3-MC and beta-naphthoflavone (Edwards, 1984).

In hepatoma cell lines, GGT is expressed at different levels as shown in Table II. Hep G2 and PLC/PRF/5 strongly express this enzyme whereas Hep 3B and SK-HEP-I exhibit very low activity.

TABLE II: Activity of gamma-glutamyltransferase in some hepatoma cell lines

Human		**Rat**		**Mouse**	
I	II	I	II	I	II
Hep G2	60-80	Fao	1-3	Hepa-1	0.5-1
Hep 3B	1-3	Faza 967	2-4	BWT G3	1-2
SK-HEP-1	1-3	Fu5	0-2		
PLC/PRF/5	65-90	H5	80-120		

I Cell lines 24 h in culture
II GGT activity expressed in nmol/min/mg protein

GGT histochemistry has been assayed on these cells according the method of Rutenburg (1969) adapted by Manson (1982) and we confirm preceding results. GGT of PLC/PRF/5 (human) is present as a weak cytoplasm gradient and shows an intense cell surface activity at cell- cell contacts. A cytoplasmic gradient of GGT activity also occurs with the highest activity in the area surrounding the nucleus (Richards et al., 1982).

SK-HEP-1 has no activity 72 h and 96 h after subculture. In Hep 3B, GGT activity is evident only in some isolated cell clusters within predominantly GGT negative cell populations. Hep G2 cells are strongly GGT positive with a typical localization of important juxtanuclear round or oval aggregates. All cells are positive, but GGT distribution seems to be heterogeneous in these last two cell populations.

In these human sells, GGT has not been induced either by PB- or 3-MC-treatments whereas these xenobiotics induce AHH activity.

The same diversity in GGT distribution can be observed among the Reuber lines tested. In Fao, no GGT activity tested by histochemistry can be detected even 120 h after subculture. In contrast H5 has an intense surface activity 24 h after sub-culture. All cells are positive and show GGT regular aggregates homogeneously distributed on the membrane. We specially tested the induction of GGT in H5 and the best inducer was ethanol. Although the induction by PB and 3-MC is late and low the induction of GGT by ethanol reflecting this enzyme behaviour in vivo., this cell line can be considered a useful model for studying the action of this xenobiotic.

In summary, hepatoma cells are useful material for xenobiotic metabolic studies. They contain many isoforms of all drug metabolizing enzymes. Some of these proteins are inducible and their regulation can be followed. Since all isoforms are not represented in all cell lines, a battery of cells with defined enzyme composition has to be used in relation to the different applications. The specificity of the protein is an important criterion for human hepatoma cells. It is possible to use these cells for toxicological screening, drug interaction studies, alcohol interferences, receptor recycling and finally for the production of metabolites, hormonal factors or specific proteins.

REFERENCES

Banerjee, D., Grieninger, G., Parkes, J.L., Mukherjee, T.K. & Redman, C.M., 1986, *Journal of Biological Chemistry*, 261, 9844.

Begue, J.M., Guguen-Guillouzo, C., Pasdeloup, N. & Guillouzo, A., 1984, *Hepatology*, 4, 839.

Benedict, W.F., Gielen, J.E., Owens, I.S., Niwa, A. & Nebert, D.W., 1973, *Biochemical Pharmacology*, 22, 2766.

Bock. K.W., Lillenblum, W., Pfeil, H. & Eriksson, L.C., 1982, *Cancer Research*, 42, 3747.

The Use of Isolated Perfused Organs

C.G. CURTIS, H.M. HUGHES and G.M. POWELL.

Department of Biochemistry, University College,
P.O. Box 78, Cardiff, Wales, CF1 1XL

INTRODUCTION

As knowledge of individual metabolic reactions becomes more complete, biochemists are turning to more complex systems in attempts to appreciate the integration and kinetics of metabolism and how these processes may be affected by toxins. The rationale for this shift in emphasis is based on the increasing amount of data showing that the whole is not necessarily the sum of its parts. In terms of the various levels of biological organisation the techniques of organ perfusion lie between whole animal studies on the one hand and whole cell preparations on the other. An organ or tissue may be studied in vitro, isolated from other tissues, by supplying oxygen and nutrients perfused in an appropriate medium through the vascular bed. One of the major advantages of such a system is that the cells are not fragmented or dispersed and by maintaining normal anatomical polarity and physiological relationships some of the cellular dynamics and cellular inter-dependence is preserved.

PERFUSED ORGANS UNDER INVESTIGATION

To date, in this department, the isolated perfused liver, kidney, lung and small intestine have been used for metabolism studies and toxicity testing.

Metabolism studies

Once it has been established that, in the whole animal, a drug, insecticide, herbicide, environmental pollutant or industrial chemical is taken up by, or becomes associated with one of these organs then the contribution of the organ to whole body metabolism of the compound is investigated by perfusion techniques. For each organ these studies provide information on (1) the nature and capacity of routes of metabolism (2) routes and rates of secretion of metabolites (3) competiton with endogenous and other exogenous molecules for uptake metabolism and secretion. Moreover, the perfusion systems are particularly useful as 'metabolite factories' for generating sufficient quantities of metabolites for structural analysis. Often this is not possible without using large numbers of animals or dose levels which may be toxic.

Toxicity testing

It is inevitable that removal of an organ from the body and perfusion *in vitro* will have some effect(s) on the tissue. Proof of this is provided by the fact that even the best perfusion systems are measured in hours rather than days. Consequently, although it is relatively easy to demonstrate metabolic conversions by perfused organs the question frequently asked is "Just how reliable is the metabolic data?" How viable are perfused organs? and how closely do they mimic the *in vivo* situation? Clearly, in order to acquire confidence in any perfusion system viability tests must be carried out simultaneously. These will vary from one tissue to another but once criteria of viability have been established then these can be utilized to monitor the effects of potential toxins. In this respect, of the four organs under investigation, the isolated liver has been assessed most thoroughly, the order of the next being lung $>$ kidney $>$ small intestine.

Liver perfusion

Perfusion of the liver through its vascular bed was reported by Claude Bernard as early as 1855 and the value of the method as a means of investigating specific problems has been demonstrated by many research groups (Miller *et al.*, 1951; 1973; Brauer, 1951; Hems *et al.*, 1966). In these laboratories liver viability is monitored routinely by (1) the rate of incorporation of radiolabelled amino acids into plasma proteins (2) incorporation of radiolabelled sugars into plasma glycoproteins (3) incorporation of ^{14}C-acetate and ^{14}C-mevalonic acid into plasma lipoproteins and (4) receptor-mediated endocytosis of radiolabelled asialoglycoproteins. Collectively these processes constitute a significant proportion of hepatic metabolism because each requires the inter-dependent operation of a number of multi-stage metabolic pathways and membrane activities. If the primary aim is to pinpoint the site(s) and mechanism(s) of action of a particular drug, industrial chemical, food additive, herbicide or pesticide, then the response of these four processes to a potential toxin may be helpful because the results may either eliminate areas of hepatic metabolism from any further consideration or the results may show which of these multi-stage processes respond to chemical challenge.

Short term versus long term toxicity testing in perfused liver

In the protocol for short term testing, the rate of incorporation of radiolabelled precursors into plasma proteins, glycoproteins or lipoproteins is allowed to reach steady-state, which is achieved within 1.5h after the onset of perfusion. The potential hepatotoxin is then added as a pulse dose and/or by continuous infusion for 6-8h. This procedure has the considerable advantage that each liver is used as its own control (prior to the addition of toxin) which overcomes the need to consider variations in rates that many arise between livers. By contrast, in long term tests, the intact animals are predosed with compound(s) at regular intervals and the livers removed and perfused at the appropriate time. Figure I shows the incorporation of ^{14}C-acetate into plasma triglycerides in control livers and test livers to which the anti-hyperlipidaemic drug gemfibrozil was added to the perfusate 3.0h after the onset of perfusion. Under these conditions, the production of ^{14}C-labelled triglycerides was greatly inhibited by gemfibrozil, whereas other anti-hyperlipidaemic drugs such as clofibrate had no effect. Similarly, in long-term experiments in which rats were dosed daily up to 17 days with either gemfibrozil or clofibrate the effects were the same viz. inhibition by gemfibrozil but no effect with clofibrate. Thus, with respect to triglyceride production, gemfibrozil has an inhibitory effect both in the short-term and after long-term dosing and the possibility that the anti-hyperlipidaemic effect of this drug is due to inhibition of triglyceride production is worthy of further investigation. By contrast, gemfibrozil has quite different effects on plasma protein production in the two experimental systems. In short-term tests gemfibrozil inhibits the incorporation of ^{14}C-leucine into plasma proteins whereas predosing over 17 days had no apparent effect. This suggests that the observed inhibition of protein synthesis by gemfibrozil in perfused liver in the short term does not explain the anti-hyperlipidaemic effect of the drug *in vivo*.

Figure I.

Effect of gemfibrozil on ^{14}C-acetate incorporation into triglycerides by the isolated perfused rat liver.

□ - Control
▨ - Gemfibrozil (1.4mM) added after 3h.

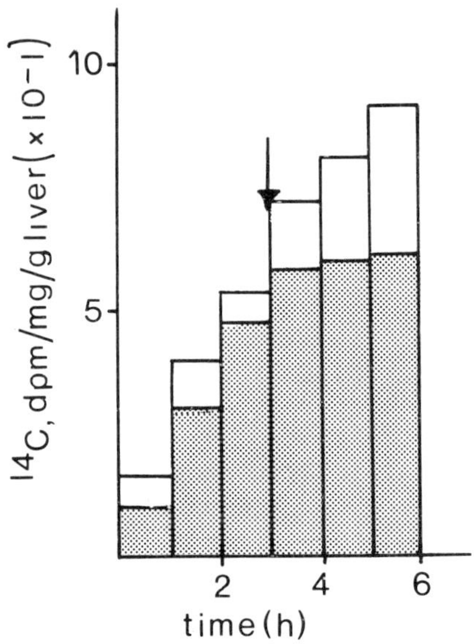

<u>Perfused liver versus hepatocytes as models for testing potential hepatotoxins</u>

Figure 2 compares the effects of the antioxidant butylated hydroxytoluene (BHT) on protein production in the isolated perfused rat liver with that in isolated rat hepatocytes. Whereas protein synthesis is inhibited, approximately 80% by 0.6mM in hepatocytes, the same concentration has no effect on the whole liver. Similar effects were observed with the anti-depressant imipramine, which at 0.1mM inhibited protein production by hepatocytes by 50% but multiple doses of 0.1mM imipramine had no effect on total protein or glycoprotein production in the perfused liver. The different responses of the two systems to BHT and imipramine might be due to the inability of hepatocytes to remove any drug and/or its metabolites from the immediate environment. In the perfused liver system, the structural integrity of the organ ensures that biliary secretion is unimpaired so that the blood level of drug equivalents drops rapidly as it would *in vivo*. In hepatocyte preparations, the polarity of the cells is lost. There is no longer, bile on the cannulicular surface and blood on the sinusoidal surface and parent compound and metabolites released into the medium are exposed to both surfaces.

The response of the whole liver and hepatocytes to other toxins such as certain lectins may also differ for other reasons. In the perfused liver very low concentrations of ricin are required to inhibit plasma protein synthesis measured by the incorporation of either ^{14}C-leucine (Fig. 3) or N-acetyl-^{3}H glucosamine. By contrast, primary hepatocyte preparations are sometimes markedly less sensitive to ricin even at relatively high concentrations. The extent of inhibition may be dependent upon the procedure adopted for cell isolation. For example, cells prepared using some collagenase preparations showed very little inhibition (20%) of ^{14}C-leucine incorporation into protein even in the presence of 10nM ricin (Fig. 3) whereas hepatocytes isolated using other commercially available collagenases showed up to 80% inhibition at the same concentration of ricin. The uptake of ricin is known to be receptor mediated (Olsnes *et al.*, 1974) and presumably these differences between different cell preparations of hepatocytes and the isolated perfused liver are due to changes in cell surface properties caused by the isolation procedures.

Perhaps even more crucial is the fact that isolated hepatocytes which are judged to be viable by dye exclusion methods are frequently compromised and more susceptible to a toxic challenge. For example in some hepatocyte preparations the initial viability value was 90% when assessed by trypan blue exclusion and this was maintained to within 10% of the initial value over 4h. However, these cells showed no incorporation of ^{14}C-leucine into protein over 4h, and it would appear that measurement of protein production, is a more sensitive and reliable indicator of functional hepatocytes. By comparing the response of cells and the whole organ to a range of drugs it is clear that the hepatocyte system is best used after it has been established that both systems respond to the same dose range of toxin.

Figure 2.

Effect of BHT on ^{14}C-leucine incorporation

By rat hepatocytes

□ - Control
▩ - BHT (0.6mM) added at zero time

By perfused liver

□ - Control
▩ - BHT (0.6mM) added after 1.5h

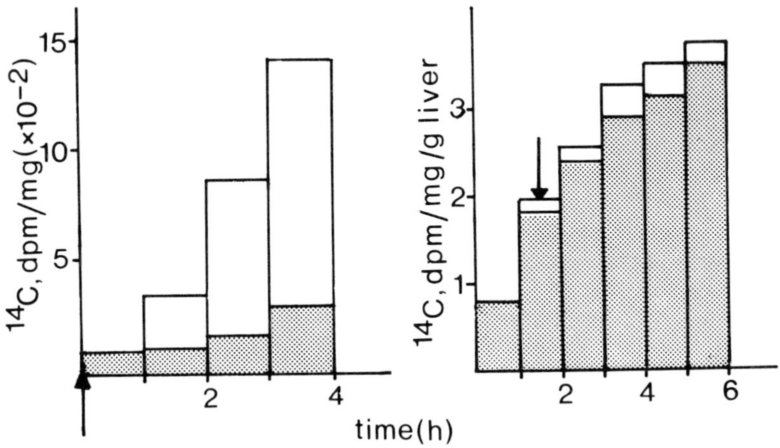

Figure 3.

Effect of ricin on ^{14}C-leucine incorporation

By rat hepatocytes

□ - Control
▩ - Ricin (10nM) added at zero time

By perfused liver

□ - Control
▩ - Ricin (1nM) added after 1.5h

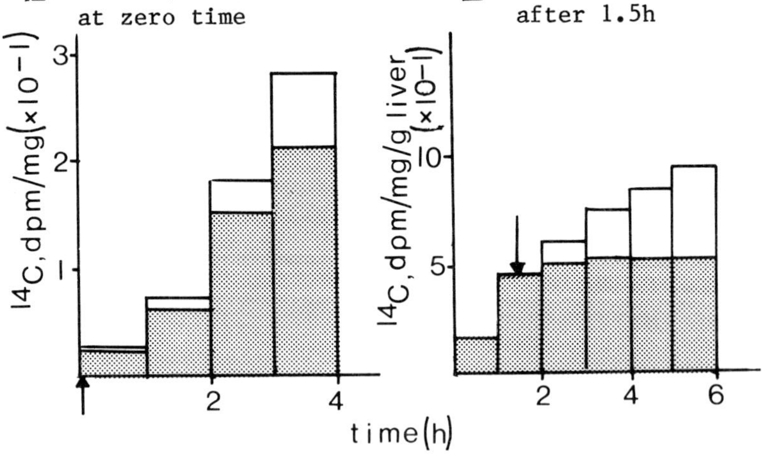

Receptor mediated endocytosis in perfused liver

The isolated perfused liver also provides an ideal model to screen for cell surface changes by measuring the gross kinetics of asialoglycoprotein uptake from the perfusate. Model substrates include horse radish peroxidase (requiring mannose receptors) ^{125}I-asialofetuin (galactose receptors) and ^{125}I-lactoferrin (fucose receptors). Although the use of specific inhibitors may assist in unravelling the mechanism(s) of hepatic uptake, the consequences of inhibiting receptor-mediated endocytosis with respect to liver and whole body functions are not understood. Nevertheless, this process is the summation of a number of complex molecular and cellular events including recognition, internalisation and receptor recycling, and chemicals which perturb this process, particularly the receptors at the cell surface, may also interfere with cell-cell interactions. It may be significant therefore that in perfused preneoplastic livers induced by aflatoxins B_1 the kinetics of asialoglycoprotein uptake from perfusate is perturbed (Al-Thamir *et al*. 1987).

PERFUSION OF ISOLATED LUNG, KIDNEY AND SMALL INTESTINE

The metabolic fates of a wide range of compounds have been investigated in these isolated organs and it is clear that such preparations are suitable for metabolism studies. However, assessments of viability in these preparations have not been investigated as fully as in the liver. Nevertheless experience with the perfused liver and isolated hepatocyte preparations has emphasised the crucial need for such assessments if these preparations are to be considered as alternatives to whole animals for metabolic studies and for toxicity testing.

REFERENCES

Al-Thamir, S.N.K., Neal, D., Connors, T.A., Powell, G.M. and Curtis, C.G. *Biochemical Society Transactions*, (1987) In Press.

Brauer, R.W., Pessotti, R.L. and Pizzolato, P. (1951) *Proceedings Society of Experimental Biology and Medicine*, 18, 174.

Hems, R., Ross, B.D., Berry, H.N. and Krebs, H.A. (1966) *Biochemical Journal*, 101, 284.

Miller, L.L. (1973) in *Isolated Liver Perfusion and its Applications*, 1-52 Raven Press, New York.

Miller, L.L., Bly, C.G., Watson, H.L. and Bale, W.F. (1951) *Journal of Experimental Medicine*, 94, 431.

Olsnes, S., Refnes, K. and Pihl, A. (1974) *Nature*, 249, 627.

Metabolism of xenobiotics in isolated cells: comparison with other *in vitro* systems and *in vivo*.

JEFFREY R. FRY

Department of Physiology and Pharmacology, Medical School, Queen's Medical Centre, Nottingham NG7 2UH, U.K.

There is a hierarchy of systems which may be used for the study of drug metabolism (Table 1), the members of which differ in a number of features, including their likely relevance to the *in vivo* situation. However, there is no single "best" system; rather, one has to choose a system that is most appropriate to the particular question posed. It is this appropriateness that defines the advantages to a system, and it is my brief in this review to discuss the advantages to the use of isolated intact cells in drug metabolism studies, with emphasis on the use of isolated hepatocytes.

Table 1. Hierarchy of drug metabolizing systems.

Whole animal
Perfused liver
Liver slices
Isolated hepatocytes
Liver homogenate and its fractions
Purified enzymes

The isolated hepatocyte system lies in the middle of this hierarchical order, and the advantages of this system must be discussed in relation to both extremes of the hierarchy. Thus, intact isolated cells may be used to assess the importance at a cellular level of phenomena observed in homogenate systems, and also as a simple cellular system for more detailed study of phenomena observed in the whole animal. In addition, intact isolated cells may be used for studies of cellular function which would be extremely difficult, if not impossible, to conduct in other cellular-based systems, including the lobar distribution of drug metabolizing activity in liver, metabolizing activity in preneoplastic nodules, and metabolizing activity in individual cell types. How well, then, does the intact isolated cell system relate to the *in vivo* and homogenate/fraction situations? What are the most appropriate uses of isolated cells? Some answers to these questions will be given in this brief review.

Comparison of drug metabolizing activity in intact isolated cells and homogenates/fractions; quantitative aspects

Examples of virtually all the principal Phase I and Phase II reactions demonstrated in liver organelles have been described in intact hepatocytes (see Table 1 in Fry 1982). For the cytochrome P450-dependent mixed function oxidase (MFO) reactions, reports have indicated that the activity towards most substrates is similar in isolated hepatocytes and hepatic microsomal fractions (see Fry 1982). However, some MFO reactions appear to be less active in hepatocytes relative to microsomes (see Fry 1982), the reasons for which are not readily apparent. Ideally, metabolism studies performed in isolated hepatocytes should use low substrate concentrations so as to minimize toxicity problems (a problem not encountered in microsomal incubations) and there is the possibility that, for enzymes exhibiting biphasic kinetics, different forms of the enzyme may be measured at the low substrate concentrations in cells and the higher concentration in microsomes. Some MFO reactions are more active in isolated hepatocytes relative to microsomes (Billings et al. 1978; Ericksson et al. 1982). In the case of ethylmorphine N-demethylase activity this has been ascribed to the involvement of an active transport system for the substrate in isolated hepatocytes (Ericksson et al. 1982).

Studies of the comparability of activities of conjugating enzymes in isolated cells and homogenate/fractions have been attempted (Andersson et al. 1978; Koster et al. 1986) but are fraught with problems, including (a) the presence of active, competing pathways of conjugation in isolated cells, and (b), in the case of UDP-glucuronosyltransferase, the known latency of this enzyme.

Comparison of drug metabolizing activity in intact isolated cells and perfused organs, and in vivo; quantitative aspects

Previous studies have demonstrated that the rates of barbiturate metabolism, 1-naphthol glucuronidation and butamoxane and amphetamine hydroxylation are similar in isolated hepatocytes and perfused liver (see Fry 1982). More recently, Stefek & Bezek (1985) have indicated that the Vmax value for pentacaine metabolism is similar in isolated hepatocytes and perfused liver.

There appear to be few reports concerning the comparability of rates of xenobiotic metabolism in isolated hepatocytes and *in vivo*, although Stewart & Inaba (1979) have demonstrated that the rate of aminopyrine N-demethylation (as judged on a gram liver basis) is comparable in the two systems, whilst Morais & Wagner (1985) have demonstrated a good agreement in the clearance values for corticosterone in these systems.

Comparison of drug metabolism in isolated hepatocytes, liver microsomes and the whole animal; qualitative aspects

A number of studies have amply demonstrated that the patterns of metabolism of particular drugs in isolated hepatocytes resemble much more closely those observed during studies *in vivo* than do those in liver microsome systems. Thus, the patterns of metabolism of 3-phenoxybenzoic acid (Huckle et al. 1984), antipyrine (Aarbakke et al. 1977), methfuroxam (Mitchell & Paulson 1982), amphetamine (Green et al. 1986), tolbutamide (Gee et al. 1984) and cyclophosphamide (Bates et al. 1981) in rat isolated hepatocytes are very similar to those in the rat *in vivo*. These findings should not be too surprising as they are a consequence of one of the principal attributes of isolated cells in drug metabolism studies, *viz.*, the retention of all the routes of metabolism operating *in vivo*, at normal physiological levels of cofactors, and under the restraint of the various rate-limiting controls that exist in intact cells. This point is illustrated by the study of de Bethizy & Rickert (1984) into the metabolism of 3-nitrotoluene by rat isolated hepatocytes and liver microsomes. The major primary metabolite produced in both systems was 3-nitrobenzyl alcohol, but only in the hepatocytes was this metabolite metabolized further to a glucuronide, and 3-nitrobenzoic acid, this latter reaction presumably catalysed by cytosolic dehydrogenases. However, it is obvious that this similarity in patterns of metabolism will hold only if the liver is the major route of metabolism *in vivo*. Furthermore, the finding of a particular modification of metabolism in isolated hepatocytes is no guarantee that such an effect will be observed in the whole animal. Thus, although enhancement of biphenyl 2-hydroxylation by betamethasone could be demonstrated in rat liver microsomes and isolated hepatocytes, no such effect could be demonstrated in the total body metabolism of biphenyl (Miller et al. 1983).

What are the most appropriate uses for isolated hepatocytes?

At least four inter-related uses for isolated hepatocytes can be suggested on the basis of current published research, each of which takes advantage of the similarity of rates and patterns of metabolism to the *in vivo* situation discussed in the previous paragraphs. These uses are: study of the balance of multiple pathways of metabolism, delineation of metabolic pathways of novel compounds, assessment of organ/species differences in drug metabolism, and study of the relation of metabolism to toxicity. Examples of these uses will be discussed briefly.

Study of balance of multiple pathways of metabolism

Cytochrome P450 exists as a family of isozymic forms of differing substrate specificity, and the possibility has been considered that the type of cytochrome P450 involved in the generation of a hydroxylated metabolite might influence the balance of sulphation/glucuronidation of the hydroxylated metabolite. The rationale that was adopted for the study of this problem was to identify two substrates which were metabolized to a common hydroxylated metabolite by different forms of cytochrome P450, and to study the patterns of metabolism of these substrates in isolated hepatocytes at similar rates of generation of the hydroxylated metabolite (Paterson et al. 1984; Paterson & Fry 1985). It should be noted that liver microsomal studies were essential for the initial experiments to establish the involvement of different forms of cytochrome P450 in the pair of reactions. The findings of these studies were that the type of cytochrome P450 did not influence the balance of subsequent conjugation, but that inducer metabolites retained within cells after isolation could influence the pattern of conjugation.

Delineation of metabolic pathways of novel compounds

Previously unidentified metabolites of ethinimate (Billings et al. 1977), 5-fluorouracil (Sommadossi et al. 1985) and cyclophosphamide (Bates et al. 1981) have been identified following metabolism studies in rat isolated hepatocytes. The novel metabolite of ethinimate (ketoethiniate) was later identified in the urine of rats dosed with ethinimate, whilst the novel metabolite of 5-fluorouracil was a glucuronide and that of cyclophosphamide was a glucuronic acid conjugate of 4-hydroxycyclophosphamide. Such studies strongly suggest that isolated hepatocyte systems could be of value in the delineation of metabolic pathways of novel compounds.

Assessment of organ/species differences in drug metabolism

Benzoic acid is conjugated predominantly with glycine in omnivores including man, with the glucuronic acid conjugate being only a very minor metabolite; in carnivores, however, the glucuronide is a more prominent metabolite in quantitative terms (Bridges et al. 1970). Studies with hepatocytes and kidney cells isolated from two omnivorous species (rat and hamster) and two carnivorous species (dog and ferret) have demonstrated that these species differences in metabolism can be explained by an absence of the glycine conjugation pathway in the liver of the carnivores, although activity of the glucuronidation pathway is similar in the livers of all four species. A high capacity for glycine conjugation was observed in the kidney cells isolated from the carnivores (Kao et al. 1979).

The patterns of metabolism of amphetamine and tolbutamide show great species variations, and recent studies by Tyson & coworkers (Gee et al. 1984; Green et al. 1986) have demonstrated that these variations are faithfully mimicked in hepatocytes isolated from these species (including man, in the amphetamine study).

These studies indicate the promise of isolated hepatocytes for the study of species differences in drug metabolism, with particular emphasis on the extrapolation of animal data to man.

Role of metabolism to toxicity

The hepatotoxicity of paracetamol is dependent upon the generation of a reactive metabolite, and the rate of this generation and the subsequent hepatotoxicity shows species variation (Davis et al. 1974). Studies with isolated hepatocytes have confirmed this species variation in both the pattern of metabolism and cytotoxicity (Moldeus 1978; Boobis et al. 1986). The study by Boobis et al. (1986) also indicated that human isolated hepatocytes were resistant to paracetamol cytotoxicity which was not due to a resistance to the reactive metabolite since a synthetic sample of this metabolite produced comparable toxicity in hepatocytes isolated from each species studied (rat, mouse, hamster and man).

Conclusions

It is apparent that the choice of drug metabolizing system should be dictated by the nature of the problem being studied. Available evidence indicates that isolated hepatocytes retain the rates and patterns of metabolism associated with such cells in perfused liver or *in vivo*. It is thus apparent that the most appropriate uses for isolated hepatocytes are those in which retention of competing multiple pathways of metabolism is of particular importance. Some examples of such uses have been described.

REFERENCES

Aarbakke, J., Bessesen, A. & Morland, J., 1977, *Acta pharmacologica et toxicologica*, 41, 225.

Andersson, B., Berggren, M. & Moldeus, P., 1978, *Drug Metabolism and Disposition*, 6, 611.

Bates, D.J., Foster, A.B. & Jarman, M., 1981, *Biochemical Pharmacology 30, 3055.*

Billings, R.E., McMahon, R.E., Ashmore, J. & Wagle, S.R., 1977, *Drug Metabolism and Disposition*, 5, 518.

Billings, R.E., Murphy, P.J., McMahon, R.E. & Ashmore, J. *Biochemical Pharmacology*, 27, 2525.

Boobis, A.R., Tee, L.B.G., Hampden, C.E. & Davis, D.S., 1986, *Food and Chemical Toxicology*, 24, 731.

Bridges, J.W., French, M.R., Smith, R.L. & Williams, R.T., 1970, *Biochemical Journal*, 118, 47.

Davis, D.C., Potter, W.Z., Jollow, D.J. & Mitchell, J.R., 1974, *Life Sciences*, 14, 2099.

de Bethizy, J.D. & Rickert, D.E., 1984, *Drug Metabolism and Disposition*, 12, 45.

Ericksson, R.R., Yudrent, P. & Holtzman, J.L., 1982, *Journal of Pharmacology and Experimental Therapeutics*, 220, 35.

Fry, J.R., 1982, *Quarterly Reviews on Drug Metabolism and Drug Interactions*, 4, 99.

Gee, S.J., Green, C.E. & Tyson, C.A., 1984, *Drug Metabolism and Disposition*, 12, 174.

Green, C.A., Le Valley, S.E. & Tyson, C.A., 1986, *Journal of Pharmacology and Experimental Therapeutics*, 237, 931.

Huckle, K.R., Hutson, D.H. & Millburn, P., 1984, *Drug Metabolism and Disposition*, 12, 264.

Kao, J., Jones, C.A., Fry, J.R. & Bridges, J.W., 1979, *Life Sciences*, 23, 1221.

Koster, A.S., Frankhuyzen-Sierevogel, A.C. & Metruip, A., 1986, *Biochemical Pharmacology*, 35, 1981.

Miller, M.S., Huang, M.T., Williams, G.M., Jeffrey, A.M. & Conney, A.H., 1983, *Drug Metabolism and Disposition*, 11, 556.

Mitchell, A.D. & Paulson, G.D., 1982, *Pesticide Biochemistry and Physiology*, 18, 57.

Moldeus, P., 1978, *Biochemical Pharmacology*, 27, 2859.

Morais, J.A. & Wagner, J.G., 1985, *European Journal of Drug Metabolism and Pharmacokinetics*, 10, 295.

Paterson, P. & Fry, J.R., 1985, *Xenobiotica*, 15, 493.

Paterson, P, Fry, J.R. & Horner, S.A., 1984, *Xenobiotica*, 14, 849.

Sommadissi, J.P., Gross, D.S., Gewirtz, D.A., Goldman, I.D., Cano, J.P. & Diasio, R.B., 1985, *Cancer Research*, 45, 2450.

Stefek, M. & Bezek, S., 1985, *Xenobiotica*, 15, 805.

Stewart, D.J. & Inaba, T., 1979, *Biochemical Pharmacology*, 28, 461.

METABOLISM ON RECONSTRUCTED MODEL SYSTEMS.

Alain FRIBOULET, Didier GUILLOCHON and Daniel THOMAS.

Laboratoire de Technologie Enzymatique.
UA 523 du CNRS.
Université de Compiègne, Compiègne 60206, FRANCE.

A wide range of in vitro techniques for toxicity assessment have now been developed, including the use of enzymes, subcellular fractions, short-term cellular systems and tissue culture. These in vitro tests are designed to replace certain animal toxicity tests, such as the LD50. Attention is now beginning to be focused on the development of tests which are capable of predicting not only the toxicity of a compound but also its metabolism and its target at the molecular level. In the present work, we have studied two model systems.

The hydroxylating enzyme systems of mammalian liver microsomes are responsible for the metabolism of toxins, drugs, carcinogens, steroids and fatty acids.These systems include an electron donor, an electron transfer flavoprotein and cytochrome P-450 as terminal oxidase. An alternative to the development of in vitro systems containing cytochrome P-450 which allow the evaluation of the metabolism of xenobiotics, it is tempting to elaborate simple model systems exhibiting cytochrome P-450-like activities. An aniline hydroxylation activity was described with a haemoglobin-cytochrome P-450 reductase-NADPH system (Mieyal et al., 1976). Similar results were obtained by Akhrem et al. (1978) with an NADPH-riboflavin-haemoglobin system, and by Tomoda et al. (1977) with red blood cells in the presence of methylene blue. Simple systems containing haemoglobin were tested for their catalytic activities, the regioselectivity and mechanism of aniline hydroxylation.

The use of insolubilized acetylcholinesterase (AChE), the key enzyme of the neuromuscular junction, allows (i) in vitro systematic screening of the potential toxicities of chemicals by coupling with an electronic sensor,the enzyme electrode (Durand & Thomas, 1984), (ii) to open new routes in understanding the pharmacology of AChE by studying reversible and irreversible phases of the reactions, synergistic and antagonist behaviours during multiinhibitor experiments, long term exposure to subtoxic doses, or evaluation of the potency of reactivators.

HYDROXYLATIONS BY HAEMOGLOBIN SYSTEMS

On the analogy of the cytochrome P-450 system, different model systems containing haemoglobin were assayed for their capacity to catalyze aniline hydroxylation (Table 1)

Table 1 : Initial appearance rates of 4-aminophenol formation by hydroxylation of aniline by haemoglobin in NADH, ascorbate, dihydroxyfumarate and red blood cell systems.

<table>
<tr><th></th><th>Methaemoglobin</th><th>Oxyhaemoglobin</th></tr>
<tr><td>Hb</td><td>0</td><td>(14 µM)</td></tr>
<tr><td>Heated Hb</td><td>0</td><td>0</td></tr>
<tr><td>NADH</td><td colspan="2">0</td></tr>
<tr><td>NADH + Hb</td><td>0.025</td><td>0.012</td></tr>
<tr><td>NADH + Heated Hb</td><td>0</td><td>0</td></tr>
<tr><td>NADH + Riboflavin</td><td colspan="2">0.10</td></tr>
<tr><td>NADH + Riboflavin + Hb</td><td>0.68</td><td>0.25</td></tr>
<tr><td>NADH + Riboflavin + Heated Hb</td><td>0.92</td><td>1.38</td></tr>
<tr><td>Ascorbic acid</td><td colspan="2">0.10</td></tr>
<tr><td>Ascorbic acid + Hb</td><td>2.13</td><td>1.13</td></tr>
<tr><td>Ascorbic acid + Heated Hb</td><td>1.08</td><td>0.45</td></tr>
<tr><td>Dihydroxyfumaric acid</td><td colspan="2">0.10</td></tr>
<tr><td>Dihydroxyfumaric acid + Hb</td><td>2.26</td><td>0.66</td></tr>
<tr><td>Dihydroxyfumaric acid + Heated Hb</td><td>1.42</td><td>2.40</td></tr>
<tr><td>Red blood cells</td><td colspan="2">0.30</td></tr>
<tr><td>Red blood cells + Methylene blue</td><td colspan="2">1.78</td></tr>
</table>

Product formation is expressed in µM/min. Experiments were conducted with 0.1mM haemoglobin and 50mM aniline in 0.1M phosphate buffer pH 6.8 at 37°C. NADH (1mM), riboflavin (0.1mM), ascorbic acid (1mM) or dihydroxyfumaric acid (1mM). Red blood cell system in isotonic solution, methylene blue (10 mM).

The aniline hydroxylase activity of native oxyhaemoglobin was always lower than that of methaemoglobin. Hydroxylations also occur, at a low level, in the absence of haemoglobin. Electrons from NADH or enediols are no longer transfered to haemoglobin but also to the oxygen of the medium in a direct or indirect way. The haemoglobin denatured by heating remained active. The higher activity levels observed with heat denatured haemoglobin when compared with native haemoglobin can be directly explained by an increase in the peroxidative activity induced by the denaturation process (Inada et al., 1961). When NADH is used as the electron donor, riboflavin increases the formation of 4-aminophenol. Riboflavin had little influence when the electron donor was ascorbic acid or dihydroxyfumaric acid. In the absence of electron donor 4-aminophenol was obtained only with oxyhaemoglobin. The stimulatory effect of methylene blue on the level of hydroxylation of aniline by erythrocytes appears to be related to its known effect on the hexose monophosphate shunt, by enhancing the production of NADPH inside the cells.

Hydroxyl radicals could be produced in the presence of trace metals in a Fenton-type reaction, from hydrogen peroxide which is produced by electron donation to oxygen. To test the specificity of the reactions catalyzed by haemoglobin, the formation rates of the aminophenol isomers were measured, using an HPLC procedure (Esclade et al., 1986).

Table 2: Regioselectivity in hydroxylation reactions. Experimental conditions as in Table 1.

	Aminophenol $\mu M.min^{-1}$			
SYSTEM	Ortho	Meta	Para	Para/Ortho
NADH + MB	0.12	-	0.04	0.3
NADH + MB + Hb^+	0.23	-	0.83	3.6
NADH + MB + HbO_2	0.15	-	0.57	3.6
AH_2	0.08	-	0.04	0.5
AH_2 + Hb^+	0.17	-	0.67	3.9
AH_2 + HbO_2	0.12	-	0.53	4.4
Erythrocytes + MB	-	-	1.17	-

MB: methylene blue; Hb^+: methaemoglobin; HbO_2: oxyhaemoglobin; AH_2: ascorbic acid.

Hydroxylations were favoured towards the para position as for cytochrome P-450 systems. Blank systems had totally different regioselectivities, hydroxylations were favoured towards the ortho positions as for Fenton type reaction.

Riboflavin or methylene blue induce NADH oxidation with molecular oxygen as the final electron acceptor, giving rise to hydrogen peroxide formation. Similarly, enediols are directly oxidized by molecular oxygen. Hydrogen peroxide production velocities were measured with each of the electron donors and a good correlation with hydroxylation velocities was observed. In a system consisting of hydrogen peroxide, aniline and methaemoglobin, 4-aminophenol appears as a short-lived intermediate changing to give more oxidized products (Figure 1).

Figure 1 :Effect of hydrogen peroxide on the aniline hydroxylation.(●) NADH-riboflavin-methaemoglobin, (▲) AH_2-methaemoglobin, (x) DHF- methaemoglobin and (o) methaemoglobin systems. Experimental conditions: 0.1 mM met-haemoglobin, 50 mM aniline with or without 1 mM NADH, AH_2 or DHF at 37°C in 0.1 M phosphate buffer, pH 6.8. The arrows indicate the addition of 1 mM H_2O_2.

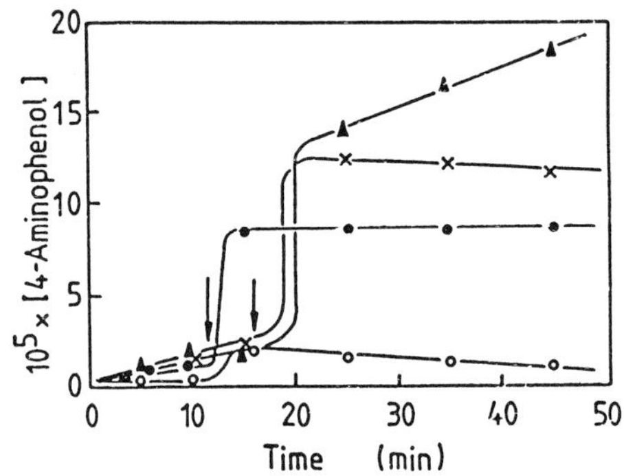

It is known that ferrylhaemoglobin is formed by reaction of methaemoglobin with hydrogen peroxide. This compound (analogous to compound I of peroxidase) has been shown to lead very shortly to an analogue of compound II of peroxidase by abstraction of an electron from the apoprotein (King & Winfield, 1963). This last species then abstracts an electron from substrates, products or reducers. In the presence of NADH, ascorbic acid or dihydroxyfumaric acid, the protection of 4-aminophenol is more important and no further oxidation occurs (Figure 2). So, NADH and enediols "protect" 4-aminophenol against further oxidation by haemoglobin by competition for the reduction of the haemoglobin species analogous to compound II of peroxidase. A similar protection was observed in the peroxidation reaction of aniline by horseradish peroxidase (Cambou et al., 1984).

These results show that in these systems, hydroxylations are intermediate reactions in peroxidations catalyzed by haemoglobin.

Figure 2 : Catalytic oxidation of 4-aminophenol by methaemoglobin in the absence of electron donor (O), or in the presence of 1 mM NADH (●), 1 mM ascorbic acid (▲) and 1 mM dihydroxyfumaric acid (x). The 4-aminophenol concentration was 70 mM. Same conditions as in figure 1.

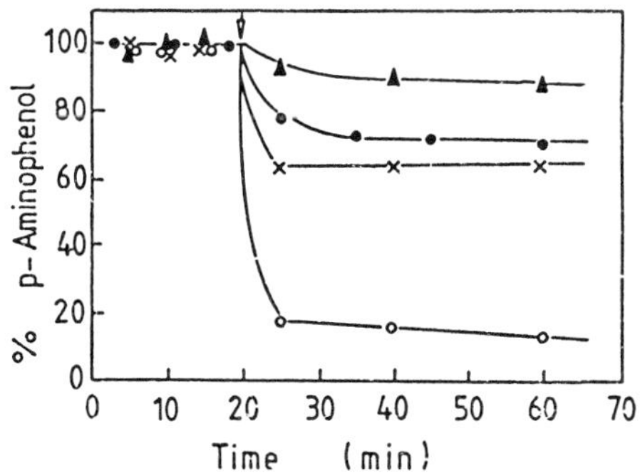

IMMOBILIZED ACETYLCHOLINESTERASE SYSTEM.

Organophosphates and carbamates are very potent inhibitors of acetylcholinesterase (AChE; acetylcholine hydrolase; EC 3.1.1.7), the key enzyme of the neuro-muscular junction. Due to their analogy in structure with the natural substrate, acetylcholine, these compounds are usually known to interact either reversibly or irreversibly with the active centre of the enzyme. Artificial AChE films can be produced by crosslinking with bovine serumalbumin as a support, using glutaraldehyde (Thomas and Broun, 1976).

Figure 3: (a) Diagram of the cholinesterase electrode: -1 perpex support; 2- pH glass electrode; 3- magnetic coil; 4- enzymatic film and 5- stainless steel disc. (b) Influence of pesticide concentration on the electrode signal; pesticide: methylparaoxon, concentrations are expressed in ppm.

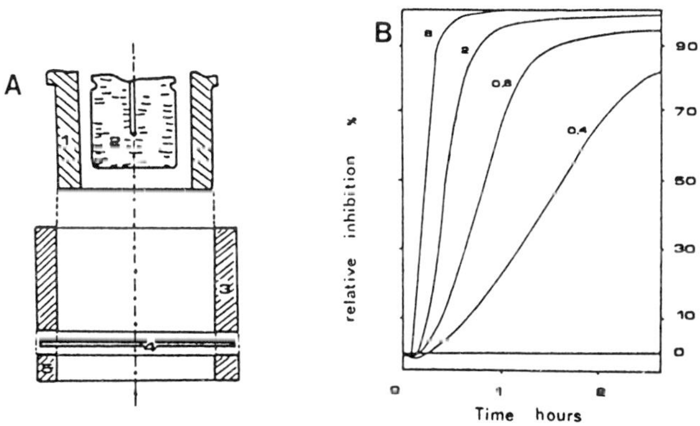

The enzymatic hydrolysis of the substrate produces protons. So, a specific biosensor was produced by coupling a pH glass electrode with such an enzymatic film (figure 3a). The biosensor detects the presence of pesticides by inhibition of the enzymatic reaction, giving rise to a decrease of the electrical response of the electrode (figure 3b). This method can be considered an indirect biological assay in which it is not the pesticide itself that is detected (as in the other physicochemical methods), but rather the toxicological effect through the inhibitory power of the pesticide.

Moreover, the insolubilization of AChE by covalent binding allows a very rapid and efficient dialysis of the enzyme by simple washing. The enzyme is not denaturated or kinetically altered by the insolubilization procedure as previously found in various kinetic studies. For example, artificial films containing AChE were exposed for 45 min to MPT (O-ethyl S2- diisopropylaminoethyl methyl phosphorothiolate), a specific phosphorylating inhibitor of AChE. The curve of residual activity of muscle AChE as a function of MPT concentration (figure 4) did not follow a classical inhibition kinetic.

Figure 4. Inhibition by MPT of insolubilized muscle AChE when the substrate was added in the incubation medium (open symbols) or after elimination of free inhibitor (full symbols) by washing 3 times 20 min each. (▲,△) crude muscle homogenate AChE, and (●, ○) 16 S isolated molecular form. Bars: SEM, 3 determinations.

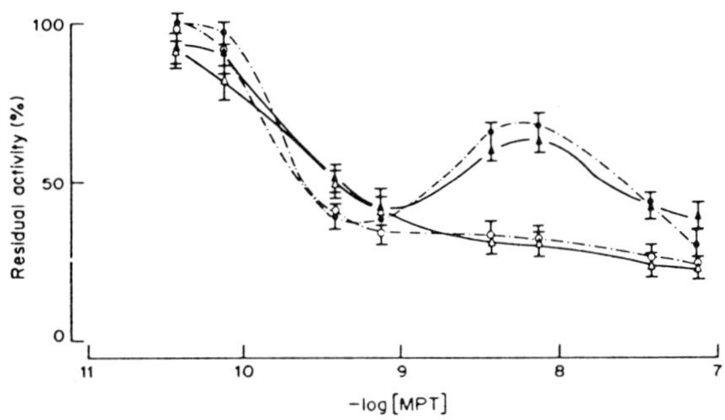

When the artificial films were exposed to the inhibitor as above and then washed (3 times, 20 min each) to remove all unbound inhibitor, before addition of the substrate, the curves exhibit an exaggerated dome shape with a significantly increased AChE activity at MPT concentrations of about 10^{-8} M. Thus, the inhibition appears to be much less efficient at higher (10^{-8} M) than at lower MPT concentrations (i.e. 10^{-9} M). There is no spontaneous reactivation of the insolubilized inactive enzyme. To explain these results, we have proposed the existence of a peripheral regulatory site of action of organophosphorus compounds (Friboulet et al., 1986 ; 1987).

Synergistic and antagonist effects between toxic compounds can also be investigated. BW 284 C 51 is a specific inhibitor of AChE, whose inhibition is totally reversible (Friboulet et al., 1986). Insolubilized AChE was preincubated for 45 min with BW, then incubated 45 min with different concentrations of MPT in the presence of BW and then washed 4 times for 45 min each (twice in the presence of BW, then twice with phosphate buffer). The protective effect of BW against MPT inhibition is presented in figure 5. For low MPT concentrations, the BW compound protects the AChE activity against irreversible inhibition, as expected for an active site-directed inhibitor. However, for MPT concentrations higher than 10^{-9} M, irreversible inhibition becomes almost total and the inhibition phase characterized by a less efficient MPT inhibition when MPT is used alone, never appears. We also find that the inhibition resulting from the use of both inhibitors together is increased over the inhibition achieved with any one of the inhibitors used alone.

Figure 5. Antagonist and agonist actions of MPT and BW on muscle AChE activity. ABW is the residual activity after inhibition by MPT in the presence of BW and AT in the absence of BW. BW concentrations were (o) 10^{-7}M, (■) 10^{-6}M, (□) 10^{-5}M and (▲) 10^{-4}M

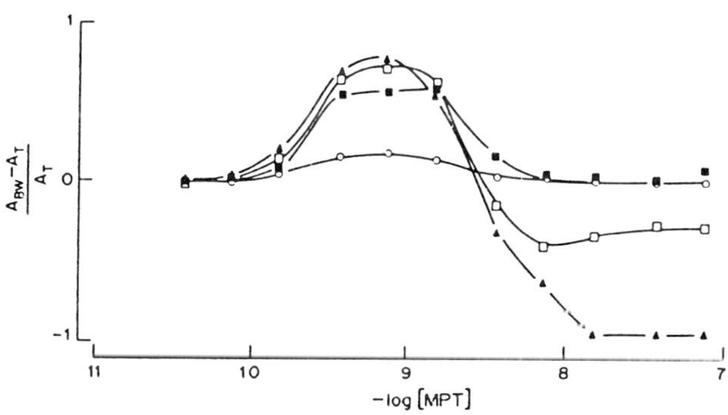

It is interesting to note that similar results were described by Tran (1984) in protection experiments by BW against MPT inhibition on whole muscle cells.

Moreover, preliminary results obtained with

co-immobilized mouse liver microsomes together with AChE indicate that such a system allows the naturally occuring oxidative bioactivation or degradation of S-alkyl phosphorothiolate pesticides to be detected.

The methodologies developped in our laboratory are not substitutive to animal testing. However, they are alternative approaches in that they allow rapid screenings of new compounds and open new routes in future approaches to understand the pharmacology of enzymes and in predicting the target of a new drug at the molecular level.

REFERENCES

Akhrem, A.A., German, S.Y. & Metelisa, D.I., 1978, Reaction Kinetic Catalysis Letters, 8, 339.

Cambou, B., Guillochon, D. & Thomas, D., 1984, Enzyme and Microbiol Technology, 6, 11.

Durand, P. & Thomas, D., 1984, Journal of Environmental Pathology, Toxicology & Oncology, 5, 51.

Esclade, L., Guillochon , D. & Thomas, D., 1986, Xenobiotica, 16, 615.

Friboulet, A., Goudou, D. & Rieger, F., 1986, Neurochemistry International, 9, 323.

Friboulet, A., Goudou, D., Taylor, P. & Rieger, F., 1987, Evidence for the interaction of acetylcholinesterase inhibitors with catalytic and extra-catalytic sites on the insolubilized enzyme. In Model systems in neurotoxicology. Alternative approaches to animal testing, edited by A. Shahar (Alan R. Liss InC.) (in the press).

Inada, Y., Kurozumi, T. & Shibata, K.,1961, Archives of Biochemistry and Biophysics, 93, 30.

King, N. & Winfield, M.E., 1963, Journal of Biological Chemistry, 238, 1520.

Mieyal, J.J., Ackerman, R.S., Blumer, J.L. & Freeman, L.S., 1976, Journal of Biological Chemistry , 251, 3436.

Tomoda, A., Yubisui, T., Ida, M., Kawaeki, N. & Yoneyama, Y., 1977, Experientia, 33, 1276.

Thomas, D. & Broun, G., 1976, Methods in Enzymology, 44, 901.

Tran, H.L., 1984 Caractérisation et localisation des formes moléculaires de l'acétylcholinestérase du muscle squelettique de souris, Thesis, Paris VI, France.

8. Enantiomers *vs* racemates

INTRODUCTION

A.G. Hildebrandt

Max von Pettenkofer-Institut des
Bundesgesundheitsamtes
Postfach 330013,
D-1000 Berlin 33, FRG.

Consideration of regioselectivity of chemical compounds and their corresponding effects have so far been of minor concern in the general safety concepts for food, pesticide and drug regulation. There are exceptions however, e.g. the German food additive regulation (Zusatzstoffverordnung) contains a regulation on the use of amino acids as taste modifiying substances. This allows for only the naturally occuring L-forms of amino acids to be used. The EEC proposals for a community list of miscellaneous food additives also contains specific regulations on certain substances e.g. malic acid and tartaric acid according to their stereoselectivity.

The importance of the effects of stereoselectivity on odour and taste qualities can be easily demonstrated by the flavouring substances that required regulation. The reason behind this is obvious: the monoterpenketon Carvon is for instance in its (S)(+)-form, the main aromatic substance of caraway oil whilst the odour of green mint is given by the (R)(-) enantiomer. The analytical proof for the presence of the required enantiomer may be important in the future in order to know whether an optically active compound represents the main component of a **naturally occuring** flavour or whether the taste relies upon the presence of a **natural identical** compound which contains the racemate only.

The problem of enantiomers versus the racemate is of more concern (yet less regulated) in the pesticide field and in the drug field and should be a matter of concern for general health and environmental aspects in other laws as well.

The main points of concern which have to be satisfied in regulations as well as under specific questions of stereoselectivity are:

(a) Whether a stereoselective characteristic of a chemical compound is capable of harming people who may be exposed to it more frequently than to the racemate.
(b) Whether humans are likely to be exposed to the chemical in ways which could be harmful.
(c) What would the magnitude of the risk of the substance be in comparison to the racemate , and what would the consequences of regulating it be?

Any regulation would at least lead to restrictions which forbid use of a toxic enantiomer whilst substituting an effective non-toxic enantiomer in its place.

The numbers of important examples of stereoselective dependent toxicity are growing, e.g.-

- DL- versus meso 3,4-dimethyl-2,5 hexane-dione for the neurotoxic action of N-hexane in industrial settings or in individuals who have inhaled the substance for its euphoric action.
- The four stereo isomeric forms of the diol epoxides of benzo[a]pyrene, the key carcinogenic product of which is (+)benzo[a]pyrene-7,8-diol-9,10 epoxide.
- The effect of thalidomide (Contergan) in teratogenesis; the (S)(-) form is teratogenic whilst the (R)(+) enantiomer has hypnotic effects only.

These few examples and those given in the accompanying texts show a need for investigation and regulation and also stress a demand for further kinetic and metabolic studies in this field.

The results and further regultion appear to be slowly progressing. The regulating toxicologist follows the descriptive toxicologist who describes the toxicity of the substance....in a practical situation however, the critical factor is not always the intrinsic toxicity but the risk or hazard associated with its use. This means that a regulator often cannot withold a decision about a problem even when the facts appear to withold judgement, or for a suspension of judgement. This creates controversy between science and regulation - it is the task of meetings like this to promote and harmonize both effects.

ENANTIOMERS VS RACEMATES: PHARMACOLOGICAL AND TOXICOLOGICAL ASPECTS

E.J. Ariëns
Institute Pharmacol. and Toxicol.
University Nijmegen
Postbox 9101
6500 HB Nijmegen
The Netherlands

INTRODUCTION

An intriguing aspect of biologically active agents, particularly xenobiotics such as drugs and pesticides is their selectivity in action, the discriminatory capacity for their molecular sites of action, specific receptors, enzymes, etc. This is based on a chemical complementarity between the xenobiotic, the exogenous messenger molecule, and the site of interaction on the receptor- or enzyme molecules. Besides the physicochemical characteristics of the groups in the molecules which participate in the interaction also their spatial arrangement, their sterical configuration, is essentially involved.

For chiral agents stereoselectivity is more rule than exception. Often only one of the isomers appears to be highly active. It may be called the "eutomer", the less active one the "distomer". The ratio of the activities (affinities, potencies, etc.)of the isomers, the eudismic ratio, gives the degree of stereospecificity (1,2,3). In the racemate the distomer, not contributing to the effect aimed at, can be considered as impurity, the "isomeric ballast". It potentially contributes, however, to undesired effects. It is a pollutant - be it of the milieu interne of man and other living organisms - or of the environment in general.

NEGLECT OF STEREOCHEMISTRY

Figure 1 and 2 show that chirality is rather common among drugs and pesticides. The use of

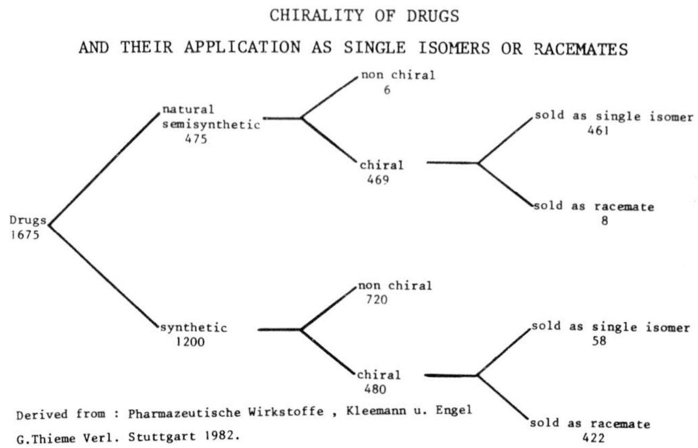

Fig.1

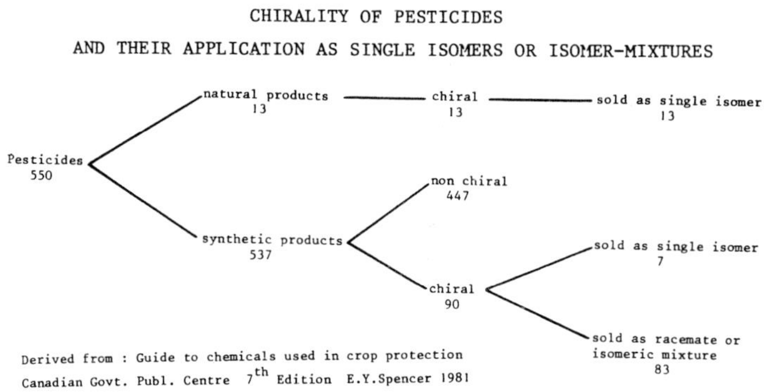

Fig.2

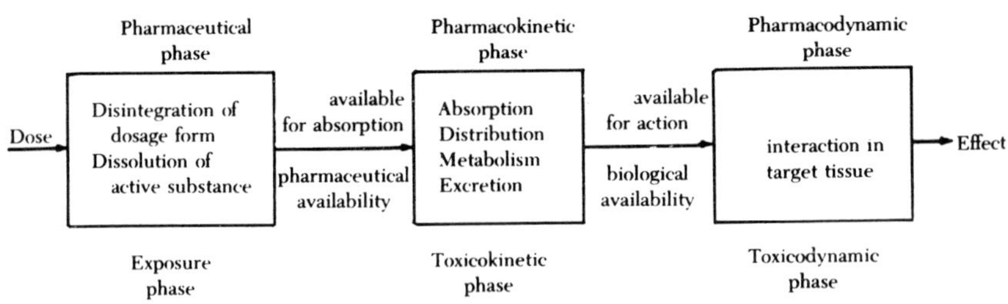

Fig.3

CHIRALITY OF DRUGS
AND THEIR APPLICATION AS SINGLE ISOMERS OR RACEMATES

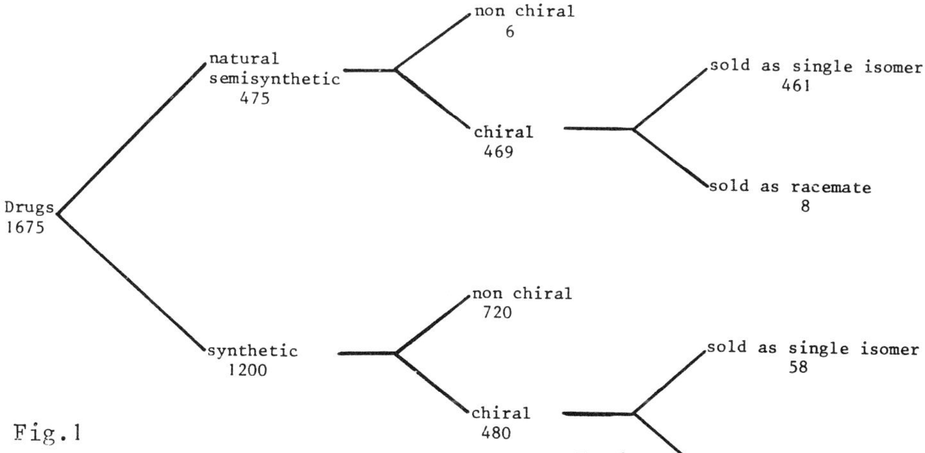

Fig.1

Derived from : Pharmazeutische Wirkstoffe , Kleemann u. Engel
G.Thieme Verl. Stuttgart 1982.

CHIRALITY OF PESTICIDES
AND THEIR APPLICATION AS SINGLE ISOMERS OR ISOMER-MIXTURES

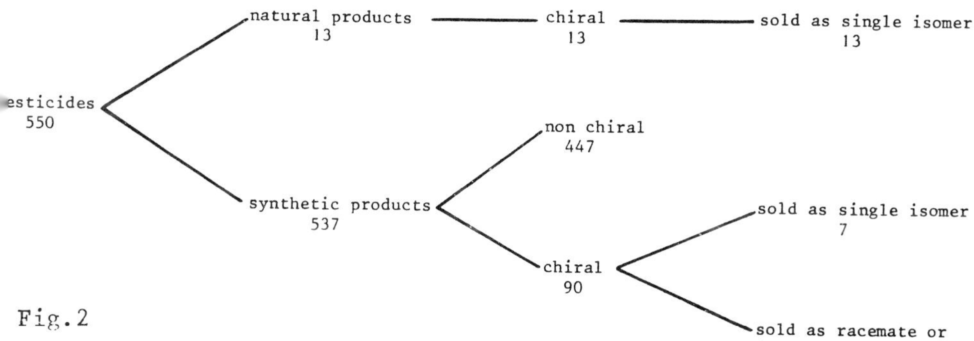

Fig.2

Derived from : Guide to chemicals used in crop protection
Canadian Govt. Publ. Centre 7th Edition E.Y.Spencer 1981

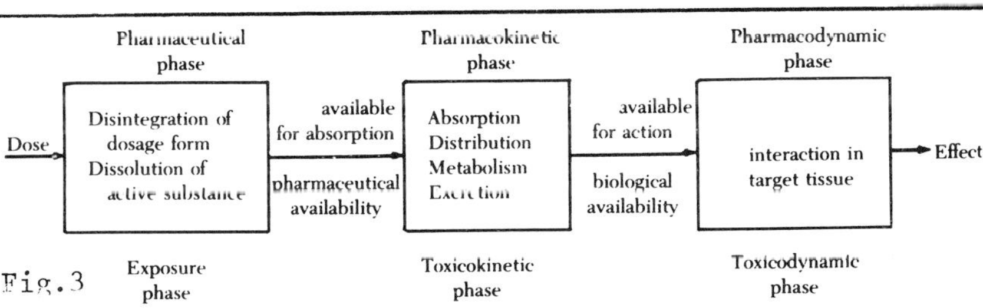

Fig.3

racemic mixtures containing 50% isomeric ballast in stead of the active isomer only is based on economic arguments. These, however, become weaker and weaker since the techniques for stereospecific synthesis and separation of isomers are rapidly developing (see in 4 the refs. 16-22). By the way, the active substance particularly in therapeutic products usually only count for a small fraction of the price.

In the use of drugs there apparently is not to much concern about applying along with the compound with the desired action an equal amount of a second compound potentially contributing to side-effects only. The implications of the use of mixtures of active and inactive isomers are even more impressive if one considers the application of pesticides. What about the presumably economically and environmentally acceptable spraying of e.g. 500 kg of an active agent, the active isomer, going hand in hand with spraying of 500 kg of a pure environmental pollutant, the isomeric ballast.

In the study of bioactive agents it is requisite to use pure compounds, with as little as possible impurities. Mixtures of compounds may be an object of study, particularly if one wants to gain information on their interaction. Too often, even without notice, in the literature data on racemic mixtures are presented as if it concerns one compound only. If such mixtures are used, e.g. because of the non-availability of the separate stereoisomers, one at least should mention explicitly that the data presented concern racemic "fixed-ratio" combinations of compounds with known, or probable, differences in biological properties. Such differences form a notable source of problems in pharmacology as well as toxicology. This holds true for racemates, composed of enantiomers as well as for mixtures of geometric isomers.

STEREOSELECTIVITY IN ACTION OF XENOBIOTICS

Figure 3 represents the main phases in biological action of xenobiotics. The stereoselectivity in action may concern each of the phases. In the dynamic phase - the desired action may be located in one, the undesired in both isomers - the desired action may be present in one, the undesired in the other (fig.4)- both isomers may show desired but different actions - one isomer may act as antagonist of the other - etc. - etc. (5,6,7). In the kinetic phase too there is a variety of possibilities particularly for metabolic conversions such as: substrate specificity, product specificity, substrate-product specificity, inversion of sterical structure, etc.(4,8,9).Even in the exposure phase stereoselectivity may count. In the case of weed killers for instance stereospecific conversions by the soil flora can take place (7) (figure 5). Recently various reviews appeared on stereoselectivity in the action of xenobiotics (1-10).

A particular aspect is the stereoselective biotoxification of which various examples are known. Remarkably little attention is paid to the biotoxification involved in e.g. the Ames tests for in vitro determination of mutagenecity and thus potential carcinogenecity. Requirement of the presence of microsomes or other enzyme preparations indicates involvement of formation of reactive metabolic intermediates. This toxification tends by its nature to stereospecificity (table 1). Such tests have been performed on innumerable compounds, many of which chiral, little attention is paid to possible and probable differences for the stereoisomers. A new product might be rejected because of a positive Ames-test although this only concerned the therapeutically or economically ineffective isomer. The final interaction of the reactive, electrophilic, metabolic intermediates and nucleophilic groups on e.g. nucleic acids as such will only exceptionally be stereospecific.

For a proper study of the pharmacology, particularly pharmacokinetics, of chiral agents stereospecific analytical methods e.g. immuno-essays are required. It should be noted that if antibodies are induced by application of a racemic mixture to the animals, the different types of lymphocytes involved will produce different antibodies against each of the chemical agents, enantiomers present. Such a mixture of antibodies is not stereoselective. If monoclonal antibodies are generated by selection of a particular lymphocyte clone, antibodies selective for one of the enantiomers can be obtained (table 2).

Fig.4

TOXICITY OF EPN

	LD_{50} µg/g topical house fly	rice stem borer
R.(+)	1	2.9
S.(-)	3.2	11.7
RS(±)	1.3	5.9

Delayed neurotoxicity (paralysis)
i.b. atropinized hens (n=3)

mg/kg	68.6	89.2
R.(+)	0	0
S.(-)	3	3
RS(±)	1	2

For the organophosphate EPN the R.isomer is mainly pesticidal, the S.isomer is mainly responsible for the neurotoxicity in mammals and birds.
Ohkawa H.e.a. Bull.Environm.Contamin. and Toxicology 18,534 , 1977.

Fig.5

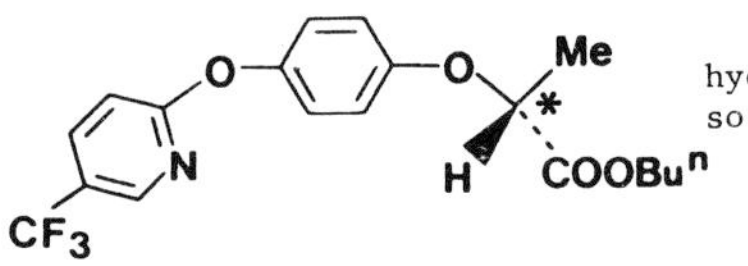

S-ester → S-acid - - - - - - - - →
inversion in fresh soil
hydrolysis in soil and plant
degradation and conjugation in fresh soil and plant
no inversion in sterilized soil
R-ester → R-acid →

STEREOSELECTIVE INVERSION OF THE WEEDKILLER FLUAZIFOP-BUTYLESTER

in vitro	: ester, R. and S. inactive	acid, R.active S.inactive
postemergence	: ester, R.active S. inactive	acid, R.active S.inactive
pre-emergence	: ester, R. and S. active	acid, R. and S. active

Dicks e.a. Brit. Crop Protection Conference-Weeds. P. 171, 1985.

Table 1 Mutagenicity of penicillamine and its enantiomeric selectivity

	Specific mutagenicity (Revertants per µmol compound)					
	Salmonella typhimurium TA100			*Salmonella typhimurium* TA92		
Test compound	Buffer	Kidney S9	Liver S9	Buffer	Kidney S9	Liver S9
L-penicillamine	12	55	27	13	70	28
D-penicillamine	1.5	7	2.3	2	11	3.3

HANSRUEDI GLATT and FRANZ OESCH , *Biochemical Pharmacology*, Vol. 34, 3725–3728, 1985.

Table 2. STEREOSELECTIVITY IN IMMUNO ESSAYS

induction with	binding to antiserum (rabbits) ID_{50}pg (a) dl-propranolol	l-propranolol	d-propranolol
dl-propranolol	--	326	314
l-propranolol	--	120	1656
induction with	**% cross-reaction with monoclonal antibody (mouse) McAb-P28 (b)**		
dl-propranolol	100	169	35

a) K. Kawashima e.a. J.P.E.T. 196, 517-523, 1976
b) L. Wang e.a. F.E.B.S. 199, 173-178, 1986.

It as a matter of fact depends on the choice of the lymphocyte used to develop the hybridoma.

No doubt the implications of stereoselectivity in action should be in the minds of those involved in design and development of drugs. Stereoselectivity restricted to only one component in the biological action indicates a difference in mechanisms of the actions involved. Then the chance to separate such actions by suitable molecular manipulation is real. It will be clear that the terms eutomer and distomer and eudismic ratio can be used only in relation to a particular biological action. The eutomer for the desired action may be, and that is not bad, the distomer for the undesired action. The eutomer for the undesired action then is the distomer for the desired action.

NEGLECT OF STEREOCHEMISTRY A SOURCE OF SENSELESS DATA

Taken into account differences in the metabolic rates of enantiomers, the proportion thereof, initially 1:1, changes with time. This holds true for the drug as such and for the metabolites. In curves for the elimination of the "racemate" from plasma or the environment one may expect a steeper part for the metabolically more labile and a more shallow part for the more stabile enantiomer. The half-lifes of the enantiomers - measured by stereoselective methods - often differ. If in the study of chiral agents stereoselectivity is neglected, computerized curve fitting may result in complex multicompartment systems with extensive sets of pharmacokinetic constants. What, however, is the meaning of the half-life, bioavailability, rate constants, etc. for a mixture of two pharmacokinetically and pharmacodynamically different agents (isomers) present in unknown and with time changing proportion.

There is a remarkable discrepancy between on one hand the high degree of purity required for pharmaceuticals and on the other hand the acceptance of 50% impurity as long as isomeric ballast is involved. Authorities responsible for the acceptance, registration, of drugs in various countries will not accept 50% of a byproduct in a drug, even it is assumed (without proof) safe. The fact that it is not easy to eliminate the impurity will hardly count. On the other hand they easily accept 50% isomeric ballast and then even require "indispensable" but senseless pharmacokinetic data on the racemates concerned. On this point there seems to be excellent agreement among FDA-type institutions, pharmaceutical industry and many scientific investigators. When will they find out the difference between an active agent and a racemic fixed-ratio combination of in their action and activity differing compounds, the enantiomers?

Without calling the situation prohibitive and requiring the use of only the active isomers, the problem should at least be recognized. Avoidance of unnecessary application of chemicals, reduction of the xenobiotic load, in the application of drugs or pesticides should count heavily both in the development of new agents and in the efforts to optimize safety and therewith acceptability for daily use. Chemistry, undoubtedly, has essentially contributed to health and to increase of standard of life in many parts of the world. The risks, however, have been underestimated. Unnecessary and uncontrolled chemical risks have been accepted. Time is ripe for "domestication" of chemistry; that is adaptation of chemistry to safe intimate association with and advantage of men, subjected to his control.

CONCLUSION

Neglect of stereochemistry results in the collection of senseless data and drawing misleading conclusions in pharmacology, toxicology and development of new crop protectants. An important role is to be played here by editorial boards of scientific journals and publishers in general. If studies on racemic mixtures are presented, at least it should be announced that the "agent" discussed is composed of two or more isomers to be regarded as different compounds each of which has its own specific properties. If kinetic data are presented on racemates, neglecting their composition, clear arguments regarding implications thereof for the value and the sense of the data presented should be required. Health authorities should be fully aware of the fact that acceptance of racemates implies acceptance of 50% or more of possibly harmful pollutants for the milieu interne of patients and the environment in general. Maintenance on, and particularly admission to, the market of racemic mixtures requires a thorough weighing up of pros and cons without exaggeration of the problems in production of clean enantiomers.

REFERENCES

Lehmann, F.P.A., Rodrigues de Miranda, J.F., Ariëns, E.J. Stereoselectivity and affinity in molecular pharmacology. In: Jucker, E., ed. *Progress in Drug Research*, 1976, 20, 101-42.

Ariëns, E.J., Soudijn, W., Timmermans, P.B.M.W.M. Stereochemistry and biological activity of drugs. Oxford: Blackwell Scientific Publications, 1982.

Series on Chirality, *Trends in Pharmacological Sciences* 1986: 7, 20-24; 60-65; 112-115; 155-158; 200-205; 227-230; 281-285.

Ariëns, E.J. Stereochemistry: A Source of Problems in Medicinal Chemistry. *Med. Res. Rev.* 1986, 6, 451-66.

Drayer, D.E. Pharmacodynamic and pharmacokinetic differences between drug anantiomers in humans: An overview. *Clin. Pharmacol. Ther.* 1986, 40, 125-33.

Ariëns, E.J. Stereochemistry, a basis for sophisticated nonsence in pharmacokinetics and clinical pharmacology. *Eur. J. Clin. Pharmacol*. 1984, 26, 663-8.

Ariëns, E.J., Rensen, J.J.S. van, Welling, W. Stereoselectivity in pesticide action. A notable source of problems. Amsterdam: Elsevier Scientific Publications, in press.

Jenner, P., Testa, B. The influence of stereochemical factors on drug disposition. *Drug Metab. Rev*. 1973, 2(2), 117-84.

Low, L.K., Castagnoli Jr, N. Enantioselectivity in drug metabolism. In: *Annual Reports in Medicinal Chemistry*, Vol.13, New York: Academic Press, 1978, 304-15.

Williams, K., Lee, E. Importance of drug enantiomers in clinical pharmacology. *Drugs* 1985, 30, 333-54.

STEREOSPECIFIC ANALYTICAL METHODOLOGY

Andrew J. Hutt and John Caldwell

Department of Pharmacy, Brighton Polytechnic, Brighton BN2 4GJ
and
Department of Pharmacology, St. Mary's Hospital Medical School, London W2 1PG, England.

The majority of synthetic drugs containing a chiral centre are used as racemic mixtures even though the pharmacological activity is frequently restricted to one enantiomer (Williams & Lee, 1985). The use of racemates may present problems due to interactions between the enantiomers during absorption, distribution, metabolism and excretion and may enhance the toxicity of the administered agent, particularly if this is associated with the 'inactive' enantiomer or does not show stereoselectivity (Ariens, 1986). There is thus a current need for investigations of the stereochemical aspects of drug disposition, and in addition to its importance for pharmacology and toxicology, the study of the chirality of metabolism of both prochiral and chiral drug molecules may also give valuable information concerning the active sites of the enzymes involved.

Until relatively recently, much of our knowledge concerning the fate of the enantiomers of a drug derived from studies involving the separate administration to the enantiomers. In such cases non-stereoselective analytical methods may be utilized in the determination of drug-related material in biological fluids. This approach has considerable limitations as (a) it does not provide information on the effect of one enantiomer upon the fate of the other, and (b) metabolic chiral inversion may occur, as in the case of the 2-arylpropionic acids (Hutt & Caldwell, 1983). It is therefore appropriate to consider the stereospecific analytical methods available for such studies.

The discrimination of enantiomers requires the interaction of the chiral substance under investigation with another chiral agent. This may variously involve plane-polarized light, as in polarimetry or circular dichroism; derivatisation with a chiral compound to produce diastereoisomers followed by achiral chromatography or NMR, or interaction with a chiral complex, solvent or surface *eg* chiral shift reagents or solvents in NMR, a chiral mobile phase for hplc, chiral stationary phases for either hplc or glc; or combinations of the above *eg* an enantioselective immunoassay could be described as resulting from the interaction between the chiral immunoglobulin to yield a diastereomeric complex on a chiral surface. Various aspects of these methods have been reviewed in recent years (Cook, 1983; Testa, 1986).

Pseudoracemates

One area of enantiomeric analysis available to the drug metabolism scientist which does not require a second chiral agent is the application of pseudoracemates. A pseudoracemate is a 1:1 mixture of enantiomers, one of which is the natural enantiomer, whilst in the other, one or more atoms have been isotopically labelled. The second compound is no longer a true enantiomer of the first but differs in some physical properties, most importantly molecular weight. Following the administration of the pseudoracemic mixture, drug-related materials in body fluids are examined conventionally *eg* by achiral chromatography, and the enantiomers differentiated by mass fragmentography (in the case of stable isotopes), or by radiochemical means. Obviously preparative chiral purification and analysis of the starting materials is required initially. Care is also required in the positioning of the label within the molecule, which must be in a metabolically stable position. Ideally the labelled and unlabelled enantiomers should be shown to be metabolically identical before administration of the pseudoracemate.

This technique, which was pioneered by Walle in his studies on propranolol (see Walle, 1985), has been used recently in an examination of the pharmacokinetics of disopyramide (Giacomini *et al*, 1986). Separate administration of the individual enantiomers of disopyramide to human volunteers indicated no differences in clearance, renal clearance and volume of distribution between the isomers. After administration of the pseudoracemate, however, d-disopyramide had decreased plasma and renal clearances, increased half-life and a lower apparent volume of distribution than its l-enantiomer.

Although this method has the obvious advantages of sensitivity and specificity and offers an ideal investigational approach for many drugs, it is unsuitable as a routine method.

Chiral Immunoassay

An area of chiral analysis which has received relatively little attention until recently is that of chiral immunoassay, although the pioneering studies of Landsteiner and van der Scheer (1929) showed that antibodies could distinguish (+), (-) and the meso isomers of tartaric acid.

More recently chiral radioimmunoassay methods have been reported for the "ephedrines", warfarin, propranolol, several narcotic analgesics and the chiral barbiturates (see Cook, 1983). Cross reactivity of the chiral antibodies with the "wrong" enantiomer in all these studies was found to be less than 3%, provided that the stereochemical purity of the drug used to prepare the antigen was sufficiently high. Small impurities in the antigen may result in disproportionately greater errors in the assay, as has been shown with warfarin. Cross reactivity with metabolites may also result in problems when the site of metabolism is far removed from the chiral centre in the drug *e.g.* 4-hydroxywarfarin (Cook *et al*, 1979a).

An advantage of chiral immunoassays is that antisera developed for the analysis of the stereoisomers of one drug may be used for the determination of the stereoisomers of a related compound. Thus, antisera developed for the chiral RIA of S-pentobarbital exhibited greater than 80% cross reactivity with S-secobarbital but only 2% with its R-antipode (Cook *et al*, 1979b; Cook, 1983).

Following from the above, complications may arise from the use of racemates for the formation of haptens and generation of antibodies. Racemic haptens may yield two enantioselective antibodies which cannot be assumed to be present in equal proportions. The use of such antisera could thus produce data of limited value, particularly if enantiomeric ratio of the drug under investigation in biological media differs from 1:1 (Cook *et al*, 1982).

Radioreceptor Assays

Radioreceptor analysis is dependent on the ability of a drug and any active metabolites to compete with a radio-labelled ligand for preparations of its biological receptors, which act as chiral surfaces. Although such assays are problematical in terms of the receptor systems employed, they do allow chiral discrimination with minimal sample preparation. The disposition of S-propranolol and its active metabolites has been determined using a radioreceptor technique (Nahorski *et al*, 1978).

Chiral Chromatography

The most significant advances over the last ten years have been in the area of chiral chromatographic techniques which enable the resolution of enantiomers on both analytical and preparative scales.

Two main approaches are available to the drug metabolism scientist: (1) formation of diastereoisomers using a chiral derivatizing agent (2) the formation of unstable diastereoisomeric complexes *eg* between chiral drugs and/or metabolites and a chiral hplc or gc column surface, or a chiral component in an hplc mobile phase. Both these approaches have advantages and limitations but any chiral chromatographic method will yield information on absolute configuration if an analogue of known configuration is available for comparison. One determinant of the sensitivity of an assay will be the order of elution of enantiomers from the column: superior performance will be achieved if the minor component elutes first. Manipulation of this important characteristic may be achieved by reversing the chirality of the stationary phase (or derivatizing reagent), which will reverse the elution order. Diastereoisomers, both covalently bonded and the unstable complexes, may also be examined by NMR which may be an additional aid in configurational determination.

Covalent diastereoisomeric derivatives may be readily prepared using a wide variety of chiral reagents (Fig. 1). However, several problems which can affect the conclusions drawn may arise from (a) the enantiomeric impurity of the reagent, (b) racemization of the analyte and/or reagent during derivatization, and (c) stereoselective derivatization *i.e.* kinetic resolution. The correct choice of derivatizing agent may increase the sensitivity of the method, depending upon the detector used.

The problems associated with the use of chiral derivatizing agents can be illustrated by the work on ketamine of Adams *et al* (1982), where the derivatization was stereoselective, gave poor yields and the acylating agent racemized. Hence the choice of a suitable chiral agent and conditions of derivatization are of great importance. Our own studies on the 'profen' Pirprofen, using S-1-(naphthen-1-yl) ethylamine as the second chiral agent, were greatly eased by the prior synthesis of the diastereoisomeric derivatives. Comparison of synthetic samples with those obtained from our derivatization method showed that the reaction was non-stereoselective, and enabled the optimisation of the conditions to give yields in excess of 90% (Hutt *et al*, 1986).

Resolutions based on the formation of limited stability diastereoisomers involve the use of chiral stationary phases (glc;

Figure 1:

Examples of chiral reagents used for the derivatization of chiral acids, alcohols and amines prior to chromatographic analysis.

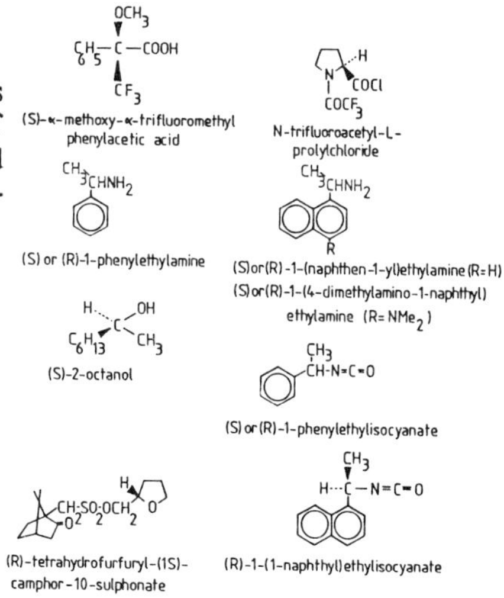

Figure 2:

Three-point interaction model for chromatographic resolutions. The enantiomer (upper) has the correct configuration for 3-simultaneous interactions between A, B and C and with 3 complimentary sites A[1], B[1] and C[1] on the resolving surface, whilst its antipode (lower) has only two interactive sites.

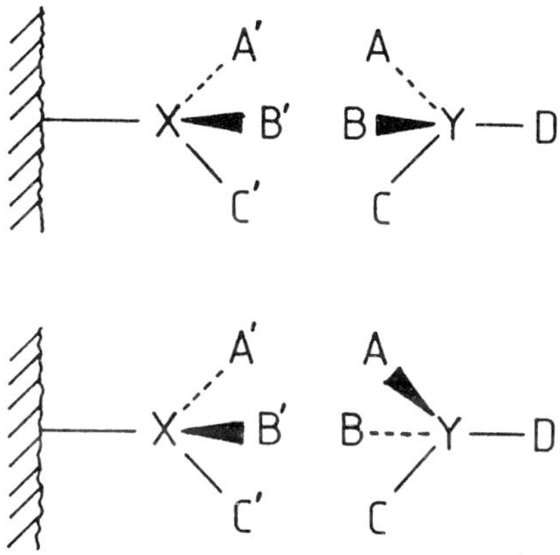

Figure 3:

Types of interaction which contribute to the resolution process of Pirkle type stationary phases.

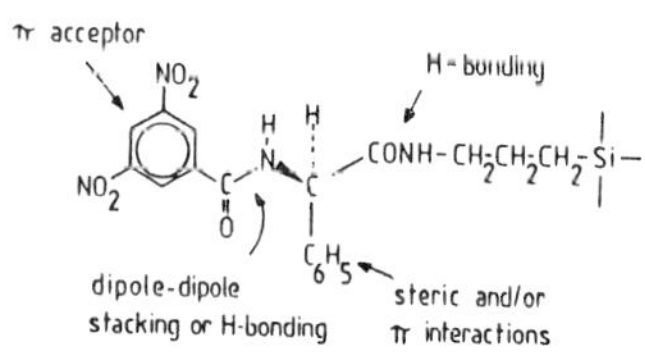

hplc) or a chiral mobile phase (hplc). Many of the constraints outlined above for the formation of covalent diastereoisomers are of much less importance with the application of chiral stationary phases and solvents. The chiral phase stationary phase need not be 100% enantiomerically pure and for preparative resolutions the use of chiral columns will increase yields as loss during regeneration of the original material is avoided. Should derivatization of the drug or metabolite be required to increase the enantiomer resolution in such cases the derivatizing agent need not be chiral.

The mechanism of resolution on a chiral stationary phase is based on the '3-point' fit model of Dalgliesh (1952). For resolution to occur the chiral stationary phase must have three simultaneous interactions with one of the enantiomers, whilst its antipode will only bind at two sites (Fig. 2). The enantiomer forming the '2-point' fit complex will be less stable and hence elute from the column first.

A variety of 'Brush type' or Pirkle phases are available for hplc (Figs. 3 & 4) which may be either covalent or ionic in nature. The ionic phases cannot be used with solvents more polar than 20% propanol in hexane, but the covalent systems may be used with aqueous based solvents, allowing more freedom in solvent choice (Dappen *et al* 1986). New chiral stationary phases are frequently reported.

We have found β-cyclodextrin to be a useful chiral resolving agent. The cyclodextrins are chiral cyclic polymers, of α-(1,4)-linked glucose units, which are "tub shaped" and open at both ends. The inside of the "tub" is hydrophobic as the hydroxyl groups are on the surface. β-Cyclodextrin consists of 7 glucose units, each of which has 5 chiral centres, so each molecule has 35 chiral centres. It has been used as both a mobile phase additive (up to <u>ca</u> 0.5% w/v) and a bonded stationary phase (Cyclobond I consists of β-cyclodextrin bonded to silica gel via a stable 6 to 10 atom spacer unit). The enantiomeric resolution is thought to be due to the formation of an inclusion complex between the solute and the cyclodextrin (Armstrong, 1984). One of the main advantages of the cyclodextrin is that aqueous based solvent systems may be used *eg* water/methanol or water/acetonitrile mixtures.

The uses of β-cyclodextrin as a mobile phase additive and as a bonded stationary phase may not be directly comparable, as illustrated by our attempts to resolve the enantiomers of mandelic acid. The partial resolution of mandelic acid using β-cyclodextrin as a mobile phase additive is shown in Fig. 5, but we were unable to reproduce this resolution on a Cyclobond I column. However, in this laboratory the Cyclobond I column gave baseline resolution of

Figure 4 : Chiral hplc stationary phases of the so-called 'Brush' or Pirkle type

N-(3,5-dinitrobenzoyl)phenylglycine (ionic)

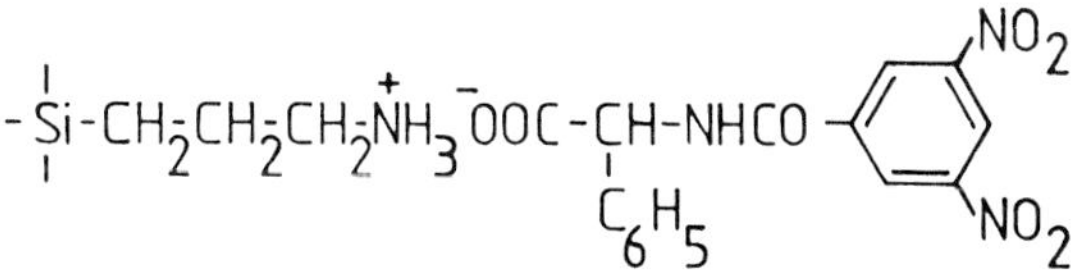

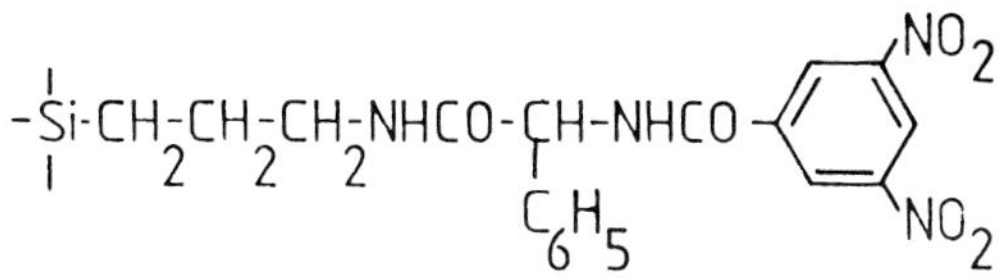

(covalent)

(S)-1-(α-naphthyl)ethylamine (covalent)

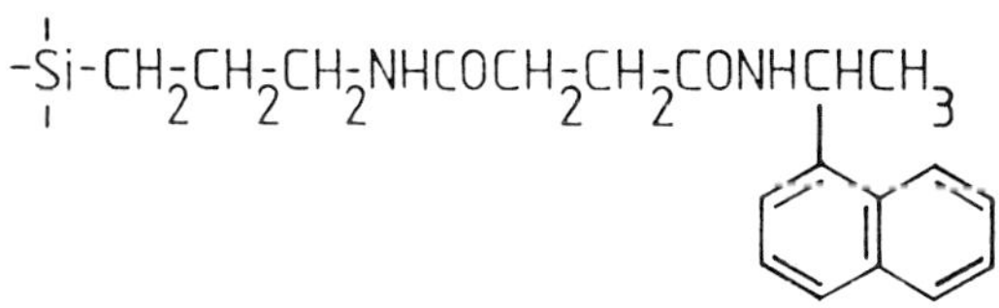

N-(S)-2-(4-chlorophenyl)isovaleroyl-(R)-phenylglycine (ionic)

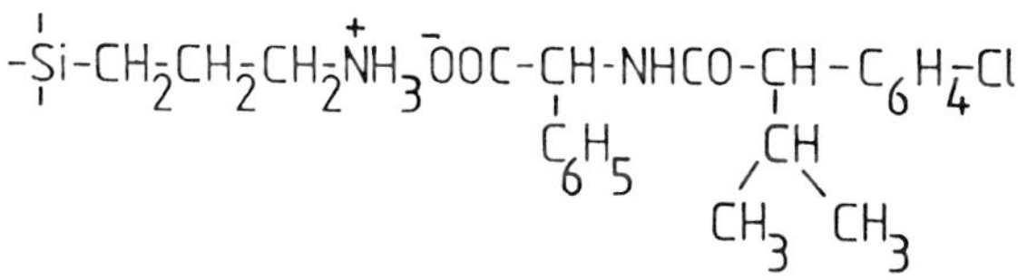

N-(1R,3R)-<u>trans</u> chrysantherioyl-(R)-phenylglycine (covalent)

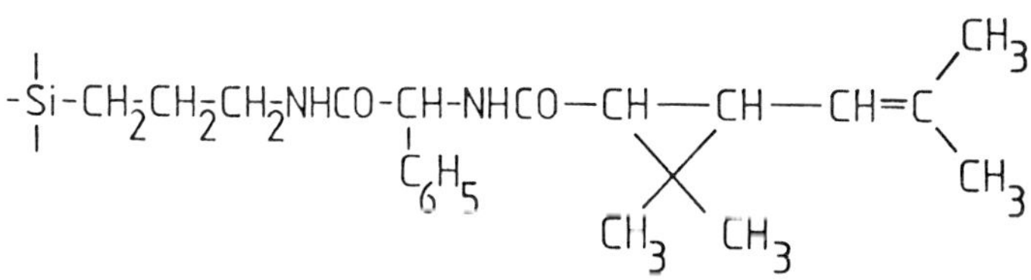

Figure 5 : Resolution of Mandelic acid enantiomers using β-cyclodextrin (0.5% w/v) and trifluoroacetic acid (0.1% v/v) in water as mobile phase components (flow rate 0.6 ml min^{-1}; column 10 um, Hypersil-ODS, 250 x 4.6mm, uv detector 254nm).

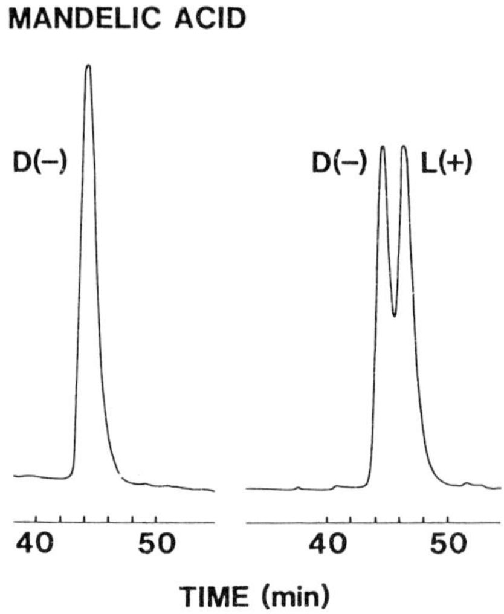

Figure 6 : Resolution of Mandelic acid enantiomers using a BSA column (Resolvosil 7) (A) 25 ug on column, abs 0.1, flow rate 2.0ml min^{-1}. (B) 2.5 ug on column, abs 0.01, flow rate 2.0ml min^{-1}. (C) 2.5 ug on column, abs 0.01, flow rate 0.2ml min^{-1}. (Column 150 x 4 mm i.d., solvent phosphate buffer 0.1M, pH 7.0, uv detector 254nm).

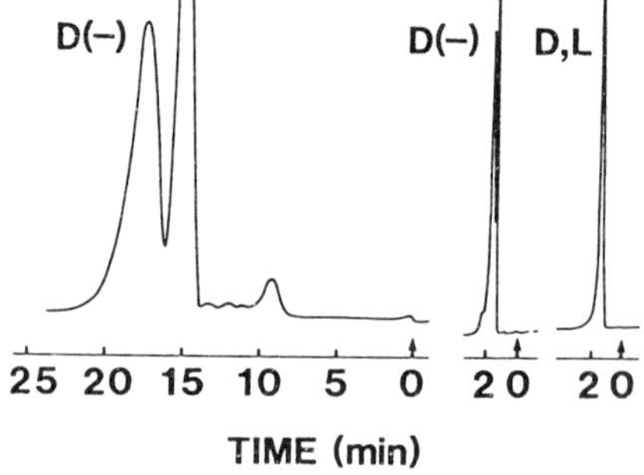

the enantiomers of the carbonyl reduced metabolite of fenofibrate and the investigational antiinflammatory agent ketorolac.

Proteins are naturally occurring chiral polymers which bind chiral molecules selectively. Commercially available columns include those based on bovine serum albumin (Resolvosil) and α_1-acid glycoprotein (EnantioPac). The mechanism of resolution of protein columns is thought to involve hydrophobic, polar and steric interactions. Selection of mobile phases is complicated as resolution depends on ionic strength, pH, the presence of low concentrations of organic modifiers and temperature (Dappen *et al*, 1986). Particular difficulties with these columns arise from the low protein loading giving low sample capacity. This is illustrated using mandelic acid in Figure 6. Other compounds successfully resolved on a Resolvosil column in our laboratories include 6-(2-hydroxypropyl)chromone 2-carboxylate and warfarin.

Chiral Detectors

HPLC in combination with uv detection is a common technique for the determination of drugs and their metabolites in biological fluids. As stated above the detection/determination of chiral compounds depends upon their interaction with another chiral agent which may be plane polarised light. Both polarimetric and circular dichroic detectors have been described for hplc instruments. The application of a micropolarimeter using laser optics coupled to hplc systems has been described (Yeung *et al*, 1980). The application of this type of methodology for biological systems has been reported and its extension to metabolic studies is eagerly awaited (see elsewhere in this volume).

Conclusion

With the increasing realisation that the enantiomers of chiral drug molecules may elicit totally different biological actions, there will be increasing demand on the drug metabolism scientist to establish analytical methods capable of distinguishing between enantiomers. The problems associated with enantiomeric analysis are many and the effective use of the newer methods requires a proper appreciation of potential sources of error. It may be necessary to use a combination of techniques to establish the stereochemistry of a metabolic product, and in cases where no standard reference compounds are available, conclusions may only properly be drawn when two or more independent methods give the same result. It is envisaged that the application and development of the methodologies described here will contribute greatly to our knowledge of drug metabolism, toxicology and clinical pharmacology in the coming years.

ACKNOWLEDGEMENTS

We are grateful to our colleagues Steven Winter, John Darbyshire, Lynn Campbell and Andre Weil for access to unpublished data and helpful discussion, and to Prof. Robert Smith for his continued encouragement. We thank Helen Edwards-Jones for expert preparation of the typescript.

REFERENCES

Adams, J.D., Woolf, T.F., Trevor, A.J., Williams, L.R. & Castagnoli, N., 1982, Journal of Pharmaceutical Sciences, 71, 658.

Ariens, E.J., 1986, Medicinal Research Reviews, 6, 451.

Armstrong, D.W., 1984, Journal of Liquid Chromatography, 7, 353.

Cook, C.E., 1983, Stereoselective Drug Analysis. In: Topics in Pharmaceutical Sciences 1983, edited by D.D. Breimer & P. Speiser (Elsevier Science BV, Amsterdam) p. 87.

Cook, C.E., Ballentine, N.H., Seltzman, T.B. & Tallent, C.R., 1979a, Journal of Pharmacology & Experimental Therapeutics, 210, 391.

Cook, C.E., Myers, M.A., Tallent, C.R., Seltzman, T. & Jeffcoat, A.R., 1979b, Federation Proceedings, 38, 742.

Cook, C.E., Seltzman, T.P., Tallent, C.R. & Wooten, J.D., 1982, Journal of Pharmacology & Experimental Therapeutics, 220, 568.

Dalgliesh, C.E., 1952, Journal of the Chemical Society, 137, 3940.

Dappen, R., Arm, H. & Meyer, V.R., 1986, Journal of Chromatography, 373, 1.

Giacomini, K.M., Nelson, W.L., Pershe, R.A., Valdivieso, Turner-Tamiyasu, K. & Blaschke, T.F., 1986, Journal of Pharmacokinetics & Biopharmaceutics, 14, 335.

Hutt, A.J. & Caldwell, J., 1983, Journal of Pharmacy & Pharmacology, 35, 693.

Hutt, A.J., Fournel, S. & Caldwell, J., 1986, Journal of Chromatography Biomedical Applications, 378, 409.

Landsteiner, K. & Van der Scheer, J., 1929, Journal of Experimental Medicine, 50, 407.

Nahorski, S.R., Batta, M.I. & Barnett, D.B., 1978, European Journal of Pharmacology, 52, 393.

Testa, B., 1986, Xenobiotica, 16, 265.

Walle, T., 1985, Drug Metabolism and Disposition, 13, 279.

Williams, K. & Lee, E., 1985, Drugs, 30, 333.

Yeung, E.S., Steenhoek, L.E., Woodruff, S.D. & Kuo, J.C., 1980, Analytical Chemistry, 52, 1399.

ENANTIOSELECTIVE DRUG METABOLISM AND ITS PHARMACOKINETIC AND PHARMACODYNAMICS CONSEQUENCES

M.Eichelbaum

Dr.Margarete Fischer-Bosch-Institut für
Klinische Pharmakologie
Auerbachstr. 112, 7000 Stuttgart 50
West Germany

Most of the drugs used today are chemical synthetised. Out of 640 synthethic drugs listed in the German pharmacopoe 266 (about 40%) contain at least one chiral centre which means that two enantiomeric configurations are possible.

In contrast to chiral drugs of natural origin which usually contain only one of two possible enantiomers, chemical synthesis generally results in the formation of both configurations unless stereospecific drug synthesis is employed. Although enantiomers contained in racemic drug preparations quite often exhibit pronounced differences in their pharmacological and toxicological properties both in quantitative and qualitative terms only 41 out of 266 racemic drugs are available as drug preparations with only one enantiomer. In order to demonstrate the contrasting effects which the two enantiomer contained in a racemic drug can elicit, thalidomide can serve as tragic example. This hypnotic drug caused ten thousands of fetal malformations in those mothers who had taken the drug during early gestational period. Later on it could be demonstrated in animal experiments that only the S (-) - thalidomide elicited the teratogenic effect, the R (+) isomer being devoid of this action. This example highlights the importance of enantioselectivity in therapeutic and toxic activity of racemic drugs (Ariens, 1984).

In addition to stereoselectivity of drug action various aspects of drug disposition (protein binding, metabolism and renal excretion) show enantioselectivity thus leading to an enantiomer composition in the organism substantially different from the one observed in vitro, that is in the drug administered. Although known for some years it was not until recently that the importance of stereoselective drug metabolism im man and its therapeutic consequences are being increasingly appreciated.

In the context of this presentation I would like to focus on four aspects of stereoselective drug metabolism in man.

1. Stereoselective first-pass metabolism
2. Stereochemical considerations of drug interactions
3. Stereochemical aspects of polymorphic drug oxidation
4. Chiral inversion of racemic drugs

1. Stereoselective First-Pass Metabolism

We became interested in stereoselective first pass metabolism during our work with the calcium channel blocker verapamil. Since its introduction more than 20 years ago clinicians realized that an i.v. dose of 5 to 10 mg was effective in terminating various supraventricular tachyarrhythymias whereas an oral dose of 80 to 160 mg was required in order to elicit a therapeutic effect comparable to i.v. administration. The cause of this pronounced differences in dose requirement became apparent when we demonstrated that despite its almost complete absorption bioavailability was only 20 to 30% due to extensive hepatic presystemic elimination (Schomerus et al.1976). Based on a bioavailability of 20 to 30% an oral dose of 25 to 50 mg should suffice to elicit a therapeutic effect comparable to an i.v. dose of 5 to 10 mg. However, analysis of the concentration-effect relationship revealed that after oral administration verapamil had less negative dromtropic potency at the same plasma concentration than after a single intravenous bolus injection. On average, verapamil plasma concentrations three times higher were required after oral administration in order to produce the same PR-prolongation as after i.v. administration. As the most plausible explanation for the different slopes of the plasma concentration - effect relationship, we proposed that the more active l- isomer is preferentially metabolized during hepatic first-pass metabolism (Eichelbaum et al., 1980). Recent studies carried out in our laboratory have demonstrated that l-verapamil (in agreement with animal experiments) is on average 8 to 10 times more potent than d-verapamil with regard to its negative dromotropic activity (Echizen et al.,1985a). In addition to these differences in pharmacodynamic activity of the l- and d- isomers, pronounced differences in the various pharmacokinetic parameters and bioavailability were observed between d- and l- verapamil. Systemic and oral clearance of l - verapamil was substantially higher than that of d- verapamil. The bioavailability of d- verapamil (50%) was 2.5 times greater than that of l - verapamil (20%) (Eichelbaum et al., 1984; Vogelgesang et al.,1984). The d to l - isomer ratio of plasma verapamil following i.v. administration was approximately 2, whereas after oral administration the d to l ratio was 5. These differences in the d to l - isomer ratio of plasma verapamil concentration in relation to the route of administration explain the observed differences in the slopes of the concentraion - effect curves (Echizen et al.,1985b). With regard to the metabolic reactions responsible for stereoselectivity both in vitro and in vivo studies demonstrated that O-demethylation was the pathway exhibiting enantioselectivity (Heuer et al.,1986).

Stereoselective first-pass metabolism has also been shown for several ß-adrenoceptor antagonists like propranolol and metoprolol. Most of the ß-blocking activity of metoprolol resides in the S(-) enantiomer. Following oral administration the R (+)- isomer had a lower bioavailability and similar results have been reported for propranolol. In this context it is interesting to note that in the case of metoprolol whose metabolism exhibits a genetic polymorphism pronounced differences in stereoselective first pass metabolism are observed between phenotypes. In contrast to EM's bioavailability of R and S-metoprolol is almost identical in PM subjects, leading to a shift in the concentration - effect curve to right in this phenotype (Lennard et al.,1986).

2. Stereochemical Considerations of Drug Interactions

Stereoselective drug metabolism may have important therapeutic implications in the case of drug interactions if pronounced differences in potency exist between enantiomers and their disposition is differently affected by the causative drug. The following example with warfarin will illustrate the importance of studying the enantiomeric disposition of drugs in drug interactions. In a very elegant study O'Reilly et al.(1980) elucidated the mechanism responsible for the augmented hypoprothrombinemia of warfarin caused by the coadministration of phenylbutazone. Although total warfarin plasma concentrations decreased during phenylbutazone treatment, yet an augmented pharmacodynamic response of warfarin was observed. In order to evaluate whether or not phenylbutazone had a differential effect on the disposition of the more potent S-isomer they studied the biological fate of the two-enantiomers by labelling the S-isomere with ^{13}C. During phenylbutazone a highly significant increase in the plasma clearance of R- warfarin and significant decrease in the clearance of S- warfarin was observed compared with the administration of warfarin alone. The authors concluded that phenylbutazone augmented the hypoprothrombinemic action of warfarin by inhibiting the metabolic disposition of the more hypoprothrombinemic S-warfarin, yet reduced total warfarin plasma concentrations by greatly augmenting the clearance of R-warfarin. Recently Toon et al.(1986) investigated the warfarin-sulfinpyrazone interaction. An enhanced hypoprothrombinemia was observed when warfarin and sulfinpyrazone were taken together. This study illustrates evenmore the necessity of monitoring the individual enantiomers of racemic drugs. Whereas one of the subjects showed an increase warfarin elimination $t_{\frac{1}{2}}$, consistent with the enhanced pharmacologic response, another subject showed a 25% decrease in warfarin elimination $t_{\frac{1}{2}}$, a result seemingly in contradiction with the observed enhanced pharmacologic response. Based on these data alone, conclusions regarding plasma concentration response relationship are meaningless, if not the $t_{\frac{1}{2}}$ for the individual enantiomer are considered and the paradox is resolved. In subjects JA the $t_{\frac{1}{2}}$ of S-warfarin increased from 25 to 49.5 hours, while that of the R-enantiomer decreased from 46 to 38 hours with sulfrinpyrazone dosing. In the case of the other subject the $t_{\frac{1}{2}}$ of S-warfarin increased from 49 to 58 hours while that of R-warfarin was so greatly decreased from 87 to 25 hours with sulfrinpyrazone dosing so that the $t_{\frac{1}{2}}$ of total warfarin decreased relative to the control value (fig 1). But in both cases the S-warfarin concentrations increased, a result in agreement with the observed enhanced pharmacologic response.

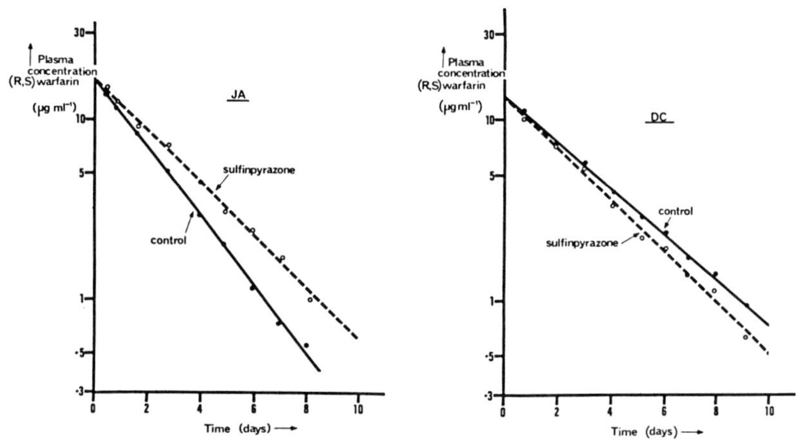

Fig.1: Plasma concentration - time profile of racemic warfarin in the presence and absence of sulfinpyrazone in subject J.A. and D.C., respectively. (from: Toon et al., (1986) Clin. Pharmacol. Ther. 39: 15-24).

3. Stereochemical Aspects of Polymorphic Drug Oxydation

Genetic factors play an important role in stereoselective metabolism of certain drugs. The oxidative metabolism of several drugs, (debrisoquine, sparteine, mephenytoin) exhibits a genetic polymorphisms

(Idle and Smith, 1984; Eichelbaum, 1984; Küpfer et al.,1982). The metabolism of several ß-adrenoceptor antagonists which are administered as racemates is controlled by the debrisoquine/sparteine polymorphism (Lennard et al.,1986; Dayer et al.,1985). Whereas in EM subjects the metabolism of these drugs exhibits a high degree of substrate stereoselectivity, PM's are characterized by a loss of stereoselectivity. Meyer and coworkers (1986) have used the stereospecific metabolism of ± bufuralol as a model reaction to characterize the molecular mechanism responsible for impaired drug oxidation in the poor metabolizer phenotype. The metabolism of bufuralol in liver microsomes of in vivo phenotyped poor metabolizers of debrisoquine or sparteine was characterized by marked increase in k_m, a decrease in the V_{max} and a virtual loss of stereoselectivity of the reaction. A cytochrome P 450 buf-I metabolized bufuralol in a highly stereoselective fashion.

Even more pronounced genetic determined differences in enantioselectivity of certain metabolic reactions are observed, if stereoselectivity of product formation is considered. Although debrisoquine has no asymmetric carbon centre, hydroxylation in position 4 leads to the formation of a new chirality centre with R and S configuration. Studies carried out in our labarotory have established the absolute configuration of the two 4-hydroxy debrisoquine enantiomers. EM subjects form predominantly the S(+)-isomere the enantiomer excess being greater 99.5%. In contrast PM subject are not only characterized by a marked decreased formation of total 4-hydroxy debrisoquine, but also by a loss of product stereoselectivity of this reaction forming up to 30% R(-)-isomer. It is also interesting to note that about 30 to 40% of all EM subjects studied showed some formatiom of the R-enantiomers. Since this number is in close agreement with the expected genotype frequency of heterozygotes in the population, this approach might be useful in identifying heterozygotes (Meese et al.,1986). Taken altogether these data seem to indicate that the mechanism responsible for impaired drugs oxidation in the poor metabolizer phenotype is more likely to be due to a cytochrome 450 with impaired catalytic properties rather than a decreased amount of enzyme.

4. Chiral Inversion of Racemic Drugs

Another stereoselective metabolic pathway in man has been demonstrated for the 2-arylpropionic acid nonsteroidal antiinflammatory drugs. These compounds are chiral, the inhibitory effect on prostaglandin synthethase being caused by the S-enantiomers. In vivo, the compounds undergo a unidirectional configurational inversion, the R-enantiomer being converted into the active S-form by an enzymatic mechanism which has not been definitely elucidated. The reverse reactions has never been detected. Thus, the R-enantiomer must be considered as prodrug of the S-enantiomer when racemates are used in therapy. For example about 2/3 of the dose of R-ibuprofen is converted to the S form in humans (Lee et al.1985).

Conclusions

The examples discussed demonstrate convincingly the importance of enantioselective drug metabolism in man and its pharmacokinetic and pharmacodynamic consequences. In view of these findings the question arises whether racemic drugs should be used as racemates or as isomers. There is no straight forward answer to this question. If only quantitative differences in therapeutic activity exist and the less active enantiomer is not predominantly responsible for side effects, the therapeutic benefit gained by using the more active enantiomer is only marginal and does not justify the substantial increase in costs involved in manifacturing such a drug preparation. But there can be exeptions form this rule. The main therapeutic action might be disadvantageous if a racemic drug is to be used for an indication where the predominant pharmacologic effects are not required and may in fact limit the therapeutic use of the drug for this indication. This can be exemplified in the case of verapamil. A number of studies both with tumor cell lines and animal tumors have demonstrated that verapamil enhances the cytotoxicity of vinca alkaloid and anthracycline cytostatics and can reverse the resistance towards these chemotherapeutic agents in resistant tumor cell lines (Tsuruo et al. 1981; Inaba and Saskurai, 1979). Calcium antagonists inhibit the active outward transport and increase intracellular content of vinblastine and anthracyclines in cells resistant to these cytostatic drugs. Based on these experiments a phase I clinical trial has been carried out to increase the cytotoxicity of vinblastine by concurrent i.v. infusion of racemic verapamil. However, no enhanced cytotoxicity of vinblastine could be observed. The verapamil plasma concentrations achieved were on average 5 times less than those which had been required in vitro to enhance cytotoxicity. Side effects due to the action of verapamil on sinus and AV-node did not allow to increase the dose to concentrations associated in vitro with enhanced cytotoxicity (Benson et al.,1985). Since the action of verapamil on the slow Ca^{++} channels seems not responsible for the cytotoxic action the use of d-verapamil might be better suited for this purpose. d-verapamil is at least ten times less active than l-verapamil with regard to its negative dromotropic action. Preliminary studies in our laboratory have shown that d-verapamil enhanced the cytotoxicity of vincristine and daunomycine in human T-lymphoma cell line (MOLT 4B) (fig 2) and Burkitt lymphoma cell line (fig 3) in a fashion similar to l-verapamil (Wolf, Schumacher and Eichelbaum, unpublished results). Therefore the use of d-verapamil for this indication might be advantageous since much higher verapamil concentrations can be achieved because it has less negative dromotropic activity than l-verapamil.

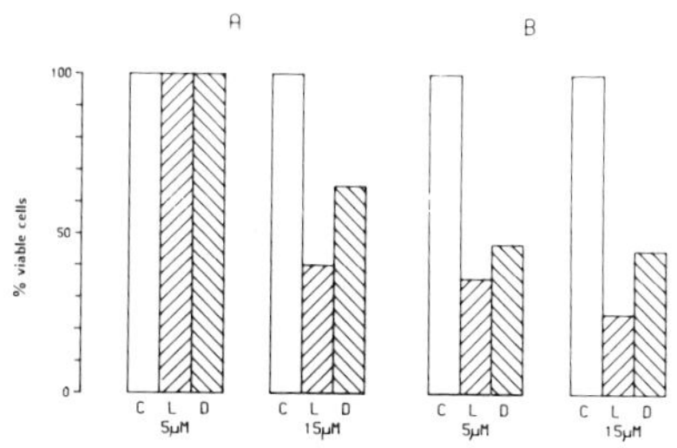

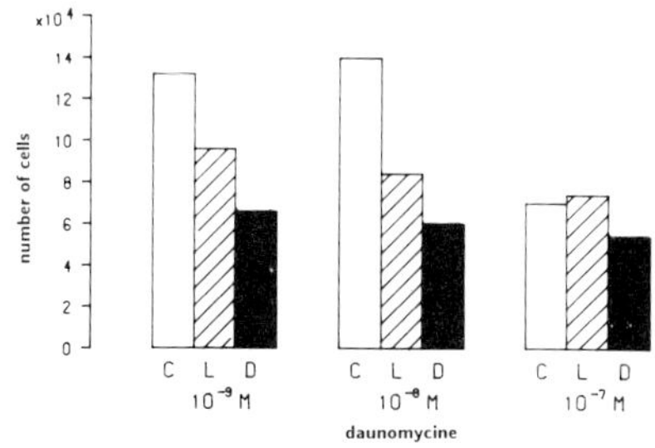

Fig.2: Enhancement of vincristine cytotoxicity at vincristine concentrations of 5 x 10^{-9}M by d-(▧) and l-verapamil (▨) in vincristine resistant (A) and sensitive (B) human T-lymphoma cell line (MOLT 4B). The open bars are the controls without verapamil.

Fig.3: Influence of d-(■) and l- (▨) verapamil on daunomycine cytotoxicity at different daunomycine concentrations in human Burkitt lymphoma cell line. The open bars are the controls without verapamil.

However, if enantioselectivity in therapeutic activity is pronounced and adverse drug reactions and side effects are caused by the enantiomer which is devoid of or has less therapeutic activity the more active enantiomer should be used (e.g. d-penicillamine). If metabolic chiral inversion occurs as in the case of 2-arylpropionic acid nonsteroidal antiinflammatory drus the use of an enantiomer is meaningless.

References

Ariens,E.J., 1984 Stereochemistry, a basis for sophisticated nonsense in pharmacokinetics and clinical pharmacology. European Journal of Clinical Pharmacology 26: 663-668.

Benson,A.B. et al. 1985 Phase I study of vinblastine and verapamil given by concurrent iv infusion. Cancer Treatment Reports 69, No.7-8, 795.

Dayer,P. et al. 1985b Steric configuration and polymorphic oxidation of lipophilic beta-adrenoceptor blocking agents: In vivo- in vitro correlations 34,399.

Echizen,H. et al. 1985a The effect of dextro, levo and racemic verapamil on atrioventricular conduction in man. American Heart Journal 109, 210-217.

Echizen,H. et al. 1985b Effects of d, l-verapamil on atrioventricular conduction in relation to its stereoselective first-pass metabolism. Clinical Pharmacology and Therapeutics 38, 71-76.

Eichelbaum,M. et al. 1980 Effects of verapamil on PR intervals in relation to verapamil plasma levels following single i.v. and oral administration and during chronic treatment. Klinische Wochenschrift 58, 919-925.

Eichelbaum,M. et al. 1984a Pharmacokinetics of (+)-, (-)- and (±)-verapamil after intravenous administration. British Journal of Clinical Pharmacology 17, 453-458.

Eichelbaum,M. 1984b Polymorphic drug oxidation in humans. Federation Proceedings 43, 2298-2302.

Heuer,B. et al. 1986 In vitro and in vivo metabolism of the optical isomers of verapamil. Abstr.562, III World Conference on Clinical Pharmacology and Therapeutics. Stockholm.

Idle,J.R., and Smith,R.L. 1984 The debrisoquine hydroxylation gene: A gene of multiple consequence. In: Lemberger,L., Reidenberg,M.M.-(Hrsg.) Proceedings of the Second World Conference on Clinical Pharmacology and Therapeutics. ASPET, Bethesda 148-164

Lee,E.J.D. et al. 1985 Stereoselective disposition of ibuprofen enantiomers in man. British Journal of Clinical Pharmacology 19, 669-674.

Lennard, M.S. et al. 1986 Debrisoquine polymorphism and the metabolism and action of metoprolol, timolol, propranolol and atenolol. Xenobiotica, 16, No 5, 435-447.

Meese,C. and Eichelbaum 1986 Stereochemische Aspekte der polymorphen 4-Hydroxylierung von Debrisoquin beim Menschen. Naunyn-Schmiedeberg's Archive of Pharmacology. Supplement 332 R 95, 377.

Meyer,U.A. et al. 1986 The molecular mechanisms of two common polymorphisms of drug oxidation-evidence for functional changes in cytochrome P-450 isozymes catalysing bufuralol and mephenytoin oxidation. Xenobiotica, 16, No.5, 449-464.

O'Reilly,R.A.et al. 1980 Stereoselective interaction of phenylbutazone with ($^{12}C/^{13}C$) warfarin pseudoracemates in man. Journal of Clinical Investigation 65, 746-753.

Toon,S. et al. 1986 The warfarin-sulfinpyrazone interaction: stereochemical considerations. Clinical Pharmacology and Therapeutics 39, 15-24.

Vogelgesang,B. et al. 1984 Stereoselective first-pass metabolism of highly cleared drugs: studies of the bioavailability of L- and D-verapamil examined with a stable isotope technique. British Journal of Clinical Pharmacology 18, 733-740.

TOXICITY-RELATED STEREOSELECTIVE BIOTRANSFORMATION

Nico P.E. Vermeulen

Department of Pharmacochemistry (Molecular Toxicology),
Free University, De Boelelaan 1083,
1081 HV Amsterdam (The Netherlands).

Introduction

During the last two decades there has been an increased interest among toxicologists to explain toxic effects of chemicals more and more mechanistically. Much clearer than before the development of toxicity is being unraveled in different stages; namely: a) kinetics (absorption, distribution and elimination, b) activating or inactivating biotransformation, c) reversible or irreversible interaction with cellular or tissue components, d) chemical or biochemical protection - or repairmechanisms and e) nature and consequences of toxicity for the organism. The approach at which explanations at the molecular level are searched for is called molecular toxicology (Vermeulen (1986a)). In this toxicological approach it is more and more recognized that stereochemical factors play a significant role in the biological action of drugs and other xenobiotics on living organisms (Ariens (1983), Albert (1985)). Apart from the differences in intrinsic biological activity, desired and undesired effects of xenobiotics ultimately may also be influenced by stereoselectivity at all other stages mentioned above (Vermeulen (1986b), Testa (1986a)).

Stereoisomerism however is a rather broad phenomenon and manifests itself in various forms, such as those related to enantiomers, epimers, diastereoisomers, meso compounds, geometrical isomers etc. Generally speaking the consequences of stereoisomerism for disposition and biological action of xenobiotics in living organisms are still difficult to predict, because they are complex and of a multifactorial origin. Nevertheless, there is a growing interest among researchers to set up experiments in such a way that beneficial or detrimental consequences of stereoselectivity can become clear as early as possible. Recent developments in analytical techniques, enabling the simultaneous separation of stereoisomers with HPLC (Special issue, J. Liq.Chrom. (1986)), GLC (Testa (1986b)), chiral antisera (Cook (1985)) and GLC-MS with the use of stable isotopes (Baillie (1981)), as well as in stereocontrolled synthesis (Beld and Zwanenburg (1986)) certainly have contributed to the increased interest in studying stereoselective aspects of biotransformation and biological activity of drugs and other xenobiotics.

In this contribution a number of examples of stereoselectivity in the biotransformation and toxicity of xenobiotics is discussed. Special attention is paid to those examples, which can illustrate the stereoselective action of important enzymes, consequences for the toxicity of xenobiotics and to examples in which stereoselectivity is used as a tool to study mechanisms of biotransformation in relation to toxicity.

Stereoselectivity and toxicity

Relevance and pertinent role of biotransformation.

Possible consequences of toxicity-related stereoselectivity might be illustrated with the almost classical, but as yet as to the underlying mechanism not completely elucidated example of thalidomide. End 50's the drug was put on the market as an hypnotic agent and early 60's taken off again because of suspected embryotoxic and teratogenic effects. Only in more recent years it has become clear that both S-(-)-thalidomide and the R-(+)-enantiomer are transformed in vivo into 1-N-phtaloylglutamine and 1-N-phtaloylglutaminic acid in various species. Although there have been published conflicting reports on the sensitivity of different mice and rat strains as to thalidomide toxicity, in SWS mice only the glutaminic acid metabolite derived from the S-(-)-enantiomer and not the one derived from the R-(+)-isomer was shown to be embryotoxic and teratogenic (Ockzenfelz *et al.* (1976)). The recognition of such complications during drug development, however, is considerably hindered by the large species differences generally encountered in the biotransformation of xenobiotics. In addition to that, species dependent stereoselectivity can hinder the search for a model species being representative for the human ultimately aimed at.

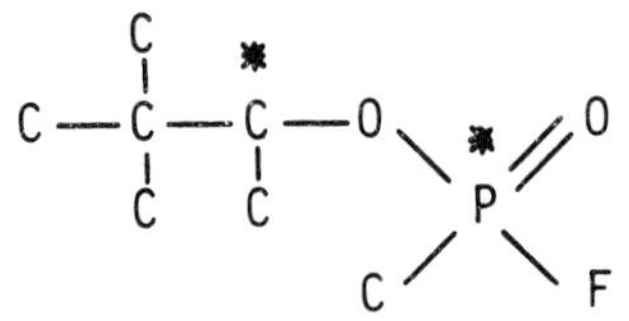

C(-) SOMAN	C(-) P(-) :	1.8 x 10^8 $mol^{-1}min^{-1}$
	C(-) P(+):	<5 x 10^3 $mol^{-1}min^{-1}$
C(+) SOMAN	C(+) P(-):	2.8 x 10^8 mol^{-1} min^{-1}
	C(+) P(+):	<5 x 10^3 $mol^{-1}min^{-1}$

Fig 1a: Chemical structure (, chiral center) of the nerve gas agent Soman. Due to two centers of asymmetry racemic Soman consists of four stereoisomers. (Benschop et al.,1984). Fig. 1b: Reaction rates for the inhibition of acetylcholinesterase from electric eel with the stereoisomers of Soman.*

Other important examples of stereoselective toxicity are represented by certain organophosphates, such as organophosphorus pesticides and so-called nerve agents. Their toxicity is mainly based on their ability to inhibit acetylcholinesterase by phosphylating the enzyme at its active site. Soman (figure 1), a nerve gas agent, is a racemic mixture of four stereoisomers, due to the presence of two centers of asymmetry, viz at a carbon atom in the pinacolyl moiety and at the phosphorus atom. The resolution of soman into the pure stereoisomers (Benschop *et al.* (1984)), has various investigators enabled to elucidate the influence of stereoselectivity on their toxicity, on the reactivation of soman inhibited acetylcholinesterases in various species by Hagedorn-oximes and on the ability of monoclonal antibodies to protect in vitro against soman induced inhibition of acetylcholinesterase (Brimfield *et al.* (1985)). From these studies, it may be derived that much care has to be taken with the extrapolation of the pronounced stereoselective effects observed in vitro to the in vivo situation. For example, the differences in anti-cholinesterase activity, measured in vitro, (figure 1b) did not reflect at all, acute toxicity nor delayed neurotoxicity data observed in vivo. Factors, such as (i) rates of transport through membranes (e.g. blood-brain barrier), (ii) rates of detoxication (e.g. by inhibition of hydrolases) and (iii) actual rates of inhibition of membrane-bound acetylcholinesterase at critical sites, may complicate this type of in vitro - in vivo extrapolation. Further knowledge into the mechanisms of toxicity, however, are still needed (e.g. to find leads better treatments of this type of intoxications). Generally speaking, it seems that chirality of the phospate moiety in this type of compounds is of more influence on the binding to the acetylcholinesterase than chirality at e.g. an α-carbon atom of an alkoxy moiety bound to phosphorons.

As to pharmacological consequences, the example of hexobarbital (HB), at present mainly used as model-substrate, can be looked upon as illustrative. Apart from a large difference between the intrinsic hypnotic activities of the enantiomers of this highly lipophilic chiral drug, the S-(+)-enantiomer being far the most active enantiomer in most species, substrate- and product-stereoselective metabolism is involved. Using a pseudoracemic mixture of HB, consisting of a mixture of S-(+)- and N_1-trideutero -R-(-)-HB, and an analytical procedure based on mass fragmentography (Van der Graaff *et al.* (1986)), recently, the stereoselective disposition of HB-enantiomers could be studied upon simultaneous administration to the rat. The difference in intrinsic clearances between S-(+)- and R-(-)-HB, as reflected by the difference in the areas under their respective blood concentration time curves after oral administration to the rat (AUC_{oral}) was about sevenfold. This was, however, far larger than the difference between the corresponding elimination half-lives ($t_{1/2}$) or systemic clearances (CL_S) as estimated upon intra-arterial administration. The observed discrepancies between the oral and intra-arterial pharmacokinetic parameters were attributed to hepatic bloodflow limited metabolism of HB, a phenomenon which was further substantiated by the relatively high hepatic extraction ratios of the enantiomers in the rat, *viz* E = 0.68 for R-(-)- and 0.95 for S-(+)-HB. Considering the pharmacokinetic and the pharmacodynamic data of the hexobarbital enantiomers, in relation to its use as a model-substrate, at least for the rat one might suggest to use the intrinsic clearance (CL_{int}) of R-(-)-HB as the preferred parameter reflecting (phenobarbital-inducible) hepatic cytochrome P-450 activity and, the intrinsic clearance (CL_{int}) of the S-(+)-enantiomer (or even the sleeping time induced by it) as a simultaneous reflection of hepatic bloodflow.

There exist many other examples illustrating various toxicological or pharmacological consequences of stereoselectivity in the biotransformation of drugs and other xenobiotics (Vermeulen (1986b)). Apart from direct substrate-stereoselective effects of the unchanged compound, stereoselective bioactivation or bioinactivation by enzymes seems to be of major importance.

Stereochemical balast

In recent years, on various occasions (e.g. Ariëns (1984)) the use of mixtures of stereoisomers has been made a matter of debate. Especially in those cases, where a great difference in biological activity (e.g. in the case of pesticides or herbicides; Ariëns (1984)) between the active and the inactive stereoisomers exists, the use of mixtures of stereoisomers has been qualified as undesirable and as an unnecessary burdening of the organism and pollution of the environment. Along with the development of more suitable chemical and biotechnological methods for the synthesis and separation of optical and geometric isomers the initial aversion against this thesis seems to diminish at present. It is too simple, however, to reject the use of mixtures of stereoisomers categorically without knowing reasons and consequences of stereoselectivity.

Stereoselective bioactivation and bioinactivation

Mixed-Function Oxidases (MFO)

One of the most important drug and xenobiotic metabolizing enzyme systems in mammalians and non-mammalians is the MFO-system, consisting of a family of cytochrome-P_{450} isoenzymes which, in general, exhibit a broadly ranging substrate- and product selectivity. The multiplicity and the widely varying substrate selectivity complicate considerably the study of the stereoselectivity as such, as well as the correlation of stereoselectivities in different species. Regio- and stereoselective hydroxylation-reactions of R-(+)- and S-(-)-warfarin, nevertheless, have been suggested to be useful as a probe for the functional characterization of the multiplicity of hepatic cytochrome P-450. As such this biochemical tool was used to study post mortem microsomal fractions of human livers of renal donors and surgical cancer patients (Kaminsky *et al.*, 1984). Mechanistical studies, e.g. on the stereochemistry of the 1'-hydroxylation of (R)- and (S)-1'-deuterated phenylethane by a single isolated enzyme, P-450_{LM2}, have demonstrated that the product-stereoselectivity most probably must rely on constraints of the substrate binding site provided by the protein environment rather than on the intrinsic hydrodroxylation mechanism of cytochrome P-450 (White *et al.*, 1986).

Among the best documented examples illustrating the stereoselective action of cytochrome-P_{450} isoenzymes as well as approaches to use stereoselectivity in biotransformation as a tool for different purposes are provided by studies on the stereoselective bioactivation of polycyclic aromatic hydrocarbons to carcinogens by cytochrome-P_{450c} (Jerina *et al.* (1985)). This isoenzyme amongst others was found to catalyze highly stereoselectively the epoxidation of benzo(a)pyrene to (+)-7R,8S-arene oxide, which upon hydrolysis by the epoxide hydrolase to (-)-7R,8R-dihydrodiol- benzo(a)pyrene is converted by the same cytochrome P-450 isoenzyme to (+)-benzo(a)pyrene-7R,8S-dihydrodiol-9S,10R-epoxide, in which the benzylic hydroxyl group and epoxide oxygen are *trans*, in over 85% diastereomeric excess (Fig. 2).

By studying the stereospecificity of various polycyclic aromatic hydrocarbons in detail, Jerina and coworkers were able to propose a model for the steric and spatial requirements of the catalytic site of the cytochrome-P_{450c} involved. This model was demonstrated to be also valid in predicting the stereoselective metabolism of other polycyclic aromatic hydrocarbons like phenanthrene, chrysene and benzanthracene (e.g. Van Bladeren *et al.* (1984)). Interestingly, the model also seems to predict the stereochemical course preferred in the oxidative metabolism of benzoring dihydrodiols of PAH's to diol-epoxides, thus suggesting that the cytochrome-P_{450c} ignores the presence of the hydroxyl groups. The model developed for polycyclic aromatic hydrocarbons is as yet not applicable, however, to the biotransformation of other non-polycyclic aromatic compounds.

As to stereoselectivity in the biological activity of PAH's, mutagenicity (Conney (1982)) and tumorigenicity (Thakker *et al.* (1982)) studies have shown that those activities of PAH's are also strongly dependent on their relative and absolute configuration. For example, the (-)-7R,8R- dihydrodiol derivative of benzo(a)pyrene has a roughly 10-fold higher skin tumor-initiating activity in female CD-1 mice than the (+)-7S,8S-enantiomer and it also produced greater than 14-fold more lung tumors in newborn mice. Among the four isomeric

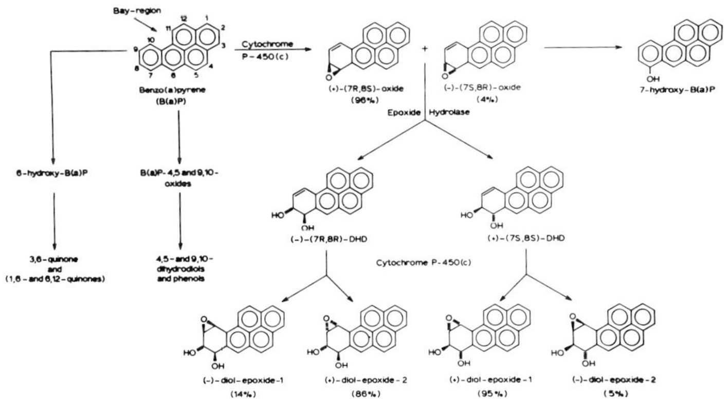

Fig. 2: Stereoselective biotransformation of benzo(a)pyrene by cytochrome-P_{450} and epoxide hydrolase to optically active bay-region 7,8-diol-9,10-epoxides. Non-bay-region pathways to quinones and phenols are also indicated (adapted from Jerina et al., 1985)

diol-epoxides, the (+)-7R,8S- dihydrodiol-9S,10R-epoxide was severalfold more mutagenic to chinese hamster V79 cells and, in addition, it was the only isomer with high tumorigenic activity on mouse skin and in newborn mice (Table 1). Thus this enantiomeric diol-epoxide was established as the ultimate carcinogen of this PAH. At the molecular level, stereoselectivity in adduct-formation between the diol-epoxides and the exocyclic 2-aminoguanine of DNA has been suggested to be responsible for the observed stereoselectivity in this type of toxicity. From comparative investigations on the tumorigenicity of various polycyclic aromatic hydrocarbons (benzo(a)pyrene, benz(a)anthracene, chrysene) it has been derived that a "bay-region" diol-epoxide functionality is of importance in the expression of tumorigenicity and, furthermore, that common stereochemical factors such as relative configuration (pseudo-diequatorial hydroxyl-groups) and absolute configuration (R-configuration at benzylic carbon atom) appear to be far more important than chemical reactivity in this regard (Jerina *et al.* (1985)). As far as tumorigenicity and mutagenicity of dibenz (c, h) acridine is concerned recent data further support the idea that the highest biological activity is attributable to a bay-region diol-epoxide that is superimposable on the highly active [R, S, S, R] bay-region diol epoxides of the polycyclic aromatic hydrocarbons mentioned above (Wood *et al.*, 1986).

In recent years, much effort has been given to the development of immunochemical techniques for sensitive detection of DNA-damage in relation to exposure of animals or humans to genotoxic agents (Lohman *et al.* (1985)). The interesting aspect of this approach is that, in principle, the toxicologically most important adduct between a stereoisomeric biotransformation-product and DNA can be determined, e.g. with monoclonal or polyclonal antibodies. A problem observed, however, is cross-reactivity with adducts of other stereoisomers. The immunochemical detection technique has been applied to DNA adducts of benzo(a)pyrene diol-epoxide metabolites. Investigations (Rojas and Alexandrov, 1986) have shown that the (+)-anti-diol-epoxide deoxyguanosine DNA-adduct formed in vivo was indeed more persistent in mouse epidermis than in rat epidermis, an observation which correlates with the relative resistance of the rat to the carcinogenic action of benzo(a)pyrene.

Table 1 Mutagenic activity expressed as revertants/nmol/plate for the S. typhimurium strains and as 8-azaguanine-resistant colonies/nmol/10^5 surviving cells for the Chinese hamster V-79 cells (Conney, 1982).

Compound tested	Mutagenic activity		
	S. typhimurium		Chinese hamster V-79 cells
	Strain TA 98	Strain TA 100	
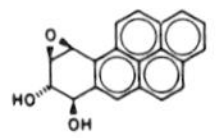 (−)-BP 7,8-diol-9,10-epoxide 1	5200	9500	60
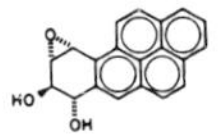 (+)-BP 7,8-diol-9,10-epoxide 1	3900	5200	34
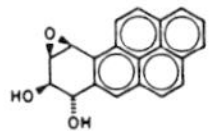 (−)-BP 7,8-diol-9,10-epoxide 2	1800	1000	22
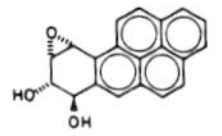 (+)-BP 7,8-diol-9,10-epoxide 2	2500	6000	400

Chirality and oxidation polymorphisms

Biotransformation by hepatic cytochrome-P_{450} containing mono-oxygenases is a major determinant of inter-individual differences in the rate of elimination of numerous drugs and other xenobiotics and, consequently, in their pharmacological or toxicological response. Amongst compounds whose oxidation has been reported to be impaired in poor metabolizer phenotypes (representing approximately 10% of the European population) is the β-adrenoceptor antagonist Bufuralol (Buf). It is a chiral drug for which 1'-hydroxylation (Fig.3) is under genetic control and selective for the (+)-isomer. Aromatic Buf 4- and 6-hydroxylations are under the same genetic control but selective for the (-)-isomer. The selectivity for the aliphatic and aromatic oxidations is virtually abolished in poor metabolizer phenotypes. Apart from these oxidation reactions, glucuronidation of the hydroxyl group in the side chain and renal elimination appeared to be stereoselective for (+)-Buf and particularly important in poor metabolizers.

Since there is no overlap between V_{max}- and K_m-values for the 1'-hydroxylation of (+)-Buf as to poor and extensive metabolizers, it was suggested to use these two parameters in combination with the enantiomeric ratio, $V_{max}(-)/V_{max}(+)$, as a tool to phenotype individuals in vitro. Various recent investigations (Dayer et al., (1984, 1985)) (including those with a purified human isoenzyme) have provided evidence for the hypothesis that 1'-hydroxylation of Buf is mediated by a polymorphic cytochrome-P_{450} isozyme, which is also catalyzing 4-hydroxylation of Debrisoquine, oxidation of Spartein, E-10-hydroxylation of Nortriptyline, 0-demethylation of Dextrometorphan, trans-4'- hydroxylation of Perhexiline, α-hydroxylation of (+)-Metoprolol and several others (e.g. Boobis *et al.* (1985); Distlerath *et al.* (1985)).

5-Substituted 5-phenylhydantoins represent another class of drugs, showing an oxidation polymorphism involving stereoselectivity. In the case of mephenytoin (Kupfer *et al.* (1981)) aromatic 4-hydroxylation is the preferred metabolic reaction in man in S-mephenytoin ($t_{1/2}$ ~ 1 hr), whereas N-demethylation is preferentially taking place in the R-isomer. Only, S-mephenytoin 4-hydroxylation is genetically deficient. The R-enantiomer was found to be

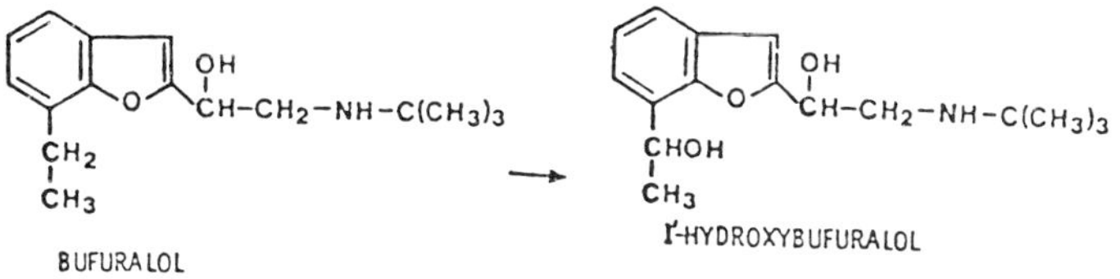

Fig.3: Chemical structure of Bufuralol and the 1'-hydroxylated metabolite, the formation of which is under genetic control and stereoselective for the (+)-enatiomer (adapted from Boobis et al., 1985)

excreted much slower ($t_{1/2}$ ~ 70 hr) and is therefore likely to contribute the most to the well-known accumulation of 5-phenyl-5-ethylhydantoin during chronic anticonvulsant therapy.

In this type of studies stereoselective metabolism has been used as a tool to phenotype inidividuals for (iso)enzymes or enzyme systems which, in principle, can activate xenobiotics into chemical carcinogens.

Epoxide hydrolases

Epoxide hydrolases are enzymes which catalyze the hydrolysis of alkene oxides into diols and of arene oxides into dihydro-diols (Oesch (1979)). Meanwhile, two different epoxide hydrolases have been isolated and identified, namely a microsomal membrane bound (Oesch (1979)) as well as a cytosolic soluble one (Hammock *et al.* (1980)). Substrate selectivities of both hydrolases is large and largely overlapping, although the cytosolic hydrolase seems to possess a larger activity towards aliphatic epoxides. simple Mechanistically, the enzymatic hydration of epoxides most probably proceeds according to a base-catalyzed nucleophilic addition of "activated water" (Hanzlik *et al.* (1976)). A electrophilic (acid-catalyzed) mechanism was ruled out by experiments with $^{18}OH_2$, which demonstrated regiospecific hydration at the 2-position of unlabelled styrene- and nafthaleneoxides (Hanzlik *et al.* (1976)).

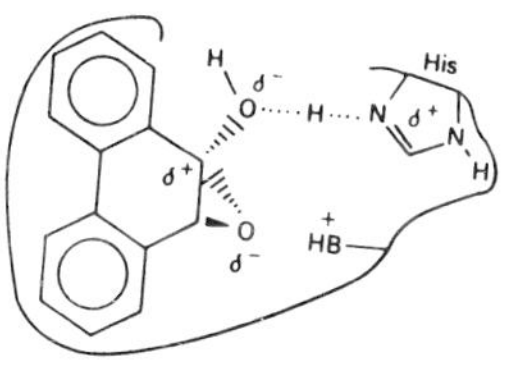

Fig.4: Proposed transition state for the reaction of the epoxide hydrolase-substrate-water complex (adapted from Armstrong et al., 1980). Apart from a certain hydrophobic pocket directing the stereoselective orientation of binding of substrates, a base-catalysed nucleophilic attack of "activated" water is generally believed to be important in this enzymatic reaction.

Stereochemical studies have shown that epoxide hydrolases hydrate epoxides of cyclic olefines including arene oxides, in such a way that *trans*-diols with a varying degree of enantiomeric homogeneity are formed (Armstrong *et al.* (1981)). Geometrical isomers of aliphatic epoxides have also been shown to undergo *trans*-hydration, which means that *trans*-epoxides yield *erytho*-glycols and *cis*-epoxides *threo*-glycols (Hammock et al., 1980). In the literature low and high substrate enantioselectivity have been described for microsomal epoxide hydrolases. For example, for 4,5-benzo(a)pyrene oxide a biphasic first-order kinetic behaviour reflecting a 40-fold difference in the rates of hydration of the (+)- and (-)enantiomers was observed under certain *in vitro* conditions (Armstrong *et al.* (1980)). The enantioselectivity and positional selectivity of the microsomal epoxide hydrolase have been studied in greater depth with stereoisomeric 3-*tert*-butyl-1,2-epoxy cyclohexanes (Belluci *et al.* (1982)) as well as with tetrahydro- and diol-epoxides derived from benz(a)-anthracene (Sayer *et al.* (1985)). From these and other studies authors have deduced a geometry of the active site where a hydrophobic pocket is directing the binding of the stereoisomers in a proper orientation for the nucleophilic attack of water (Fig. 4).

Recently, sterically differently substituted epoxides, such as reactive metabolites of the pesticides vinclozolin, rotenone and phenothrin, were investigated as to their ability to inhibit epoxide hydrolase. Mono- and di-substituted oxiranes were good substrates and strong non-competitive inhibitors of hepatic epoxide hydrolase, whereas tri-substituted epoxides were virtually inactive in this regard (Cova *et al.* (1986)). Obviously, selective inhibition of epoxide hydrolase by epoxide metabolites could interfere with the natural protection of the organism against other toxic epoxides. Intrinsically, epoxides have been shown to be able to exert various kinds of toxicity. Bay-region diol-epoxides are the most well-known ultimately carcinogenic metabolites of polycyclic aromatic hydrocarbons (Jerina *et al.* (1985)). With respect to aliphatic epoxides it has been shown that the following decreasing order of mutagenicity exists: mono->cis-1,2-di->>1,1-di->trans-1,2-di∞tetra-substituted oxiranes (Wade *et al.* (1978)). Generally speaking, both steric and electronic factors will determine the reactivity and the toxicity of oxiranes.

Glutathion-s-transferases (GSH-t)

[Xenobiotics possessing an electrophilic center]. Apart from aliphatic and aromatic epoxides, GSH-s-transferases catalyze the conjugation of the optically active tripeptide glutathione (GSH, γ-Glu-Cys-Gly) to many other hydrophobic and electrophilic substrates possessing leaving groups, such as phosphates, sulphates and halogenides. The mechanism of the conjugation reaction, which is generally catalyzed by a cytosolic system of GSH-s-transferases, is consistent with a S_{N2}-type single displacement substitition mechanism involving a direct attack of the sulfhydryl group of GSH at the electrophilic atom.

With regard to the stereoselectivity of GSH conjugation to rigid epoxides it was, for example, found by identifying and quantifying mercapturic acids excreted in urine of rats treated with the model compound cyclohexene oxide, that only two *trans*-2-hydroxycyclohexyl-mercapturic acids and no *cis*-isomers were *in vivo* found (Van Bladeren *et al.* (1981), Vermeulen *et al.* (1980)). GSH-conjugation of chiral α-Bromo isovalerylurea, recently proposed as a possible model substrate for the study of kinetics of GSH-conjugation in vivo (Te Koppele *et al.*, (1987)), in the rat was also shown to proceed with a high degree of stereoselectivity. In alkylhalogenides rat liver cytosolic GSH-s-transferases were found to conjugate chiral α-phenylethyl-chloride and -bromide with a high degree of substrate-stereoselectivity (Mangold and Abdel-Monem (1980)). S-enantiomers were far better substrates than R-enantiomers and the chloride-analogue showed a higher stereoselectivity than the bromide-analogue. A *trans*-addition mechanism involving S_{N2}-substitution was also found for the enzymatic conjugation of (±)-benz(a)pyrene-4,5-oxide using rat liver cytosol as a source of transferase activity. Both positional isomers (at C_4 and C_5) were produced, however, with a preference for two diastereoisomers. Subsequent investigations with optically active (+)-4S,5R and (-)-4R,5S-benzo(a)pyrene-4,5-oxides (Armstrong *et al.* (1981) have shown that the rat liver cytosol GSH-transferases preferentially catalyze the formation of the 5-glutathionyl-isomer (4S,5S) from the (+) and the 4-gluthionyl-isomer (4S,5S) from the (-)benzo(a)pyrene-4,5-oxide isomer. Apparently, these GSH-transferases prefer to attack the oxirane carbon of the benzo(a)pyrene-4,5-oxide, which has the absolute R-configuration.

Unless different isoenzymes possess the same kind of stereoselectivity towards a substrate, it may be anticipated that a mixture of isoenzymes will exhibit a diminished stereoselective metabolism. In the case of GSH-s-transferases the stereoselection is even more complicated since one isoenzyme may exist as a homo- or heterodimeric protein of two subunits, each of the subunits potentially having structurally different active sites apart from their GSH-binding site. By studying the stereoselectivity of a heterodimeric isoenzyme C towards various K-region arene oxides and azarene analogues, Cobb *et al.* (1983) confirmed a high stereoselectivity with predominant (>95%) attack at the oxirane carbon of R-absolute configuration to give S,S-products. Their results further suggested that hydrophobic interactions between the substrate and the enzyme surface distal to the oxirane ring, rather than electronic differences between the two oxirane carbons, are important in determining the stereoselectivity of the isoenzyme C. (Fig. 5).

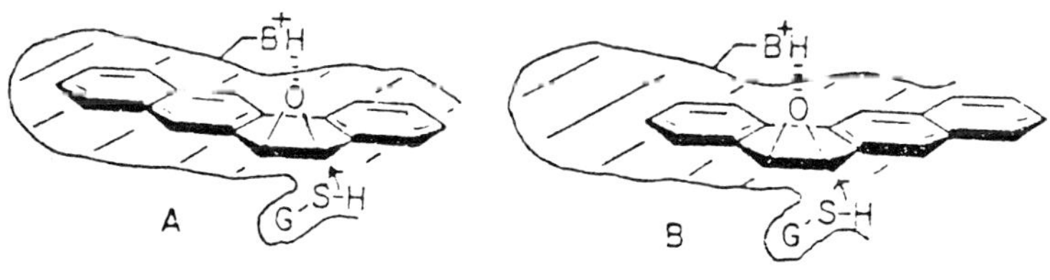

Fig.5: Illustration of possible asymmetries in the active site of the C subunit of GSH-transferase isoenzyme C. Differences in hydrophobic overlap between enzyme and substrate and/or in efficiency of protonation of the leaving group dictate the stereo- and regioselectivity of the GSH-attack (Cobb et al., 1983).

Recently it was shown that cytosolic GSH-s-transferases from rat hepatic and extra-hepatic tissues varied markedly in their stereoselectivity towards a number of polycyclic arene and alkene oxide substrates. This stereoselectivity was found to correlate roughly with known tissue differences in isoenzyme composition and it was suggested to use this stereo- and enantioselectivity for the functional characterization of GSH-s-transferase isoenzymes in different tissues (Dostal *et al.* (1986)).

Stereoselective metabolism by cytosolic GSH-transferases may be important from a toxicological point of view. This was for example illustrated by experiments in which the mutagenic behaviour of *cis*- and *trans*-1,2-dichlorocyclohexane with and without metabolic activation was investigated (Van Bladeren *et al.* (1979)). Using the Ames-test with Salmonella typhimurium cells it was shown that, in contrast to the *trans*-isomer, the *cis*-isomer demonstrated mutagenic activity that was significantly increased upon addition of 9000 g and 100,000 g supernatant of a rat liver homogenate (Fig. 6).

The explanation of this stereoselective effect was given in terms of a stereospecific action of glutathione transferases present in the liver homogenate fractions and catalyzing the substitution of the vicinal chlorine atoms according to a S_{N2}-substitution mechanism. Only

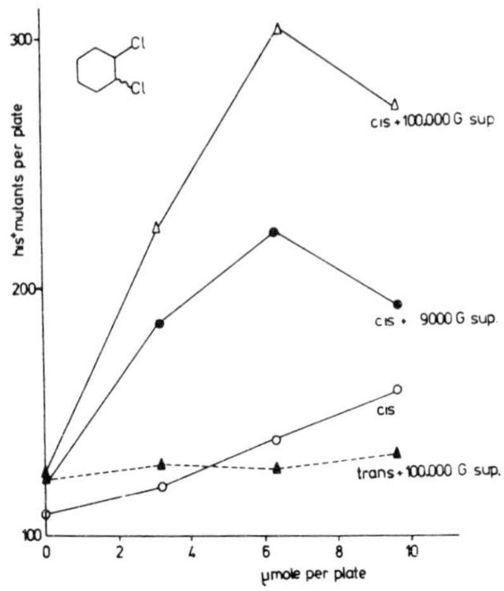

Fig.6: Mutagenicity in Salmonella Typhimurium TA100, induced by cis- and trans-1,2-dichlorocyclohexanes with and without the addition of homogenated rat liver fractions

in the *cis*-1,2-dichlorocyclohexane this conjugation reaction can lead to the formation of a reactive thiiranium-ion, which is suspected to be responsible for the mutagenic activity. Apart from stereoselectivity in the bioactivation, stereoselectivity in the bioinactivation may be important too from a toxicological point of view. Thus, it was shown recently that (in contrast to the basic (α-ε)) both the human near neutral (μ) and acidic (π) classes of GSH-transferases were efficient in the conjugation of anti-benz(a)pyrene diol-epoxides and in particular the carcinogenic (+)-enantiomer (Table 2, Robertson *et al.*, (1986)).

Table 2. Kinetic parameters for the human GSH transferases μ and π with the (+)- and (-)-enantiomers of anti-BPDE as substrate

Isoenzyme	substrate	V_{max}(nmol $mg^{-1}.min^{-1}$)	K_M(μM)	Catalytic efficiency ($mM^{-1}.s^{-1}$)
Near neutral (μ)	(+)-*anti*-BPDE	690 ± 130	50 ± 18	11
	(-)-*anti*-BPDE	500 ± 90	45 ± 15	9
Acidic (π)	(+)-*anti*-BPDE	2900 ± 500	85 ± 24	28
	(-)-*anti*-BPDE	ND[a]		

[a] ND, no activity detected (< 1% of added *anti*-BPDE, (Robertson et al, 1886).

More recently, the existence of microsomal GSH-transferases has been established firmly (Morgenstern *et al.* (1983). Apart from the usual substrates for the cytosolic GSH-transferases, compounds like the nephrotoxins hexachloro-1,3-butadiene and tetrafluorethene seem to be the better substrates for the microsomal enzymes (Wolf *et al.*

(1984)). Dohn *et al.* (1985) were the first to show with ^{19}F-NMR a stereochemical control of an enzymatic addition (and no addition-elimination) reaction of chlorotrifluoroethene with GSH. By a microsomal rat liver fraction predominantly one diastereomeric GSH-conjugate was formed, whereas a cytosolic fraction produced an equimolar fraction of two diastereomeric S-(2-chloro-1,1,2-trifluoroethyl) glutathione conjugates. Further studies on the (regio- and) stereospecificities of GSH-transferases might reveal information on the respective mechanisms of the reactions.

Cysteine-conjugate β-lyase

Several cysteine-conjugates are metabolyzed by β-lyase to produce thiols, ammonia and pyruvate. Cytosolic β-lyases have been isolated from the kidney, liver and from intestinal microflora. Since it has become clear that β-lyases can play a decisive role in the bioactivation of cysteine conjugates, such as those from hexachloro-1,3-butadiene or other halogenated alkenes, to nephrotoxic agents, the scientific interest in this enzyme has increased considerably (Elfarra and Anders (1984), Commandeur *et al.* (1986)).

As to its stereoselectivity relatively little is know as yet except that the natural S-configuration in the cysteine residue is a prerequisite for cysteine-conjugates to be a substrate of β-lyases. This fact has been used as a tool to ascertain the role of β-lyase in the development of nephrotoxicity by cysteine conjugates. No data are available as yet with regard to substrate-stereoselective effects of the non-cysteine part of the thioether substrates of β-lyase.

Glucuronyl-transferases

β-D-glucuronic acid is an important optically active cofactor for the microsomal UPD-glucuronyl-transferases, which catalyse the detoxifying conjugation of this glucuronic acid to substrates containing O-, N- or C-functional groups. In a number of cases, however, glucuronidation is thought to play a significant role in the production of toxic effects (Mulder *et al.* (1983)). Apart from increasing the instability and/or reactivity of pro-carcinogens (e.g. O-glucuronide of N-hydroxy-2-acetamidofluorene) it has been suggested that glucuronides may serve as transport forms of pro-carcinogens (e.g. N-glucuronide of N-hydroxy-2-naphtylamine) to various tissues.

Apart from substrate-stereoselective glucuronidation of hydroxylated hexobarbital, considerable enantioselective differences and species differences have been shown in vitro for propranolol (refs. in Vermeulen (1986)), fenoterol (Koster *et al.* (1986)) and oxazepam (Table 3) (Sisenwine *et al.* (1982)). In vivo, enantioselectivity is often less pronounced when compared to in vitro.

Table 3 In vitro glucuronidation of oxazepam (Sisenwine et al. 1982).

Species	S(+)	R(−)	Ratio S/R
	nmol/hr/g liver		
Rhesus monkey	238	596	0.4
Dog	826	43	19.1
Miniature swine	41	29	1.4
Rabbit	178	92	1.9
Rat	424	22	19.3

It is conceivable that such differences may be a result of other competing stereoselective reactions or of biliary excretion of glucuronides, subsequent enterohepatic circulation and de-/reconjugation in the intestine and/or intestinal mucosa. The lack of an in vivo - in vitro correlation as well as the observed species dependent variations in stereoselectivity considerably complicate the selection of a proper model system for glucuronidation in humans. 3-Methylcholanthrene, β-naphtoflavone, usually seen as inducers of a so-called GT_1-isoenzyme, and ethanol have been shown to increase the enantioselectivity in the formation of diastereomeric glucuronides from racemic oxazepam in hepatic microsomes of rabbits and produced a large increase in enantioselectivity, whereas inducers of the GT_2-isoenzyme, such as phenobarbital only increased oxazepam glucuronidation activity without affecting enantioselectivity. Inducers of forms other than GT_1 and GT_2, such as trans-stilbeneoxide and clofibric acid generally caused increases in activities coupled with increases in R/S ratios. Measurement of enantiomeric selectivity in the glucuronidation of racemic oxazepam was suggested to be a useful tool to characterize the nature and selectivity of inducers of the glucuronyltransferase system (Yost and Finley (1985)). Possible racemization of oxazepam in aqueous solution, however, is a complicating factor in using the compound for this purpose.

Sulfo-transferases

Generally speaking, conclusions regarding stereoselective sulfation in vivo are difficult to draw, because of the fact that mostly a competition exists between (stereoselective) glucuronidation and sulfation of the same substrates. Recently, however, stereoselective sulfation of 4'-hydroxypropranol enantiomers was demonstrated in vitro in hepatic tissue of various species (Christ and Walle (1985)). Enantiomeric (-/+)- 4'-hydroxypropranolol sulfate ratios varied from 1,07 in the rat and 0,73 in the dog to 0,62 in the hamster. Both the species-dependent preference as well as the degree of apparent stereoselectivity may be due to the activity of multiple sulfotransferase isozymes present in the supernatant preparations. At least three isozymes have been isolated from rat liver.

No examples are known as yet, demonstrating a causal relationship between sulfation and stereoselective toxicity.

Stereoselectivity and prevention of toxicity by cysteine

Remarkably, the naturally occurring L-cysteine was found to be transformed by rat liver and rat kidney post-mitochondrial (S9) homogenate into a mutagen responding in Salmonella TA92 and TA100 bacterial strains. D-cysteine did not show mutagenicity under any experimental conditions (Glatt *et al.* (1985)). However, it was strongly bacteriotoxic. The mechanism of this remarkable toxicity of cysteine and of the apparent stereoselectivity is as yet unknown. It seems not to be irrelevant, however, since other thio-compounds (e.g. L- and D-penicillamine) apparently show a similar toxicity.

L-cysteine is utilized for the bio-synthesis of co-substrates for several conjugation reactions, such as glutathione, sulfate and taurine. The unphysiological isomer D-cysteine has been used frequently to investigate mechanistical aspects of physiological processes involving cysteine. In rats, sulfoxidation rates of L- and D-cysteine as well as sulfation rates of the test substrate harmol to inorganic sulfate were found to be very similar, so that stereoselectivity for the amino acid seems not to play a role in these reactions (Glazenburg *et al.* (1984)). Since D-cysteine, in contrast to the L-isomer, did not increase taurine concentration in serum, this type of stereoselectivity can be used to selectively enhance sulfate availability in vivo.

Glutathione, as the main intracellular non-protein sulfhydryl, plays an important role as a co-substrate or a reductance in the detoxication of electrophilic compounds in organisms as well as in the repair of various kinds of cellular injury. Consequently, increased levels of glutathione may exert beneficial effects in some cases. N-acetyl-L-cysteine, which is rapidly hydrolyzed to L-cysteine, compared to L-cysteine itself more successfully promotes glutathione synthesis in vivo and is known to protect more efficiently against paracetamol induced hepatotoxicity. Alternatively, however, 2-alkyl- or 2-aryl-substituted thiazolidine-4-R-carboxylic acids - especially those derived from the condensation of L-cysteine with even alkyl carbon aldehydes, i.e. aldehydes that are readily metabolizable to endogenous or nontoxic products - can more successfully serve as prodrugs of L-cysteine and can also protect against paracetamol toxicity (Fig. 7; Nagasawa *et al.* (1984)). Incorporation of L-cysteine into glutathione and not the liberation of sulfhydryl groups per se appears to be important, since analogues with a 4-S-configuration, which dissociate to the unphysiological D-cysteine, were found to be totally ineffective as a protecting agent.

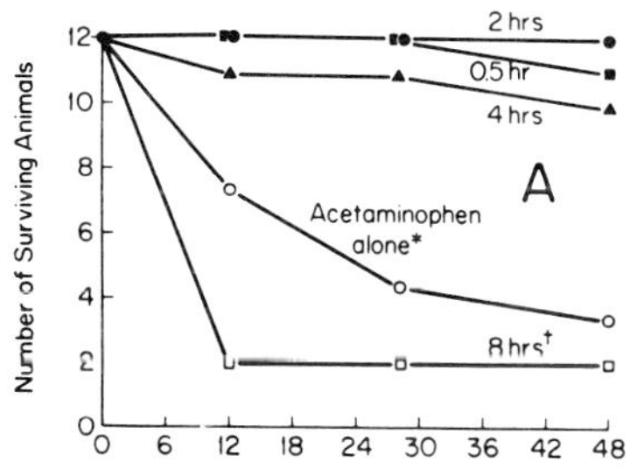

Fig. 7: Effect of post-administration of 2-methyl-thiazoline-4-(R)-carboxylic acid on paracetamol lethality in mice. I.p. dose 4,97 mmol/kg. The corresponding 4-(S)-isomer did not protect against paracetamol induced lethality (Nagasawa et al. 1984)

Stereoselectivity as a tool in bio-monitoring

Apart from using stereoselectivity as a tool to elucidate biotransformation and toxicity-mechanisms (examples mentioned before) in principle, it might also be interesting to consider stereoselectivity as a tool in biological monotoring studies, notably in those cases where toxicity is stereo-controlled. For example, from styrene it is known that optical activity is introduced by the formation of two enantiomeric 7,8-styreneoxides. In the rat, oxygenation with a 4:1 preference for the less mutagenic R-(+)-styreneoxide has been demonstrated (Van Bladeren (1981)). In principal, an accurate estimation of the balance between both unstable isomeric epoxides is only possible when the excretion in urine of two possible diastereomeric pairs of mercapturic acids (Delbressine *et al.* (1985)), two enantiomeric phenylethylene glycols and two enantiomers of mandelic acids (refs. in Korn *et al.* (1986)) is determined. The determination of only one type of stereoisomers, as has been suggested (Korn *et al.* (1986)), not necessarily will reflect accurately the stereoselectivity in the formation of the enantiomeric styrene-oxides.

Recently, we developed a stereoselective analytical procedure using gas chromatography, amongst others with mass spectrometric detection, for the two (3-substituted) mercapturic acids, both in rat and humans formed as major metabolites, from the isomers of the nematocide Z- and E-1,3-dichloropropene (Onkenhout *et al.* (1986)). Previously, it had been suggested that the Z-isomer was considerably more directly mutagenic than the corresponding E-isomer (Eder *et al.* (1982)). This so-called stereoselective effect, however, was more recently due to mutagenic impurities (most probably 1,2-epoxidized derivatives) in 1,3-dichloropropene preparations (Watson *et al.* (1987)). The former and the latter example given here illustrate that, in principle, it is possible to use stereoselectivity as a tool in toxicological studies. However, they also illustrate the great carefulness which has to be taken when stereoselectivity is used for this purpose.

General Conclusions

This review has demonstrated that, at present, it is more and more recognized that stereochemical factors play a significant role in the disposition and the pharmacological or toxicological action of drugs and other xenobiotics. As to toxicity [of xenobiotics], stereoselectivity in biotransformation (i.e. bioactivation or bioinactivation) reactions, is probably the factor of major importance. Consequences of this for the biological action of xenobiotics in general are difficult to predict because of the complex regulation of the biological activities.

In recent years, however, considerable progress has been made in the elucidation of stereochemical mechanisms of several important biotransformation enzymes, despite the fact that the multiplicity, a widely varying substrate-selectivity as well as secondary metabolism (which in itself can be stereoselective) complicate considerably the study of such mechanisms. In principle, the same factors complicate the correlation of data on stereoselective effects obtained in vitro with those obtained in vivo, even though it concerns the same species. Prediction of stereoselective effects from one species to another or from one chemical to another is even more difficult. As this review also has demonstrated, in some case further insights in stereochemical mechanisms at a molecular level (i.e. at the level of binding of substrate molecules to active (or binding) sites of isolated and purified (iso-)enzymes (or other proteins)) provided a simplified model or a working hypothesis that might be helpful to predict stereoselective processes. Progress in research along these lines will be most promising, not only from an academic but also from a more practical point of view, namely directed to predictability. From a toxicological point of view it is important to stress that knowledge on stereoselective effects at the different levels of the development of biologically active drugs or other chemicals should be obtained as early as possible. Without this knowledge it is almost impossible to interpret the toxicodynamics and toxicokinetics of a chiral compound.

References

- Albert, A.,"Steric Factors" (1985) In: Selective toxicity. The physicochemical basis of therapy. 7th Ed. A. Albert (ed.) 490.
- Ariens, E.J. (1983) In: Stereochemistry and biological activity of drugs. E.J. Ariens, W. Soudijn and P.B.W.M.M. Timmermans (eds.). Blackwell Scientific Publications. Oxford, 11.
- Ariëns, E.J., (1984) Drug Metab.Rev., 15, 425.
- Armstrong, R.N., Kedzierski, B., Levin, W. and Jerina, D.M. (1981) J. Biol. Chem. 256, 4726.

- Armstrong, R.N., Levin, W. and Jerina, D.M. (1980) In "Microsomes, Drug Oxidations and chemical Carcinogenesis" (M.J. Coon, A.H. Conney, R.W. Estabrook, N.V. Gelboin, J.R. Gillette and P.J. O'Brien, eds.). Academic Press Inc., New York.
- Armstrong, R.N., Levin, W., Ryan, D.E., Thomas, P.E., Duck Mah, H. and Jerina, D.M. (1981) Biochem. Biophys. Res. Commun., 100, 1077.
- Baillie, T.A. Pharmacol. (1981) Rev. 33, 81.
- Beld, A.J. and Zwanenburg, B. (1986) In: Innovative Approaches in Drug Research. A.F. Harms (ed.). Elsevier Science Publishers B.V., Amsterdam, 331.
- Belluci, G., Berti, G., Bianchini, R., Cetera, P. and Mastrorilli, E., (1982) J. Org.. Chem. 47, 3105.
- Benschop, H.P., Konings, C.A.G., Van Genderen, J. and De Jong, L.P.A., (1984) Fundam. and Appl.Toxicol., 4, S84.
- Boobis, A.R., Murray, S., Hampden, C.E. and Davies, D.S., (1985) Biochem. Pharmacol., 34, 65.
- Brimfield, A.A., Hunter K.W., Lenz, D.E., Benschop H.P., Van Dijk, C. and de Jong L.P.A., (1985) Molec.Pharmacol., 28, 32.
- Christ, D.D. and Walle, T., (1985) Drug Metab. Dispos., 13, 380.
- Cobb, D., Boehlert, C., Lewis D. and Armstrong, R.N., (1983) Biochem. 22, 805.
- Commandeur J.N.H., Oostendorp R.A.J., Schoofs P.R. and Vermeulen N.P.E., (1986) Biochem. Pharmacol., in press.
- Conney, A.H. (1982) Canc. Res., 42, 4875.
- Cook, C.E. (1985) TIPS, 6, 302.
- Cova D., Arnoldi, A., Colombo, R. and Rossini, l. (1986) Toxicol.Lett., 30, 273.
- Cox, J.W., Cox, S.R., Van Giessen, G. and Ruwart, M.J., (1985) J. Pharmacol. Exp. Ther., 232, 636.
- Dayer, P., Gasser, R., Gut, J., Kronbach, T., Roberts, G.-M., Eickelbaum, M. and Meyer, U.A. (1984) Biochem. Biophys. Res. Comm., 125, 374.
- Dayer, P., Leemann, T., Gut, J., Kronbach, T., Kupfer, A., Francis, R. and Meyer, U. (1985) Biochem. Pharmacol., 34, 399.
- Distlerath, L.M., Reilly, P.E.B., Martin, M.V., Wilkinson, G.R. and Guengerich, F.P. (1985) In: Microsomes and Drug Oxidations. (Eds. A.R. Boobis, J. Caldwell, F. De Matters and C.R. Elcombe). Taylor and Francis, London, 380.
- Dohn, D.R., Quebbeman, A.J., Borch, R.F. and Anders, M.W. (1985) Biochemistry, 24, 5137.
- Dostal, L.A., Aitio, A., Harris, C., Bhatia, A.V., Hernandez, O. and Bend, J.R. (1986) Drug Metab. Dispos., 14, 303
- Eder, E., Neudecker, T., Lutz D. and Henschler, D. (1982) Chem. Biol. Interact.,38, 303.
- Elfarra, A.A. and Anders, M.W. (1984) Biochem., Pharmacol. 33, 3729.
- Glatt, H. and Oesch, F. (1985) Biocem. Pharmacol. 34, 3725.
- Glazenburg, E., Jekel-Halsema, I.M.C., Baranczyk-Kuzma, A., Krijgsheld, K.R. and Mulder, G.J., (1984) Biochem. Pharmacol., 33, 525.
- Hammock, B., Ratcliff M. and Schooley, D.A. (1980) Life Sci. 27, 1635.
- Hanzlik, R.P., Edelman, M., Michaely, W.J. and Scott, G. (1976) J. Am. Chem. Soc. 98, 1952.
- Jerina, D.M., Sayer, J.M., Yagi, H., van Bladeren, P.J., Thakker, D.R., Levin, W., Chang, R.L., Wood, A.W. and Conney, A.H. (1985) In. Microsomes and Drug Oxidations. Taylor and Francis, London, 310.

- J. Liq. Chromatogr. 9 (1986) Special issue.
- Kaminsky, L.S., Dunbar, D.A., Wang, P.P., Beaune, P., Larrey, D., Guengerich, F.P., Schnellmann, R.G. and Sipes, I.G. (1984) Drug Metab. Dispos. U12, 470
- Kupfer, A., Roberts, R.K., Schenker, S. and Branch, R.A. (1981) J. Pharmacol. Exp. Ther., 218, 193.
- Lohman, P.H.M., Baan, R.A., Fichtinger, A.M., Muysken, M.A., Lansbergen, R.J. and Berends F. (1985) T.I.P.S., november pg. 5.
- Mangold, J.B. and Abdel-Monem, M.M. (1980) Biochem. Biophys. Res. Commun. 96, 333.
- Morgenstern, R., Guthenberg, C., Mannervik, B. and Depierre, J.W. (1983) FEBS 160, 264.
- Mulder G.J. and Meerman J.H.N. (1983). In: Extra-hepatic drug metabolism and Chemical Carcinogenesis, Elsevier Science Publishers (Rydström *et al.* eds.) pg 143.
- Nagasawa, H.T., Coon, D.J.W., Muldoon, W.P. and Zera, R.T., (1984) J. Med. Chem., 27, 591.
- Ockzenfels, H., Köhler F. and Meise, E. (1976) Drug Res., 31, 492
- Oesch, F. (1979). In "Progress in Drug Metabolism", Part 3, p. 253 (J.W. Bridges and L.F. Chasseaud, eds.). Wiley, Chichester.
- Onkenhout, W., Mulder, P.P.J., Boogaard, P.J., Buys, W. and Vermeulen, N.P.E. (1986) Arch. Toxicol., 59, 235.
- Rojas, M. and Alexandrov, K. (1986) Carcinogenesis, 46, 1553.
- Robertson, I.G.C., Guthenberg, C., Mannervik, B. and Jernström, B. (1986) Canc. Res. 46, 2220.
- Sayer, J.M, Yagi, H., van Bladeren, P.J., Levin W. and Jerina, D.M. (1985) J. Biol. Chem. 260, 1630.
- Sisenwine, S.F., Tio, C.O., Hadley, F.V., Lin, A.L., Kimmel, H.B. and Ruelius, H.W., (1982) Drug Metab. Dispos., 10, 605.
- Te Koppele, J.M., Dogterom, P., Vermeulen, N.P.E., Meijer, D.K.F., Van Der Gen, A. and Mulder G.J. (1986) J. Pharmacol. Exp. Ther., 239, 905.
- Testa, B. (1986a) TIPS, 7, 60.
- Testa, B. (1986b) Xenobiotica, 265.
- Thakker, D.R., Levin, W., Yagi, H. Conney, A.H. and Jerina, D.H. (1982). In: Biol. Reactive Intermediates - II part A (R. Snyder *et al.* eds) Plenum Press, New York, pg 525.
- Van Bladeren, P.J., van der Gen, A., Breimer, D.D. and Mohn, G.R. (1979) Biochem. Pharmacol., 28, 2521.
- Van Bladeren, P.J., Breimer, D.D., van Huijgenvoort, I.A.T.C.M., Vermeulen, N.P.E. and van der Gen, A. (1981) Biochem. Pharmacol. 30, 2499.
- Van Bladeren, P.J., Vyas. K.P., Sayer, J.M., Ryan, D.E., Thomas, P.E., Levin, W. and Jerina, P.M. (1984) 259, 8966.
- Van der Graaff, M., Vermeulen, N.P.E., Hofman, P.H., Breimer, D.D., Knabe, J. and Schamber, L., (1985) Biomed. Mass Spectrom. 12, 464.
- Vermeulen, N.P.E. (1986a) Chemisch magazine, October 727.
- Vermeulen, N.P.E. and Breimer, D.D. (1983). In: Stereochemistry and biological activity of drugs. E.J. Ariens, W. Soudijn and P.B.W.M.M. Timmermans (eds.). Blackwell Scientific Publications. Oxford, pg.33.
- Vermeulen, N.P.E., Cauvet, J., Luijten W.C.M.M. and van Bladeren, P.J. (1980) Biomed. Mass Spectrom. 7, 413.

- Vermeulen, N.P.E., Danhof, M., Setiawan, I and Breimer, D.D. (1983) J. Pharmacol. Exp. Ther., 226, 201.
- Vermeulen, N.P.E. (1986) In: Innovative Approaches in Drug Research. A.F. Harms (ed.). Elsevier Science Publishers B.V., Amsterdam 393.
- Watson, W.P., Brooks, T.M., Huckle, K.R., Hutson, D.H., Lang, K.L., Smith, R.J. and Wright, A.S. (1987) Chem. Biol. Interact. 61, 17.
- White, R.E., Miller, J.P., Favreau, L.V. and Bhattacharyya, A. (1986) J. Am. Chem. Soc., 108, 6024.
- Wolf, C.R., Berry, P.N., Nash, J.A. and Lock, E.A. (1984) J. Pharmacol. Exp. Ther., 288, 202.
- Wood, A.W., Chang, R.L., Kumar, S., Shirai, N., Jerina, D.M., Lehr, R.E. and Conney, A.H., (1986) Canc. Res., 46, 2760.

Index